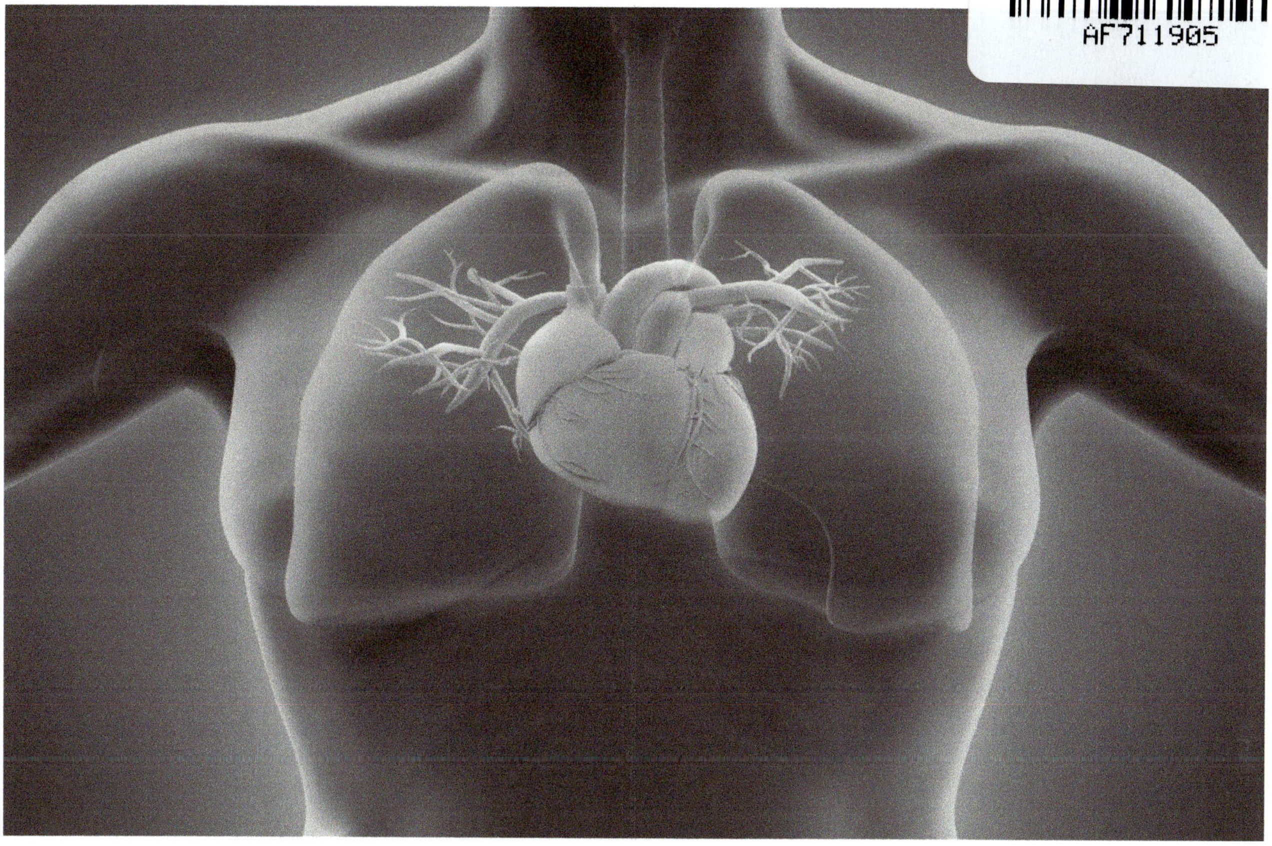

BMJ Clinical Review:

Cardiology and Respiratory Medicine

Edited by
Babita Jyoti & Michail A. Karvelis

BPP
UNIVERSITY
SCHOOL OF HEALTH

First edition August 2015

ISBN 9781 4727 3889 9
eISBN 9781 4727 4409 8
eISBN 9781 4727 4417 3

British Library Cataloguing-in-Publication Data
A catalogue record for this book is available from the British Library

Published by
BPP Learning Media Ltd
BPP House, Aldine Place
London W12 8AA

www.bpp.com/health

Printed in the United Kingdom by
Ashford Colour Press Ltd.

Unit 600, Fareham Reach
Fareham Road
Gosport, Hamphire
PO13 0FW

Your learning materials, published by BPP Learning Media Ltd, are printed on paper sourced from sustainable, managed forests.

The content of this publication contains articles from The BMJ which have been selected, collated and published by BPP Learning Media under a licence.

About the publisher

BPP Learning Media is dedicated to supporting aspiring professionals with top quality learning material. BPP Learning Media's commitment to success is shown by our record of quality, innovation and market leadership in paper-based and e-learning materials. BPP Learning Media's study materials are written by professionally-qualified specialists who know from personal experience the importance of top quality materials for success.

About The BMJ

The BMJ (formerly the British Medical Journal) in print has a long history and has been published without interruption since 1840. The BMJ's vision is to be the world's most influential and widely read medical journal. Our mission is to lead the debate on health and to engage, inform, and stimulate doctors, researchers, and other health professionals in ways that will improve outcomes for patients. We aim to help doctors to make better decisions. BMJ, the company, advances healthcare worldwide by sharing knowledge and expertise to improve experiences, outcomes and value.

Contents

About the editors

Dr Babita Jyoti is a Radiation Oncologist with a special interest in Paediatric Proton Therapy. She graduated in Medicine in India followed by training in UK and obtained MRCP (UK) & FRCR (UK). She trained as a Clinical Oncologist at Clatterbridge Cancer Centre. She is currently working at the University of Florida Health Proton Therapy Institute in Paediatric Proton Therapy. She has been a PBL tutor and an OSCE examiner at Manchester Medical School.

Dr Michail A. Karvelis is a Pain Fellow at the Royal Liverpool and Broadgreen University Hospitals. He qualified from the Medical School of the Aristotle University of Thessaloniki, Greece in 2003. He trained as an anaesthetist both in Greece and the UK and he obtained his CCT in 2011. He was awarded a Masters degree in Pain management from Leicester University in 2011. He has worked as a consultant anaesthetist in the Naval Hospital of Athens and since 2014 he has been developing his special interest in regional anaesthesia and pain medicine in the NHS.

Introduction to Cardiology and Respiratory Medicine

Cardiology and Respiratory Medicine are an integral part of every day clinical medicine in both primary, as well as secondary care. New pharmaceutical products are being discovered and relevant guidelines are constantly under review. In this book, we have made every effort to refresh and update knowledge by carefully selecting clinical reviews on cardiology and respiratory medicine published in The BMJ in the past 7 years.

Clinical reviews from The BMJ provide a clear, up to date account of the topic in a collaborative venture including general physicians, cardiologists and chest physicians as well as general practitioners, epidemiologists, surgeons, gastroenterologists, radiologists and pharmacists.

We have attempted to select and include the clinical reviews that provide a thorough, useful, ready-to-use knowledge on common cardio-respiratory conditions. Our intention is to cover some of the major topics in the field and provide answers to clinical questions relating to everyday clinical practice situations. However, there is no book that can compete with the pace of literature. This book provides the reader with relevant references to further their knowledge and understanding. The reader should use this book as their starting point of their challenging journey into the world of evidence based medicine rather than an answer to every clinical question.

Preparticipation screening for cardiovascular abnormalities in young competitive athletes

Michael Papadakis, cardiac research registrar[12], Greg Whyte, professor of sports sciences[3], Sanjay Sharma, consultant cardiologist, and director of heart muscle diseases[12]

[1]King's College Hospital, London SE5 9RS

[2]University Hospital Lewisham, London

[3]CRY Sports Cardiology Centre, Olympic Medical Institute, Northwick Park Hospital, Middlesex

Correspondence to: S Sharma ssharma21@hotmail.com

Cite this as: BMJ 2008;337:a1596

‹DOI› 10.1136/bmj.a1596
http://www.bmj.com/content/337/bmj.a1596

The cardiovascular benefits of regular physical exercise are well established.[1] However, a small proportion of young (≤35 years) athletes with unsuspected heart disease are at increased risk of exercise related sudden cardiac death.[2] The majority of such deaths are attributable to cardiac anomalies,[2 3 4] most of which can be identified during life. A range of therapeutic strategies can be implemented to prevent fatalities, raising support for screening young athletes in medical and sporting communities.[5 6 7 8 9] The efficacy, cost effectiveness, and impact of false positive tests of preparticipation screening strategies are, however, controversial. This article provides a factual overview of preparticipation screening, as more general practitioners are likely to be confronted with the questions relating to cardiovascular screening in athletes in countries where systematic screening programmes are currently not available.

Epidemiology and demographics of sudden cardiac death in young athletes

Sudden cardiac death in young athletes is uncommon. In the United States a retrospective review of 650 000 competitive high school athletes aged 15-17 reported an incidence of 0.5 per 100 000 per year.[10] In Italy, a prospective population based observational study reported the higher incidence of 2.1 per 100 000 per year in athletes aged 14-35.[2] The absence of systematic registries precludes data relating to the incidence of sudden cardiac death in young athletes in most other European countries.

Over 90% of sudden cardiac deaths in young athletes occur during or shortly after exercise.[2] A sex and sport related predilection exists, with a predominance in males (male to female ratio 9:1) and the largest number of deaths reported in soccer and basketball. Higher participation rates provide the most plausible explanation. The mean age of sudden cardiac death in young athletes ranges from 17.1 to 23.[2 3]

A broad spectrum of congenital, inherited, and acquired cardiovascular diseases causes sudden cardiac death (fig 1). Inherited cardiomyopathies are the commonest cause, with hypertrophic cardiomyopathy accounting for over one third of cases of sudden cardiac deaths in athletes in the United States[5] and arrhythmogenic right ventricular cardiomyopathy predominating in Italy.[4] Congenital coronary artery anomalies and premature atherosclerosis account for almost 20% of cases of sudden cardiac death.[4]

What is the objective of preparticipation screening?

The potential for preventing sudden cardiac death in young athletes by abstinence from exercise of moderate to high intensity, pharmacotherapy, or implantation of a cardiovertor defibrillator has prompted the medical and sporting community to recommend preparticipation cardiovascular screening to permit identification of potentially fatal disorders. Both the American Heart Association and the European Society of Cardiology agree that the justifications for providing preparticipation screening to protect athletes are compelling.[5 6] Given the low prevalence of the disorders implicated in sudden cardiac death during sport, several thousand athletes would need to be screened to identify a small number at risk, therefore the emphasis is on providing the most cost effective method for minimising sudden cardiac death.[11]

What are the current practices?

Most countries do not offer systematic programmes for preparticipation screening. In the United States the American Heart Association recommends such screening using a health questionnaire and physical examination (box 1).[5] This strategy seems cheap and easy to carry out but has limited value as 80% of athletes who die as a result of sudden cardiac death are asymptomatic and physical examination identifies few implicated disorders. The lack of sensitivity of the American model was highlighted in a series of 115 reported cases of sudden cardiac deaths in young athletes who had been screened. A correct diagnosis was identified in only one athlete (0.9%), who was allowed to compete. The limited sensitivity of this strategy has been further highlighted by prospective observational studies in the United Kingdom and Italy.[12 13]

In Italy a unique state sponsored, national preparticipation screening programme has been in operation for over 25 years. The programme, which evaluates several million athletes annually, comprises a history, examination, and electrocardiography. Athletes with abnormalities on

SOURCES AND SELECTION CRITERIA

We searched PubMed and Medline from 1980 onwards using the search terms "pre-participation screening", "sudden death", "electrocardiogram", "athletes", "black athletes", and "cost-effectiveness". Although we scrutinised and selected the highest quality articles, comprising original papers, reviews, recommendations, and consensus reports, the studies are all population based, prospective or retrospective observational reports. To our knowledge the efficacy of preparticipation screening programmes in young athletes has not been subjected to controlled trials, as they would be challenging to do both ethically and technically.

SUMMARY POINTS

- Regular exercise is beneficial and only a small number of athletes with silent cardiovascular disease are at increased risk of sudden cardiac death during exercise
- Preparticipation screening using health questionnaires and physical examination only has poor sensitivity whereas elaborate screening programmes are cost prohibitive
- Screening with 12 lead electrocardiography prevents sudden cardiac death from channelopathies and cardiomyopathies but not from coronary artery disease
- Electrocardiography may vary depending on athletic activity, age, race, and sex, and skilled doctors are required to avoid a large number of false positive test results
- Implementation of preparticipation screening is currently hampered by the lack of resources and infrastructure and cannot be regarded as cost effective in most countries

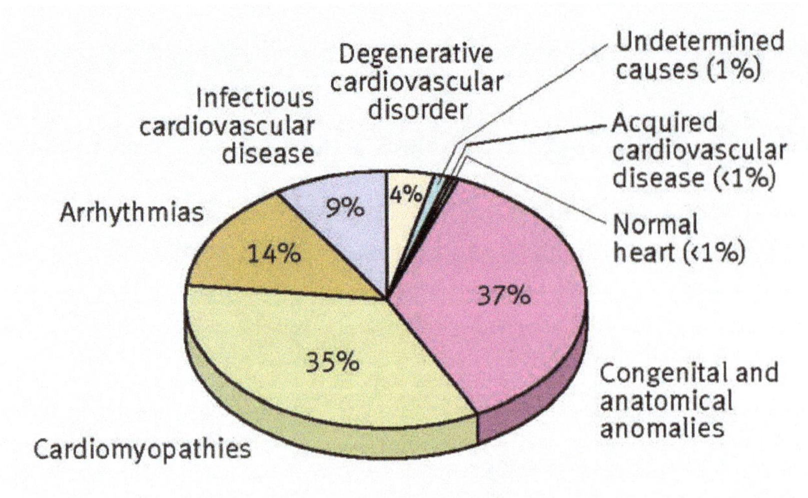

Fig 1 Causes of sudden cardiac death in young athletes

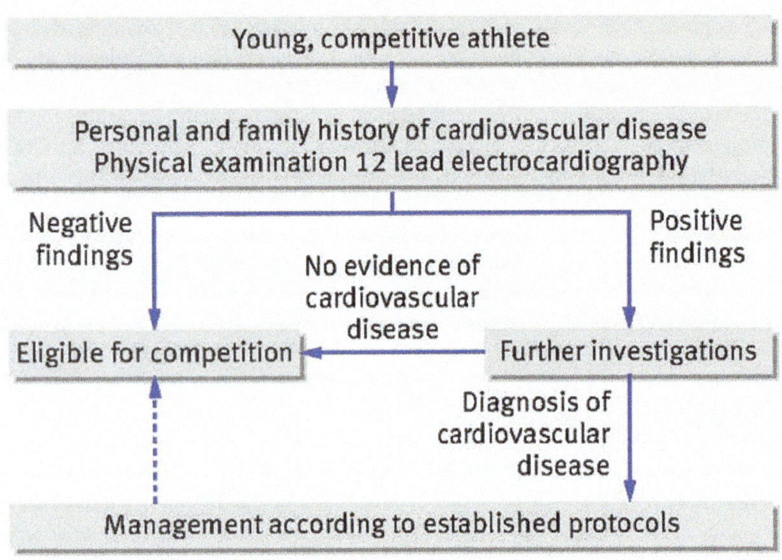

Fig 2 Italian preparticipation screening protocol endorsed by International Olympic Committee, Fédération Internationale de Football Association, European Football Associations, and European Society of Cardiology. Reproduced from Corrado et al[6] with permission of the European Society of Cardiology

initial evaluation are investigated further and those with potentially serious abnormalities are disqualified (fig 2).[13 14] The additional electrocardiography increases the sensitivity of the programme, enabling the diagnosis of a large proportion of cardiomyopathies and disorders of accessory pathways and ion channels. Although the definitive diagnosis of cardiomyopathies depends on cardiac imaging, electrocardiographic abnormalities are exhibited by 95% of people with hypertrophic cardiomyopathy and 80% of those with arrhythmogenic right ventricular cardiomyopathy.[15 16]

Is the Italian model effective in identifying cardiovascular disorders in young athletes?

The efficacy of the Italian screening programme in the identification of cardiomyopathies is established. Evidence suggests, however, that the strategy is not effective in detecting athletes with congenital coronary anomalies or premature coronary atherosclerosis.[17]

In a large population based study of screening outcomes in 33 735 young athletes in the Veneto region of Italy, 621 (1.8%) were disqualified because of an identified cardiovascular disorder. Of these, 22 (0.07%) were considered to have

BOX 1 AMERICAN HEART ASSOCIATION GUIDELINES FOR PREPARTICIPATION CARDIOVASCULAR SCREENING OF YOUNG, COMPETITIVE ATHLETES

Medical history*

- Chest pain or discomfort on exertion
- Unexplained syncope or near syncope†
- Excessive exertional dyspnoea or fatigue
- Prior recognition of a heart murmur
- Raised systemic blood pressure

Family history

- Premature death (<50 years) from heart disease, in one or more relatives
- Disability from heart disease in a close relative aged less than 50
- Specific knowledge of certain cardiac conditions in family members: hypertrophic and dilated cardiomyopathy, long QT syndrome or other ion channelopathies, Marfan's syndrome, or clinically important arrhythmias

Physical examination

- Heart murmur‡
- Femoral pulses to exclude aortic coarctation
- Physical stigmata of Marfan's syndrome
- Brachial artery blood pressure (sitting position, taken in both arms)

**Parental verification is recommended for high school and middle school athletes*

†Judged not to be vasovagal; of particular concern when related to exertion

‡Auscultation should be done both while supine and while standing or with Valsalva manoeuvre, specifically to identify murmurs of dynamic left ventricular outflow tract obstruction

hypertrophic cardiomyopathy, predominantly (73%) on the basis of an abnormal electrocardiogram.[13] This frequency is similar to that observed in a population based study in the United States, which used echocardiography, suggesting that the Italian model performs as well as echocardiography in detecting hypertrophic cardiomyopathy.[18] The specificity of the Italian programme in excluding the diagnosis of hypertrophic cardiomyopathy was also assessed in a study of 4450 elite athletes who were initially judged eligible for competition after preparticipation screening using 12 lead electrocardiography. The athletes underwent echocardiography to assess previously undetected hypertrophic cardiomyopathy.[19] After an average follow-up of eight years hypertrophic cardiomyopathy was diagnosed in only one (0.02%) athlete indicating that a normal electrocardiogram has a high negative predictive value (99.98%), excluding hypertrophic cardiomyopathy in most athletes. More recent experience from the Italian programme suggests that screening using 12 lead electrocardiography is also effective in detecting athletes with arrhythmogenic right ventricular cardiomyopathy.[17]

Does the Italian model reduce the number of sudden cardiac deaths in young athletes?

Although hypertrophic cardiomyopathy is the commonest cause of exercise related sudden cardiac death in the United States, in Italy it is responsible for a much smaller proportion of deaths. Although antagonists of preparticipation screening argue that this might reflect a lower genetic cluster of people with hypertrophic cardiomyopathy in the Mediterranean region, these figures probably reflect the efficacy of the Italian programme in identifying athletes with hypertrophic cardiomyopathy and minimising deaths through disqualification from sport; none of the 22 athletes identified with hypertrophic cardiomyopathy in the Veneto region between 1979 and 1996 died during a mean follow-up of 8.2 years. Of the 49 deaths recorded among young athletes during the same period, only one had hypertrophic cardiomyopathy (2%)—lower than the incidence of 7.3% recorded in 220 sudden deaths among non-athletes.[13]

The most compelling evidence for the Italian preparticipation screening model reducing the incidence of sudden cardiac death in sport is derived from a subsequent prospective study by the same group. The group compared the incidence of sudden cardiac death between the prescreening era and a 25 year period of screening and showed a reduction in incidence of sudden cardiac death from 3.6 per 100 000 person years before screening to 0.4 per 100 000 person years in 2003-4 (fig 3).[17] These figures represent a 90% reduction in mortality since preparticipation screening was implemented and predominantly result from fewer cases of sudden cardiac death from cardiomyopathies, particularly arrhythmogenic right ventricular cardiomyopathy—a relatively novel entity in the early screening era which cardiologists have become more effective at diagnosing. Of concern, however, was the unchanged incidence of sudden cardiac death from coronary disorders.

What are the limitations of 12 lead electrocardiography as a screening tool?

Electrocardiography is unable to identify premature coronary artery disease and congenital coronary anomalies, which account for a major proportion of sudden cardiac death in young athletes.[4, 17] Testing might also fail to detect people with long QT syndrome and arrhythmogenic right ventricular cardiomyopathy with incomplete phenotypic expression.

Electrocardiographic changes associated with physical conditioning often overlap with those observed in cardiomyopathy, resulting in unnecessary investigations or false disqualification of athletes. Therefore preparticipation screening should be done by cardiologists with knowledge of cardiovascular adaptation to exercise as well as the broad phenotypic manifestations of the cardiomyopathies. Even in the most experienced hands, the false positive rate may be unacceptably high. An observational study of 1005 selected Italian athletes reported an incidence for mildly or distinctly abnormal electrocardiogram findings of 40%, only 5% of which were eventually diagnosed as a cardiovascular abnormality. The investigators reported an electrocardiographic sensitivity of 51%, specificity of 61%, positive predictive value of 7%, and negative predictive value of 96%, raising concerns about the value of such testing in preparticipation screening.[20] A large Italian study of 42 386 young athletes screened over 22 years and using more conventional electrocardiographic criteria (box 2) found a false positive rate of 7%, with only 2% of athletes being disqualified because of cardiovascular disease.[4]

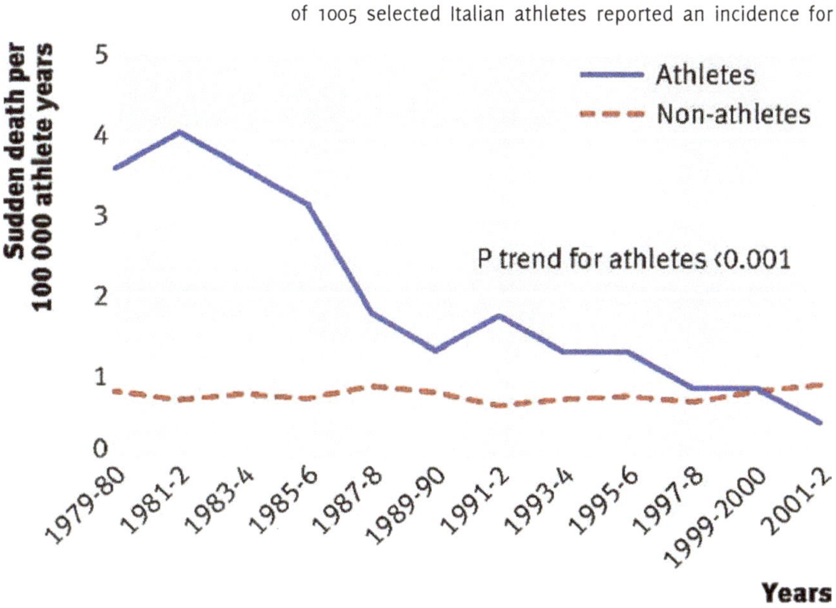

Fig 3 Annual incidence of sudden cardiovascular death in screened competitive athletes compared with non-athletes in Veneto region, Italy, 1979-2004. Reproduced from Corrado et al[17] with permission of *JAMA*

The impact of ethnicity on cardiovascular adaptation in athletes has not been studied in detail; however, evidence is emerging that noticeable repolarisation changes, similar to those observed in people with cardiomyopathies, are more commonly exhibited by Afro-Caribbean athletes. Further data relating to the spectrum of physiological electrocardiographic changes in this cohort are required.[21, 22]

What is the psychological impact of preparticipation screening?

No data have been published on the psychological impact of preparticipation screening in young athletes. On the basis of studies on established screening programmes[23, 24] it is reasonable to assume that athletes with a false positive test result will be anxious until further investigations can provide reassurance. The psychological burden is even greater in young athletes with a diagnosis of a potentially life threatening condition and who are excluded from competing. This highlights the need for prompt evaluation of athletes who fail the initial screening, as well as the need for expert psychological support if preparticipation screening in athletes is to be adopted.

Is preparticipation screening of young athletes cost effective?

Few data exist on the cost effectiveness of preparticipation screening in young athletes, and these are not easily comparable. The American model is cheap but relatively ineffective. A cost effectiveness analysis of a prospective observational study of 5615 high school athletes in the United States, which compared history with electrocardiographic examination (assuming that 10% of the athletes identified as being at risk would live an additional 40 years and 90% an additional 20 years), showed that electrocardiography was more cost effective than history and electrocardiographic examination combined, costing $44 000 (£24 897; €30 921) per year of life saved compared with $84 000 per year of life saved.[25, 26]

An Italian cost effectiveness analysis of 33 735 athletes compared the screening cost of the Italian model with that of the American model. Using a more conservative approach (10% of affected athletes would live an additional 20 years) the study estimated the cost per year of life saved at €14 220 for the Italian model and €37 750 for the American model.[27] These estimates were in the context of a well organised, national setting where preparticipation cardiovascular screening was part of a wider screening programme. In countries such as the United Kingdom, however, where the health service is already burdened by limited finances and resources, the implementation of a national screening programme to identify silent cardiac diseases in athletes cannot be regarded as cost effective.

BOX 2 CRITERIA FOR POSITIVE 12 LEAD ELECTROCARDIOGRAPHY ACCORDING TO EUROPEAN SOCIETY OF CARDIOLOGY CONSENSUS STATEMENT[13]

P wave

- Left atrial enlargement: negative portion of P wave in lead V1 of 0.1 mV or less depth and duration of 0.04 or more seconds
- Right atrial enlargement: peaked P wave in leads II and III or V1 of 0.25 mV or more amplitude

QRS complex

- QRS axis deviation: right 120° or more or left −30° to −90°
- Increased voltage: amplitude of R wave or S wave in a standard lead of 2 mV or more, S wave in lead V1 or V2 of 3 mV or more, or R wave in lead V5 or V6 of 3 mV or more
- Pathological Q waves: duration 0.04 seconds or more, or 25% or more of the height of the ensuing R wave, or QS pattern in two or more leads
- Right or left bundle branch block with QRS duration of 0.12 seconds or more
- R or R′ wave in lead V1 0.5 mV or more in amplitude and R/S ratio of 1 or more

ST segment, T waves, and QT interval

- ST segment depression, T wave flattening, or inversion in two or more leads
- Prolongation of heart rate corrected QT interval of more than 0.44 seconds in males and more than 0.46 seconds in females

Rhythm and conduction abnormalities

- Premature ventricular beats or more severe ventricular arrhythmias
- Supraventricular tachycardias, atrial flutter, or atrial fibrillation
- Short PR interval (<0.12 seconds) with or without "delta" wave
- Sinus bradycardia with resting heart rate 40 beats/min or less*
- First (PR ≥0.21 seconds†), second or third degree atrioventricular block

**Increasing less than 100 beats/min during limited exercise test*
†Not shortening with hyperventilation or limited exercise test

BOX 3 WHO CRITERIA FOR SCREENING[28]

- The condition should be an important health problem
- There should be an accepted treatment or useful intervention
- The natural history of the disease should be adequately understood
- There should be a latent or early symptomatic stage
- There should be a suitable and acceptable screening test
- Facilities for diagnosis and treatment should be available
- There should be an agreed policy on who to treat as patients
- Earlier treatment should be beneficial
- Case finding should be a continuing process and not a once and for all project
- The cost should be economically balanced in relation to possible expenditure on medical care as a whole

ARGUMENTS FOR AND AGAINST PREPARTICIPATION SCREENING

Arguments in favour

- Highly visible events affecting young, fit people
- Association between exercise and sudden death
- Identifiable conditions with acceptable interventions that can prevent sudden cardiac death
- Life years lost
- Acceptable screening test
- The Italian experience

Arguments against

- Sudden cardiac death in athletes is rare; 0.5-2.1 per 100 000 per year
- Low risk even in affected athletes
- Screening for several rare disorders, with diverse pathology
- Cost prohibitive
- Limitations of electrocardiography as a screening test
- Population based observational studies

Does preparticipation screening comply with the World Health Organization screening criteria?

Critics highlight that preparticipation screening does not fulfil most of the WHO criteria (box 3). Although sudden cardiac deaths of athletes may be regarded as an important health problem by some, it is uncommon and is caused by rare disorders, the clinical course of which are not always fully understood. Deaths are the result of diverse diseases and therefore no single investigation can identify all disorders capable of causing sudden cardiac death. Moreover, most countries have limited facilities for the diagnosis and treatment of athletes. Finally, even the most optimistic estimates, as reported by the Italian group, suggest that the cost of preparticipation cardiovascular screening exceeds that of established screening programmes for breast and cervical cancer.[29]

Conversely, evidence suggests that electrocardiography is a suitable and acceptable screening test (simple, safe, precise, and validated) for the identification of the cardiomyopathies and cardiac conduction tissue diseases. A long latent stage is also recognised as well as effective intervention for improved outcomes.

Conclusion

Preparticipation cardiovascular screening of young competitive athletes is recommended by both the American Heart Association and the European Society of Cardiology.[5 6] The European recommendations have been endorsed by the International Olympic Committee and the football governing bodies, with the Union of European Football Associations advocating mandatory screening of all players participating in European championships.[7 9] These recommendations are based on Italy's experience of preparticipation screening for 25 years, which has shown that screening is effective in reducing sudden cardiac death from cardiomyopathies at the expense of some false positive test results. Implementation of preparticipation screening is hampered in most countries by lack of expertise, resources, and infrastructure. Concerns are also justified that further research is required on the efficacy and cost effectiveness of preparticipation screening. The studies from Italy, however, provide the best available evidence to date, supporting the implementation of systematic preparticipation screening for the prevention of sudden cardiac death in young athletes. Although such programmes are effective at minimising deaths from cardiomyopathies and cardiac conduction tissue disorders, they have no impact on deaths from coronary anomalies or premature coronary atherosclerosis.

Contributors: MP, GW, and SS carried out the literature search, analysed and interpreted the data, drafted the article and revised it critically for scientific content, and approved the final version for publication. SS is guarantor.

Funding: None. SS and MP work in the NHS and GW for Liverpool University.

Competing interests: MP is funded by a research grant from the charitable organisation Cardiac Risk in the Young, which support preparticipation screening in young athletes. CRY has provided facilities, including necessary staffing and electrocardiography and echocardiography machines for screening many national sporting squads, including rugby, tennis, boxing, swimming, athletics, and football. The data from the screening programme have resulted in several publications in major peer reviewed journals; GW is a CRY trustee. SS is consultant cardiologist to CRY and a CRY trustee.

Provenance and peer review: Not commissioned; externally peer reviewed.

1 Bernadet P. Benefits of physical activity in the prevention of cardiovascular diseases. *J Cardiovasc Pharmacol* 1995;25(suppl 1):S3-8.
2 Corrado D, Basso C, Rizzoli G, Schiavon M, Thiene G. Does sport activity enhance the risk of sudden death in adolescents and young athletes? *J Am Coll Cardiol* 2003;42:1959-63.
3 Maron BJ, Shirani J, Poliac LC, Mathenge R, Boberts WC, Mueller FO. Sudden death in young competitive athletes. Clinical, demographics and pathological profiles. *JAMA* 1996;276:199-204.

ONGOING RESEARCH AND UNANSWERED QUESTIONS

Ongoing research

- Electrocardiographic and echocardiographic characteristics of athletes of Afro-Caribbean origin to identify the spectrum of electrocardiographic changes and the upper limits of physiological left ventricular hypertrophy in this cohort to facilitate the differentiation between athlete's heart and cardiomyopathy
- Charity funded prospective evaluation of a large cohort of British athletes to identify the prevalence of disorders capable of causing sudden cardiac death in athletes to support arguments for or against preparticipation screening in the United Kingdom
- Molecular genetics of cardiomyopathies and ion channel diseases to facilitate early diagnosis of these disorders in the future

Unanswered questions

- What is the precise significance of noticeable repolarisation changes, specifically deep T wave inversions in the presence of a structurally normal heart?
- What is the precise false negative rate of electrocardiographic screening in different ethnic groups and can the same criteria of electrocardiographic abnormality that warrants further investigation be used for all athletes?

ADDITIONAL EDUCATIONAL RESOURCES

Review articles on preparticipation screening

- Corrado D, Thiene G. Protagonist: routine screening of all athletes prior to participation in competitive sports should be mandatory to prevent sudden cardiac death. *Heart Rhythm* 2007;4:520-4
- Viskin S. Antagonist: routine screening of all athletes prior to participation in competitive sports should be mandatory to prevent sudden cardiac death. *Heart Rhythm* 2007;4:525-8
- Chaitman BR. An electrocardiogram should not be included in routine preparticipation screening of young athletes. *Circulation* 2007;116:2610-5
- Myerburg RJ, Vetter VL. An electrocardiogram should be included in routine preparticipation screening of young athletes. *Circulation* 2007;116:2616-26
- Crawford MH. Screening athletes for heart disease. *Heart* 2007;93:875-9
- Maron BJ, Pelliccia A. The heart of trained athletes. Cardiac remodelling and the risks of sport, including sudden death. *Circulation* 2006;114:1633-44

Information for patients

- Cardiac Risk in the Young (www.c-r-y.org.uk/)—subsidises cardiovascular screening in the United Kingdom, provides information and support to families of victims of sudden death, and funds research and educational events
- The Cardiomyopathy Association (www.cardiomyopathy.org/index.html)—provides information and support to families with cardiomyopathy and funds research and educational events
- Sudden adult death (www.patient.co.uk/showdoc/580/) and When a young person dies suddenly (www.sads.org.uk/)—information on, for example, causes of sudden death and support groups

TIPS FOR NON-SPECIALISTS

- Symptoms, clinical signs, and electrocardiographic abnormalities of significant importance that should raise concern about young athletes and initiate a referral to a specialist are:
- Chest pain or discomfort on exertion
- Unexplained syncope or near syncope during exertion
- Dyspnoea that is disproportional to the amount of exercise being performed
- Palpitations associated with any of the above
- A family history of hereditary cardiac disorder or sudden cardiac death in a first degree relative when young (≤40 years)
- Marfanoid phenotype
- Left parasternal, systolic heart murmur that increases in intensity when standing or with Valsalva manoeuvre
- Electrocardiographic abnormalities (see box 2)
- Athletes with clinical symptoms and signs of an infection—for example, flu-like symptoms, should be advised against intense exercise until they have made a complete recovery owing to the risk of myocarditis

4 Maron BJ. Sudden death in young athletes. *N Engl J Med* 2003;349:1064-75.

5 Maron BJ, Thompson PD, Ackerman MJ, Balady G, Berger S, Cohen D, et al. Recommendations and considerations related to preparticipation screening for cardiovascular abnormalities in competitive athletes: 2007 update. *Circulation* 2007;115:1643-55.

6 Corrado D, Pelliccia A, Bjørnstad HH, Vanhees L, Biffi A, Borjesson M, et al. Cardiovascular pre-participation screening of young competitive athletes for prevention of sudden death: proposal for a common European protocol. Consensus Statement of the Study Group of Sport Cardiology of the Working Group of Cardiac Rehabilitation and Exercise Physiology and the Working Group of Myocardial and Pericardial Diseases of the European Society of Cardiology. *Eur Heart J* 2005;26:516-20.

7 Bille K, Fiquiras D, Schamasch P. Sudden cardiac death in athletes. The Lausanne recommendations. *Eur J Cardiovasc Prev Rehabil* 2006;13:859-75.

8 Estes NAM III, Link MS, Cannom D, Naccarelli GV, Prystowsky EN, Maron BJ, et al. Expert consensus conference of arrhythmias in the athlete of the North American society of pacing and electrophysiology. Report of the NASPE policy conference on arrhythmias and the athlete. *J Cardiovasc Electrophysiol* 2001;12:1208-19.

9 De Ceuninck M, D'Hooghe M, D'Hooghe P. FIFA and UEFA Sports Medical Committee. Sudden cardiac death in football. 2008. http://eur.i1.yimg.com/eur.yimg.com/i/eu/fifa/do/commi.pdf and www.uefa.com/uefa/keytopics/kind=64/newsid=686439.html.

10 Maron BJ, Gohman TE, Aeppli D. Prevalence of sudden cardiac death during competitive sports activities in Minnesota high school athletes. *J Am Coll Cardiol* 1998;32:1881-4.

11 Basavarajaiah S, Wilson M, Whyte G, Shah A, McKenna W, Sharma S. Prevalence of hypertrophic cardiomyopathy in highly trained athletes. Relevance to pre-participation screening. *J Am Coll Cardiol* 2008;51:1033-9.

12 Wilson MG, Basavarajaiah S, Whyte GP, Cox S, Loosemore M, Sharma S. Efficacy of personal symptom and family history questionnaires when screening for inherited cardiac pathologies: the role of electrocardiography. *Br J Sports Med* 2008;42:207-11.

13 Corrado D, Basso C, Schiavon M, Thiene G. Screening for hypertrophic cardiomyopathy in young athletes. *N Engl J Med* 1998;339:364-9.

14 Pellicia A, Maron BJ. Preparticipation cardiovascular evaluation of the competitive athlete: perspectives from the 30-year Italian experience. *Am J Cardiol* 1995;75:827-9.

15 Maron B J. Hypertrophic cardiomyopathy: a systematic review. *JAMA* 2002;287:1308-20.

16 Marcus FI. Electrocardiographic features of inherited diseases that predispose to the development of cardiac arrhythmias, long QT syndrome, arrhythmogenic right ventricular cardiomyopathy/dysplasia and Brugada syndrome. *J Electrocardiol* 2000;33(suppl):1-10.

17 Corrado D, Basso C, Pavei A, Michieli P, Schiavon M, Thiene G. Trends in sudden cardiovascular death in young competitive athletes after implementation of a preparticipation screening program. *JAMA* 2006;296:1593-601.

18 Maron BJ, Gardin JM, Flack JM, Gidding SS, Kurosaki TT, Bild DE. Prevalence of hypertrophic cardiomyopathy in a general population of young adults; echocardiographic analysis of 4111 subjects in the CARDIA study. *Circulation* 1995;92:785-9.

19 Pelliccia A, Di Paolo FM, Corrado D, Buccolieri C, Quattrini FM, Pisicchio C, et al. Evidence for the efficacy of the Italian national pre-participation screening programme for identification of hypertrophic cardiomyopathy in competitive athletes. *Eur Heart J* 2006;27:2196-200.

20 Pelliccia A, Maron BJ, Culasso F, Di Paolo FM, Spataro A, Biffi A, et al. Clinical significance of abnormal electrocardiographic patterns in trained athletes. *Circulation* 2000;102:278-84.

21 Magalski A, Maron BJ, Main ML, McCoy M, Florez A, Reid KJ, et al. Relation of race to electrocardiographic patterns in elite American football players. *J Am Coll Cardiol* 2008;51:2250-5.

22 Basavarajaiah S, Boraita A, Whyte G, Wilson M, Carby L, Shah A, et al. Ethnic differences in left-ventricular remodelling in highly-trained athletes. Relevance to differentiating physiologic left ventricular hypertrophy from hypertrophic cardiomyopathy. *J Am Coll Cardiol* 2008;51:2256-62.

23 Brewer NT, Salz T, Lillie SE. Systematic review: the long-term effects of false-positive mammograms. *Ann Intern Med* 2007;146:502-10.

24 McNaughton-Collins M, Fowler FJ Jr, Caubet JF, Bates DW, Lee JM, Hauser A, et al. Psychological effects of a suspicious prostate cancer screening test followed by a benign biopsy result. *Am J Med* 2004;117:719-25.

25 Fuller CM, McNulty CM, Spring DA, Arger KM, Bruce SS, Chryssos BE, et al. Prospective screening of 5615 high school athletes for risk of sudden cardiac death. *Med Sci Sports Exerc* 1997;29:1131-8.

26 Fuller CM. Cost effectiveness analysis of screening of high school athletes for risk of sudden cardiac death. *Med Sci Sports Exerc* 2000;32:887-90.

27 Corrado D, Basso C, Schiavon M, Maron BJ, Thiene G. Cost-effectiveness analysis of preparticipation screening strategies for the prevention of sudden death in young competitive athletes. American Heart Association scientific sessions. 2004 [abstract 3213].

28 Wilson JMG, Jungner G. Principles and practice of screening for disease. *WHO Chronicle* 1968;22:473.

29 Beral V, Ellis IO, Emery J, Faulkner K, Given-Wilson R, Law M et al. *Screening for breast cancer in England: past and future. NHS Cancer Screening Programmes* . NHSBSP publication No 61. Sheffield: NHS Breast Screening Programme, Feb 2006.

Hypercholesterolaemia and its management

Deepak Bhatnagar, honorary clinical senior lecturer [1], consultant in diabetes and metabolism [2], Handrean Soran, consultant physician [1], Paul N Durrington, professor of medicine [1]

[1]University of Manchester Cardiovascular Research Group, Core Technology Facility, Manchester M13 9NT

[2]Diabetes Centre, Royal Oldham Hospital, Oldham OL1 2JH

Correspondence to: D Bhatnagar, Diabetes Centre, Royal Oldham Hospital, Oldham OL1 2JH d.bhatnagar@man.ac.uk

Cite this as: *BMJ* 2008;337:a993

<DOI> 10.1136/bmj.a993
http://www.bmj.com/content/337/bmj.a993

Hypercholesterolaemia is one of the major causes of atherosclerosis. Although there are many causes, hypercholesterolaemia is the permissive factor that allows other risk factors to operate.[1] The incidence of coronary heart disease is usually low where population plasma cholesterol concentrations are low.[2] In Britain coronary heart disease is a major cause of mortality, and a recent Department of Health survey suggested that the average plasma cholesterol concentration in the United Kingdom was 5.9 mmol/l, much higher than the 4 mmol/l seen in rural China and Japan, where heart disease is uncommon.[3] Many studies before and after the introduction of statins have indicated that reducing the prevalence of hypercholesterolaemia is an important means of decreasing coronary risk.

What is hypercholesterolaemia?

Cholesterol plays an important role as the precursor for steroid hormones and bile acids and it is essential for the structural integrity of cell membranes. It is transported in the body in lipoproteins. Figure 1 shows the role of cholesterol in lipoprotein metabolism.

Conventionally the upper limit for laboratory reference ranges is based on the 95th or 90th centile for a healthy population. This does not apply to plasma cholesterol, however, as several studies show that the epidemiological relation between plasma cholesterol and risk of coronary heart disease extends to the lower end of the cholesterol distribution. Although the relation becomes progressively steeper, there is no obvious threshold below which it ceases to exist.[5] Therefore, it is more rational to base a desirable or healthy concentration of plasma cholesterol on the value at which coronary risk is considered unacceptably high. Most patients developing coronary heart disease have plasma cholesterol concentrations that are likely to be between the 30th and 90th centile for their population of origin.[6] A population is considered to be unhealthy when its average plasma cholesterol concentration exceeds 5 mmol/l (equivalent to low density lipoprotein (LDL) cholesterol of 3 mmol/l).[7]

The Joint British Societies (JBS2) guidelines on prevention of cardiovascular disease recommend that the optimal levels of plasma cholesterol should be ≤4 mmol/l (LDL cholesterol ≤2 mmol/l) in patients with pre-existing atherosclerotic disease or diabetes or in those who have a combination of other risk factors that produce a risk of cardiovascular disease (coronary heart disease and stroke) of 20% or more over the next 10 years.[8] These risk factors include male sex, increased age, cigarette smoking, high blood pressure, impaired fasting glucose concentration, low concentrations of high density lipoprotein (HDL) cholesterol, raised triglycerides, Indian subcontinent ancestry, and low socioeconomic class.

Who gets hyperlipidaemia?

Hypercholesterolaemia usually results from nutritional factors such as obesity and a diet high in saturated fats combined with an underlying polygenic predisposition. There is overproduction of LDL,[9] and its genetic component is unlikely to be monogenic, unless it is extreme. Hypercholesterolaemia can also have an entirely genetic cause. A common example of this is monogenic familial hypercholesterolaemia, an autosomal dominant disorder in which the LDL cholesterol is raised from birth (table 1).[10] It is characterised by a dominant pattern of inheritance of premature coronary disease and/or tendon xanthomata.[11]

Raised plasma triglyceride concentration in association with hypercholesterolaemia is common (table 2) and poses an additional risk of coronary heart disease.[12] Usually such patients have an increase in both low density lipoprotein (VLDL) cholesterol and LDL cholesterol and a decrease in HDL cholesterol. This condition is called combined hyperlipidaemia or, if there is a strong familial tendency, familial combined hyperlipidaemia. Usually the disorder is polygenic with a strong overlap with glucose intolerance, diabetes, and the metabolic syndrome and may precede the onset of diabetes.[13]

Occasionally patients with hypercholesterolaemia have a plasma triglyceride concentration of >10 mmol/l owing to an increase in both chylomicrons and VLDL. The plasma has a milky appearance and eruptive xanthomata, and other features such as acute pancreatitis may occur. Such patients should be referred to lipid clinics for treatment.

Remnant removal disease (type III hyperlipoproteinaemia) leads to combined hyperlipidaemia.[14] Although rare, it carries a high risk of both coronary heart disease and peripheral vascular disease early in life. Typically striate palmar and tuberoeruptive xanthomata occur.[15] Chylomicron remnants accumulate in the circulation owing to homozygosity for the apo E2 isoform of apolipoprotein E, the ligand important for their hepatic clearance. It has variable penetrance, suggesting that some other cause such as obesity or insulin resistance is necessary for its expression.

SOURCES AND SELECTION CRITERIA

We selected references if they included a recent meta-analysis or provided a useful, objective, and comprehensive account including extensive recent references. We chose them from a search of PubMed, personal reference lists, and three textbooks[26 27 28]

SUMMARY POINTS

- The relation between plasma cholesterol concentration and coronary heart disease is curvilinear and without threshold
- Hypercholesterolaemia is a leading cause of atherosclerosis
- Hypercholesterolaemia can result from eating a diet high in saturated fat, primary disorders of lipid metabolism, and conditions that lead to hypercholesterolaemia
- The Joint British Societies (JBS2) charts and guidelines can be used to assess coronary risk, but they may underestimate risk in certain comorbid conditions. Therefore a clinical approach to estimate overall risk is important
- Statins represent a relatively safe way to lower cholesterol
- Abnormal liver function tests can occur in dyslipidaemia, and statins should not be stopped, especially in high risk patients, without good cause

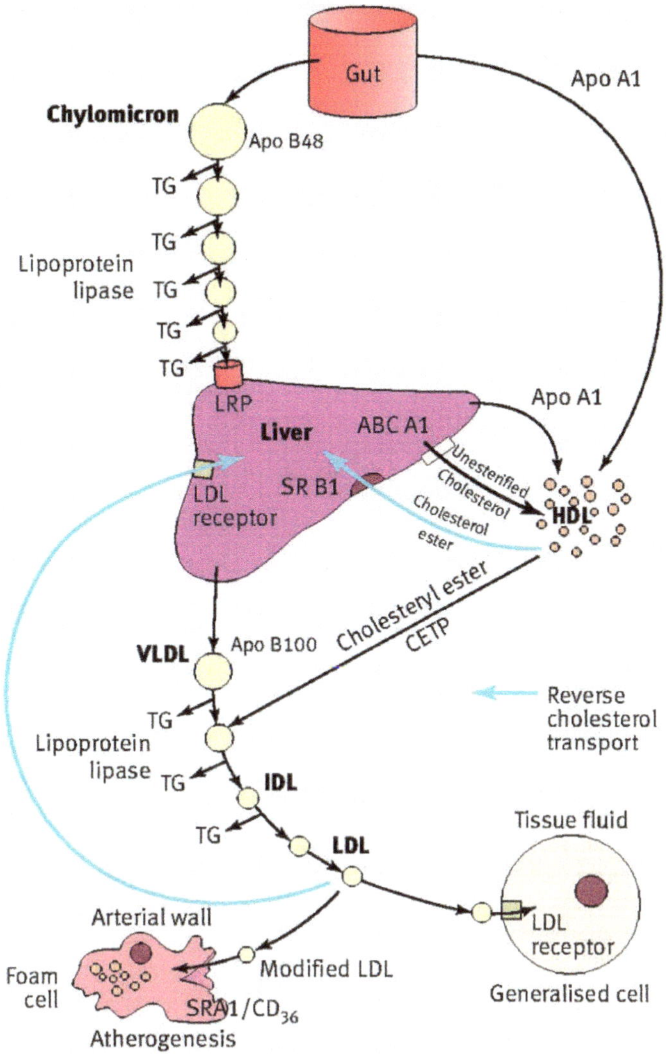

Dietary cholesterol absorbed in the gut is transported to the liver in chylomicrons, which are rich in triglyceride. Cholesterol is also synthesised de novo in the liver, gut, and central nervous system. Cholesterol in the liver is packaged along with triglycerides and secreted as VLDL, which is then converted into LDL in the circulation. LDL delivers cholesterol to most tissues, and the uptake of cholesterol is facilitated by LDL receptors. Excess cholesterol is removed from cells by HDL and is then either transferred to LDL and VLDL, whence it can return to the liver via hepatic LDL receptors or be taken up directly from HDL via the hepatic class B scavenger receptors. Cholesterol is also excreted in bile both as free cholesterol and as bile acids, which are both subject to enterohepatic circulation. Most of the plasma cholesterol is present in LDL, with smaller amounts in VLDL and HDL. Total plasma cholesterol mainly reflects LDL cholesterol. In the fasting state, plasma triglyceride generally indicates the VLDL concentration.

LDL = low density lipoprotein
HDL = high density lipoprotein
VLDL = very low density lipoprotein
IDL = intermediate density lipoprotein
CETP = cholesteryl ester transfer protein
ABCAI = ATP binding cassette transporter 1
SRB 1 = class B scavenger receptors
LRP = lipoprotein related receptor
TG = triglyceride
Apo = apolipoprotein
SRA1 = steroid receptor RNA activator
CD_{36} = thrombospondin receptor

Fig 1 The role of cholesterol in the metabolism of lipoprotein. Adapted from Charlton-Menys[4]

Table 1 Diagnostic criteria for heterozygous familial hypercholesterolaemia, taken from the Simon Broome familial hypercholesterolemia register (www.primarycare.ox.ac.uk/research/vascular/research/simon_broome)

Criterion	Description
A	Total cholesterol concentration >7.5 mmol/l (adults) or >6.7 mmol/l (children aged <16 years); *or* low density lipoprotein cholesterol concentration >4.9 mmol/l in adults or >4.0 mmol/l in children
B	Tendinous xanthomata in the patient or a first degree relative
C	DNA based evidence of an LDLR mutation, familial defective apo B100, or a PCSK9 mutation
D	Family history of myocardial infarction before age 50 years in a second degree relative or before age 60 years in a first degree relative
E	Family history of raised total cholesterol concentration >7.5 mmol/l in a first or second degree relative

A + B or A + C, constitutes a definite diagnosis of heterozygous familial hypercholesterolaemia.
A + D or A + E constitutes possible heterozygous familial hypercholesterolaemia.

Table 2 and box 1 outline the diagnostic classification of hypercholesterolaemia. Before primary hypercholesterolaemia is diagnosed underlying secondary causes should be excluded.

How to investigate the patient with hypercholesterolaemia

Before treatment is started for hypercholesterolaemia a detailed history, clinical examination, and baseline laboratory tests are needed to discover causes of secondary hypercholesterolaemia, manifestations of primary lipoprotein disorders, and any complications related to atherosclerosis. A family and occupational history—including a history of smoking, alcohol intake, and dietary preferences—will help to indicate the extent to which these factors contribute to hypercholesterolaemia and/or to risk of cardiovascular disease and to gauge the patient's ability to change lifestyle. The physical examination should include blood pressure, body weight, height, waist circumference,

Table 2 Most commonly encountered causes of primary hypercholesterolaemia

Diagnosis	Prevalence (%)	Inheritance	Clinical features	Biochemistry
Common hypercholesterolaemia*	70	Polygenic	Usually none (sometimes corneal arcus, xanthelasmata)	Raised cholesterol owing to low density lipoprotein
Heterozygous familial hypercholesterolaemia	0.2	Monogenic	Cholesterol raised from childhood. In adulthood often tendon xanthomata or Achilles tenosynovitis; sometimes corneal arcus and xanthelasmata	Raised cholesterol owing to low density lipoprotein
Familial defective apoplipoprotein B	0.2	Monogenic	Usually none. Occasionally familial hypercholesterolaemia phenotype	Raised cholesterol owing to low density lipoprotein
Combined hyperlipidaemia†	10	Polygenic	Usually none (sometimes corneal arcus, xanthelasmata); overlap with dyslipidaemia of type 2 diabetes and metabolic syndrome	Raised triglycerides and cholesterol owing increased very low density lipoprotein
Type III hyperlipoproteinaemia (dysbetalipoproteinaemia; remnant removal disease)	0.02	Monogenic	Striate palmar xanthomata; tuberoeruptive xanthomata	Raised triglycerides and cholesterol owing to intermediate density lipoprotein and chylomicron remnants. Usually apo E2 homozygosity
Severe hypertriglyceridaemia (>10 mmol/l)	0.1	Polygenic or monogenic	Eruptive xanthomata; acute pancreatitis; milky plasma; lipaemia retinalis	Raised triglycerides owing to fasting chylomicronaemia and increased very low density lipoprotein

Prevalence is approximate and refers to the adult population in the UK (Durrington, see "Additional education resources" box).
**Defined as plasma cholesterol ≥5 mmol/l in middle age.*
†Defined as plasma cholesterol ≥5 mmol/l and fasting plasma triglycerides ≥1.7 mmol/l in the absence of diagnostic features of heterozygous familial hypercholesterolaemia (table 1).

and a search for xanthomata. A family history is essential to facilitate cascade testing in primary hypercholesterolaemia.[16]

Laboratory assessment in hypercholesterolaemia

When screening for hypercholesterolaemia it is advisable to take blood samples after a fast of at least 10 hours to avoid the postprandial contribution to plasma triglycerides. If plasma triglycerides do not exceed 4.5 mmol/l, the LDL cholesterol concentration can be calculated by the Friedewald formula (box 2). If low density lipoprotein cholesterol cannot be measured owing to hypertriglyceridaemia, then non-HDL cholesterol can be used as a target for statin treatment. Biological and laboratory variations in plasma cholesterol concentrations mean that tests should be done more than once before treatment is started. Laboratory reports should also provide HDL cholesterol values and the total cholesterol:HDL ratio to help assess risk of cardiovascular disease, but LDL cholesterol should be used as the target for treatment where possible. The targets for non-HDL cholesterol are 0.75 mmol/l higher than for LDL cholesterol.

In assessing risk of cardiovascular disease it is also essential to measure fasting glucose concentration. Before lipid lowering treatment is started, liver function tests, creatine kinase activity, serum creatinine, and dipstick urine protein should be measured. In some patients specialised assays may be needed to identify the cause of hypercholesterolaemia.

BOX 1 CAUSES OF HYPERLIPIDAEMIA

Some causes of secondary hyperlipidaemia

- Nephrotic syndrome
- Obstructive jaundice
- Hypothyroidism
- Cushing's syndrome
- Anorexia nervosa
- Thiazide diuretics
- Ciclosporin

Some causes of mixed hyperlipidaemia*

- Type 2 diabetes mellitus
- Obesity, particularly if accompanied by features of the metabolic syndrome
- Alcohol excess
- Monoclonal gammopathy
- Renal dialysis
- Glucocorticoids
- β blockers
- Retinoic acid derivatives

**Increase in plasma cholesterol and triglycerides*

BOX 2 CALCULATING LDL CHOLESTEROL AND NON-HDL CHOLESTEROL CONCENTRATIONS*

- Low density lipoprotein cholesterol = total serum cholesterol – (HDL cholesterol + (serum triglycerides/2.2))
- Non-HDL cholesterol = total cholesterol – HDL cholesterol

**All values in mmol/l*

When should treatment for hypercholesterolaemia be introduced?

The introduction of cholesterol lowering drugs should always be based on an assessment of risk of cardiovascular disease. In patients without diabetes, the pre-existing risk can be estimated using the JBS2 charts[8] or the JBS2 cardiovascular risk assessor computer program (www.heartuk.org.uk/new/pages/prof/jbs_cv_riskassessor.html) (figure 2).

Cholesterol lowering drugs are intended for use in people between the age of 40 and 70 years. The assessment tables are likely to underestimate risk in people with adverse family history, impaired fasting glucose, or impaired glucose tolerance; people from the Indian subcontinent; people with hypertriglyceridaemia or renal dysfunction; and in the presence of multiple comorbidities. The computer program makes adjustments for these. The footnote to the tables recommends multiplying the cardiovascular risk by 1.3-1.5 when one or more of these factors are present. In certain groups of patients—for example, those with inherited dyslipidaemia—treatment through diet and with appropriate drugs should be started without calculating cardiovascular risk (box 3).[8 17] The charts and computer program are designed to assist clinical judgment not to replace it. They should be used along with the clinical approach described above.

What are the targets for cholesterol lowering?

The targets to which plasma cholesterol should be lowered have changed over the years, but the near linear relation between the log of the risk and cholesterol reduction described by the Cholesterol Trialists Collaboration[18] forms part of the evidence for setting targets. The JBS2 guidelines[8] advocate an optimal total cholesterol target of <4.0 mmol/l (or a 25% reduction) or an LDL cholesterol concentration

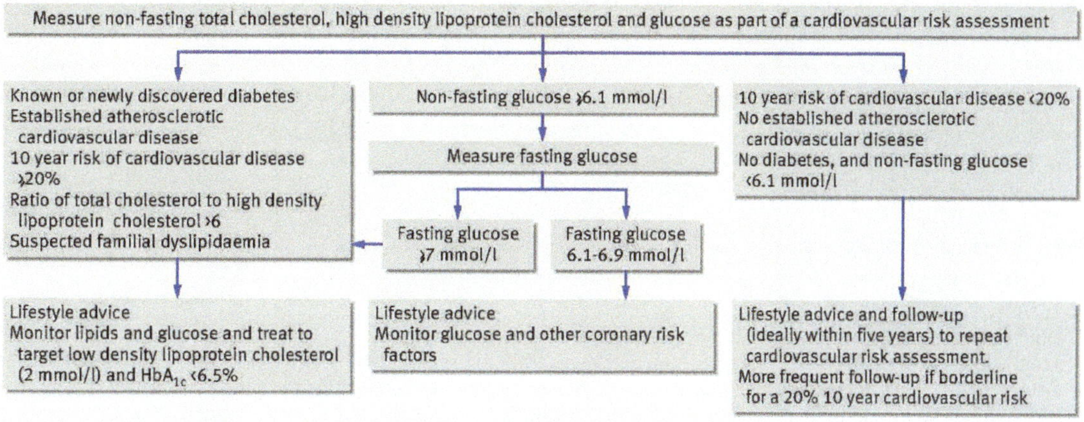

Fig 2 Summary of the Joint British Societies' guidelines on preventing cardiovascular disease in clinical practice[8]

BOX 3 STARTING STATIN TREATMENT WITHOUT FORMAL ESTIMATION OF CARDIOVASCULAR RISK

Statin treatment should be considered in the following people without formal estimation of cardiovascular risk[8 17]:

- Those with atherosclerotic cardiovascular disease including coronary heart disease, stroke, transient cerebral ischaemia, peripheral arterial disease
- Those with type 1 and type 2 diabetes mellitus who are aged ≥40 years (or younger if additional cardiovascular risk factors are present)
- Those with renal dysfunction including diabetic nephropathy
- Those with familial hypercholesterolaemia, familial combined hyperlipidaemia, or other genetic dyslipidaemias
- Ratio of total cholesterol:HDL cholesterol ≥6.0

of <2.0 mmol/l (or a 30% reduction) for both primary and secondary prevention and for people with diabetes mellitus.

The 2008 guidelines from the National Institute for Health and Clinical Excellence (NICE) on lipid modification[19] agree with the JBS2 guidelines on secondary prevention targets but do not advise any targets for primary prevention. They recommend that when the decision to prescribe a statin for primary prevention has been made patients should be given 40 mg of simvastatin without further monitoring of serum lipids, unless clinical judgment or patient preference indicate a review of drug treatment or lipid profile. The JBS2 and NICE guidelines both advise an "audit" concentration of total cholesterol of 5 mmol/l or an LDL cholesterol concentration of <3 mmol/l as the minimum standard of care for high risk individuals.

Clinicians should be aware that cholesterol lowering treatment can reduce the cholesterol content of an atheromatous plaque, which may be too small for angioplasty or bypass surgery but which can rupture, enabling clot formation, arterial occlusion, and the acute clinical syndromes associated with atherosclerosis.[20]

What treatments are available to lower plasma cholesterol?

The strength of the evidence that cardiovascular risk can be decreased by treatment with statins[18] means that the most appropriate approach to treating people at the highest risk combines lifestyle advice with use of statins.

Lifestyle measures

Lifestyle measures such as stopping smoking, decreasing excess alcohol consumption, increasing physical activity, losing weight, and following a low fat saturated diet will all decrease the risk of cardiovascular disease. However, dietary advice given by health professionals often produces inadequate lowering of cholesterol, typically by about 3%, although reductions of 10% or more have been seen in studies carried out in controlled conditions on a metabolic ward.[21]

Plant sterols

A recent systematic review suggests that margarines and drinks containing plant sterols or stanols rather than saturated fat can decrease plasma cholesterol by up to 10%.[22]

Statins

Several large trials of primary and secondary prevention of coronary heart disease using statins have established their efficacy. A meta-analysis of 14 statin trials using data from 90 056 participants showed that for each 1 mmol/l lowering of plasma LDL cholesterol coronary and stroke events fell by about 21% and this was accompanied by a decrease in all cause mortality.[18]

This linear decrease extends down to current LDL cholesterol targets of 2 mmol/l. Patients in clinical trials whose pretreatment LDL cholesterol concentrations were <3 mmol/l showed the same reduction in relative risk of cardiovascular disease with statin treatment as those with higher LDL cholesterol concentrations.[18]

Statins are generally well tolerated and efficacious. However, efficacy varies: at a maximum dose of 40 mg, pravastatin reduces LDL cholesterol by 29%, and at a maximum dose of 80 mg, simvastatin, atorvastatin, and rosuvastatin reduce LDL cholesterol by 42%, 55%, and 58% respectively.[23] Each doubling of dose with a statin results in a further 5-6% reduction in LDL cholesterol.

About 1-3% of patients complain of side effects such as tiredness, indigestion, or change in bowel habit. Some patients develop increases in liver transaminase or creatine kinase activity. Tests for liver function should be done before and about three months after statins are started. If serum transaminase activity increases to three times the upper limit of normal then treatment should be stopped.

However, a substantial number of patients with dyslipidaemia already have abnormal serum liver

ADDITIONAL EDUCATIONAL RESOURCES FOR HEALTHCARE PROFESSIONALS

- Grundy SM. Metabolic syndrome: connecting and reconciling cardiovascular and diabetes worlds. *J Am Coll Cardiol* 2006;47:1093-1100.
- Pollex RL, Hegele RA. Genetic determinants of plasma lipoproteins. *Nat Clin Pract Cardiovasc Med* 2007;4:600-9.
- Cannon CP, Steinberg BA, Murphy SA, Mega JL, Braunwald E. Meta-analysis of cardiovascular outcomes trials comparing intensive versus moderate statin therapy. *J Am Coll Cardiol* 2006;48:438-45.
- National Institute for Health and Clinical Excellence. *Lipid modification: cardiovascular risk assessment and the modification of blood lipids for the primary and secondary prevention of cardiovascular disease.* London: NICE, 2008. www.nice.org.uk/ CG67
- Durrington PN. *Hyperlipidaemia diagnosis and management.* London: Hodder Arnold, 2007.
- National Institute for Health and Clinical Excellence. *Clinical guidelines and evidence review for familial hypercholesterolaemia: the identification and management of adults and children with familial hypercholesterolaemia.* 2008 (Clinical guideline 71.) www.nice.org.uk/CG71
- Bhatnagar D. Diagnosis and screening for familial hypercholesterolaemia: finding the patients, finding the genes. *Ann Clin Biochem* 2006;43:441-56.

TIPS FOR NON-SPECIALISTS

- A desirable or healthy plasma cholesterol concentration is based on the value associated with a coronary risk that is unacceptably high
- Both the JBS 2 guidelines and the NICE guidelines advocate assessment of coronary risk based on the Framingham equation (www.framinghamheartstudy.org/risk/index.html)
- A clinical approach to hypercholesterolaemia will often identify genetic hyperlipidaemias, which are associated with premature coronary heart disease
- Patients with the following conditions should be referred to a specialist lipid clinic:
  - Suspected genetic hyperlipidaemias
  - Abnormal pretreatment liver enzymes or creatine kinase activity
  - Intolerance to or side effects from lipid lowering treatment
  - Mixed hyperlipidaemia
  - Resistance to statin treatment
  - Patients taking complex combinations of drugs with high risk of serious drug interaction with lipid modification treatment
  - Secondary hyperlipidaemia
  - Dyslipidaemia related to HIV
  - Lipodystrophy syndromes
  - Post-transplant hyperlipidaemia
- The introduction of cholesterol lowering drugs should always be based on assessment of cardiovascular risk

ADDITIONAL EDUCATIONAL RESOURCES FOR PATIENTS

- HEART UK, 7 North Road, Maidenhead SL6 1PE (www.heartuk.org.uk; helpline, tel: 0845 450 5988)—Raises awareness about the risks of high cholesterol and about better detection of those at risk; provides information and advice on preventing premature deaths, particularly in those with inherited high cholesterol
- British Heart Foundation, 14 Fitzhardinge Street, London W1H 6DH (www.bhf.org.uk; heart information line, tel: 08450 70 80 70)—Supports heart patients, invests in research, and provides information to help people reduce their risk of dying prematurely from a heart or circulatory related illness
- British Nutrition Foundation (www.nutrition.org.uk)—Provides impartial interpretation and effective dissemination of scientifically based knowledge and advice on the relation between diet, physical activity, and health
- *Cholesterol*—Information leaflet about cholesterol published by the NHS for patients (http://cks.library.nhs.uk/patient_information_leaflet/cholesterol)
- *Cholesterol*— Information leaflet about cholesterol published by Patient UK for patients (www.patient.co.uk/showdoc/23068704/)

function tests owing to non-alcoholic steatohepatitis, with increases in alanine aminotransferase and γ glutamyl transpeptidase being particularly common in patients with hypertriglyceridaemia. This is not a reason to withhold statin treatment. Fluctuations in alanine aminotransferase may create the impression that it has risen as a result of statin treatment. But hepatotoxicity induced by statins is rare, and in patients at high risk of cardiovascular disease statins should not be discontinued because of abnormal liver function tests without firm proof of causality.[24]

Myositis induced by statins is also uncommon,[24] and minor fluctuation in creatine kinase activity and in muscle discomfort should not lead to discontinuation of statins. People who are physically active or are of African origin can have creatine kinase levels as high as 1000 U/l regardless of statin treatment. Untreated hypothyroidism and certain drugs when used with statins can increase the possibility of myositis.[25] Nevertheless, when patients complain of tiredness or muscle pain then liver function tests and measuring creatine kinase activity should be part of the routine investigations. If patients are convinced that the symptoms are linked to statin use, then it is worth trying another statin.

Other pharmacological agents

For patients who are unable to tolerate statins, bile acid sequestrants or alternatives such as nicotinic acid can be used, but these are more likely than statins to cause side effects. Fibrates increase HDL cholesterol and lower plasma triglycerides but have marginal effect in lowering LDL cholesterol. Moreover, several large trials of fibrates have shown that although non-fatal cardiovascular events are decreased, total mortality increases.

Combination treatments

In patients who do not achieve target cholesterol levels when they are taking statins, combination treatment can be used. It is usual to combine a statin with ezetimibe, which will lower LDL cholesterol by a further 15%. Nicotinic acid, fibrates, and the fish oil preparation Omacor (Solvay), which have the advantage of lowering plasma triglycerides too, can also be used in combination with statins to lower LDL cholesterol. Currently large randomised controlled trials are looking at whether statins and fibrates combined are more beneficial than statins alone.

Combination treatments are associated with more side effects and must be used with caution. Gemfibrozil, in particular, interferes with the conjugation of statins, increasing the chances of myositis, and it should not be combined with statins. Combinations of statins with fibrates or nicotinic acid should not be used in secondary hyperlipidaemia, elderly people, or those being treated long term with ciclosporin, tacrolimus, macrolide antibiotics, or antifungals. Lipid lowering drugs should be stopped at least three months before a woman plans to conceive because of potential teratogenicity.

Contributors: DB, HS, and PND have contributed equally to the preparation of this article. DB and PND are the guarantors.

Competing interests: DB has received lecture fees and fees for consultancies from pharmaceutical companies making lipid lowering drugs and treatments for diabetes mellitus. HS has received lecture fees from a pharmaceutical company making insulin and lipid lowering drugs. PND has an independent research grant to the University of Manchester from Pfizer and has also received lecture fees from pharmaceutical companies.

Provenance and peer review: Commissioned; externally peer reviewed.

1 Libby P. Inflammation in atherosclerosis. *Nature* 2002;420:868-74.
2 Chen Z, Peto R, Collins R, MacMahon S, Lu J, Li W. Serum cholesterol concentration and coronary heart disease in population with low cholesterol concentrations. *BMJ* 1991;303:276-82.
3 Chaudhury M. Blood analytes. In: Sproston K, Primatesta P, eds. *Health survey for England 2003. Risk factors for cardiovascular disease.* Vol 2. London: Stationery Office, 2004:241-87.
4 Charlton-Menys V, Durrington PN. Human cholesterol metabolism and therapeutic molecules. *Exp Physiol* 2008;93:27-42.

5 Stamler J, Wentworth D, Neaton JD. "Is the relationship between serum cholesterol and risk of premature death from coronary heart disease continuous and graded?" Findings in 356,222 primary screenees of the multiple risk factor intervention trial (MRFIT)." *JAMA* 1986;256:2823-8.

6 LaRosa JC, Hunninghake D, Bush D, Criqui MH, Getz GS, Gotto AM Jr, et al. The cholesterol facts. A summary of the evidence relating dietary fats, serum cholesterol, and coronary heart disease. A joint statement by the American Heart Association and the National Heart, Lung, and Blood Institute. The Task Force on Cholesterol Issues, American Heart Association. *Circulation* 1990;81:1721-33.

7 Department of Health. *National service framework for coronary heart disease* . London: DoH, 2000.

8 Wood DA, Wray R, Poulter N, Williams B, Kirby M, Patel V, et al. JBS2: joint British guidelines on prevention of cardiovascular disease in clinical practice. *Heart* 2005;91(suppl V):v1-52.

9 Kane JP, Havel RJ. Disorders of the biogenesis and secretion of lipoproteins containing the B apolipoproteins. In: Scriver CR, Beaudet AL, Sly WS, Valle D, eds. *The metabolic and molecular bases of inherited disease* . 8th ed. New York: McGraw-Hill, 2001:2717-52.

10 Goldstein JL, Hobbs HH, Brown MS. Familial hypercholesterolaemia. In: Scriver CR, Beaudet AL, Sly WS, Valle D, eds. *The metabolic and molecular bases of inherited disease* . 8th ed. New York: McGraw-Hill, 2001:2863-913.

11 Stone NJ, Levy RI, Fredrickson DS, Verter J. Coronary artery disease in 116 kindred with familial type II hyperlipoproteinaemia. *Circulation* 1974;49:476-88.

12 Sarwar N, Danesh J, Eiriksdottir G, Sigurdsson G, Wareham N, Bingham S, et al. Triglycerides and the risk of coronary heart disease: 10,158 incident cases among 262,525 participants in 29 Western prospective studies. *Circulation* 2007;115:450-8.

13 Haffner SM, Stern MP, Hazuda HP, Mitchell BD, Patterson JK. Cardiovascular risk factors in confirmed prediabetic individuals: does the clock for coronary disease start ticking before the onset of clinical diabetes? *JAMA* 1990;263:2893-8.

14 Mahley RW, Rall SC. Type III hyperlipoproteinemia (dysbetalipoproteinemia): the role of apolipoprotein E in normal and abnormal lipoprotein metabolism. In: Scriver CR, Beaudet AL, Sly WS, Valle D, eds. *The metabolic and molecular bases of inherited disease.* 8th ed. New York: McGraw-Hill, 2001:2835-62.

15 Durrington PN. Dyslipidaemia. *Lancet* 2003;362:717-31.

16 Bhatnagar D, Morgan J, Siddiq S, Mackness MI, Miller JP, Durrington PN. Outcome of case finding among relatives of patients with known heterozygous familial hypercholesterolaemia. *BMJ* 2000;321:1497-500.

17 Durrington PN, Prais H, Bhatnagar D, France M, Crowley V, Khan J, et al. Indications for cholesterol lowering medication: comparison of risk-assessment methods. *Lancet* 1999;353:278-81.

18 Cholesterol Treatment Trialists' (CTT) Collaborators. Efficacy and safety of cholesterol-lowering treatment: prospective meta-analysis of data from 90,056 participants in 14 randomised trials of statins. *Lancet* 2005;366:1267-78.

19 National Institute for Health and Clinical Excellence. *Lipid modification: cardiovascular risk assessment and the modification of blood lipids for the primary and secondary prevention of cardiovascular disease* . London: NICE, 2008. www.nice.org.uk/ CG67

20 Rioufol G, Gilard M, Finet G, Ginon I, Boschat J, André-Fouët X. Evolution of spontaneous atherosclerotic plaque rupture with medical therapy: long-term follow-up with intravascular ultrasound. *Circulation* 2004;110:2875-80.

21 Tang JL, Armitage JM, Lancaster T, Silagy CA, Fowler GH, Neil HAW. Systematic review of dietary intervention trials to lower blood total cholesterol in free-living subjects. *BMJ* 1998;316:1213-9.

22 Katan MJ, Grundy SM, Jones P, Law M, Miettinen T, Paoletti R, et al. Efficacy and safety of plant stanols and sterols in the management of blood cholesterol levels. *Mayo Clin Proc* 2003;78:965-78.

23 Law MR, Wald NJ, Rudnicka AR. Quantifying effects of statins on low density lipoprotein cholesterol, ischaemic heart disease, and stroke: systematic review and meta-analysis. *BMJ* 2003;326:1423-30.

24 Armitage J. The safety of statins in clinical practice. *Lancet* 2007;370:1781-90

25 Ballantyne CM, Corsini A, Davidson MH, Holdaas H, Jacobson TA, Leitersdorf E, et al. Risk for myopathy with statin therapy in high-risk patients. *Archives of Internal Medicine* 2003;163:553-64.

26 Betteridge DJ, Illingworth DR, Shepherd J, eds. *Lipoproteins in health and disease* . London: Arnold, 1999.

27 Scriver CR, Beaudet AL, Sly WS, Valle D, eds. *The metabolic and molecular bases of inherited disease.* 8th ed. New York: McGraw-Hill, 2001.

28 Durrington PN. *Hyperlipidaemia diagnosis and management.* London: Hodder Arnold, 2007.

Investigation and management of congestive heart failure

Bruce Arroll, professor and head of general practice and primary health care [1], Robert Doughty, associate professor[2], Victoria Andersen, PhD candidate[1]

[1]University of Auckland, Private Bag 92019, Auckland, 1142, New Zealand

[2]Department of Medicine, University of Auckland, Private Bag 92019

Correspondence to: B Arroll b.arroll@auckland.ac.nz

Cite this as: *BMJ* 2010;341:c3657

‹DOI› 10.1136/bmj.c3657 http://www.bmj.com/content/341/bmj.c3657

Congestive heart failure is a common condition that increases in prevalence with increasing age. In 2003, guidance from the National Institute for Health and Clinical Excellence acknowledged that the "rising epidemic of heart failure" is partly the result of people living longer and the more effective treatments for coronary heart disease now available. It also acknowledged, however, that average life expectancy is only about three years after diagnosis, which is much worse than for many other serious illnesses such as cancer of the breast or colon.[1] The condition is associated with poor quality of life, frequent hospital admissions, and poor survival,[2] although this may have changed with the advent of better treatments. Community estimates of prevalence vary from 1.6 to 4.6 cases per 1000 in men aged 45-74 years and from 0.9 to 2.2 cases per 1000 in women. About 1% of men develop heart failure after age 75 and almost 2% after 80 years.[3] This review discusses the immediate management of patients who present with the clinical syndrome of heart failure (usually a combination of dyspnoea, fatigue, exercise intolerance, and fluid retention) and the management of chronic congestive heart failure. It is based on evidence from guidelines, randomised controlled trials, and population cohorts followed for many years. We also emphasise the distinction between heart failure with low ejection fraction and heart failure with preserved ejection fraction because although plenty of evidence exists on how to treat the first entity very little exists on how to treat the second.

What are the clinical features of heart failure?

Heart failure is a clinical syndrome comprising reduced cardiac output, tissue hypoperfusion, and congestion.[4] Table 1 lists the common symptoms and signs of heart failure. In hospital, patients with heart failure typically present with shortness of breath, exercise intolerance, and leg swelling, and they may have most of the signs in table 1. Dyspnoea, fatigue, exercise intolerance, and fluid retention are common, but some of the other features may not be present. In the community, patients often present with less acute symptoms and fewer clinical signs, and the clinical diagnosis of heart failure can be difficult.

SOURCES AND SELECTION CRITERIA

As well as using our personal reference collections, we searched the Cochrane database, Clinical Evidence and Best Practice (*BMJ* electronic textbook), and the US National Guideline Clearing House up to 18 March 2010. We also reviewed guidelines from the National Institute for Health and Clinical Excellence, Scottish Intercollegiate Guidelines Network, European Society of Cardiology, and the American College of Cardiology Foundation/American Heart Association. We selected systematic reviews and meta-analyses and when not available we used large randomised controlled trials.

SUMMARY POINTS

- Perform echocardiography in patients with certain or probable heart failure to refine the diagnosis and plan treatment
- Measure brain natriuretic peptide (BNP) in patients with an uncertain diagnosis
- A normal BNP result is better than electrocardiography for diagnosing heart failure and rules out heart failure; if raised perform echocardiography
- Echocardiography can determine the underlying structure and function of heart failure
- It is crucial to distinguish heart failure with low ejection fraction from that with preserved ejection fraction because most high quality evidence on treatment is for patients with low ejection fraction
- While waiting for echocardiography (or if not available) give an angiotensin converting enzyme inhibitor and β blocker (where possible) and uptitrate to maximum doses

Fluid overload

Fluid retention may be present in patients who have dyspnoea, an increase in weight from baseline of more than 2 kg in under three days, raised jugular venous pressure, crepitations on chest auscultation, hepatomegaly, or signs of peripheral oedema.

Exercise tolerance

The degree of exertion needed to elicit symptoms such as breathlessness can be used to grade the severity of symptoms into one of four New York Heart Association functional classes (table 2). Functional class does not define the cause of heart failure or the underlying cardiac abnormality that contributes to the syndrome but the categories are associated with different prognoses. Disease classification may change—for example, during an acute exacerbation a patient may have class IV disease but have class I disease (asymptomatic) after recovery.

Left ventricular ejection fraction

Patients with heart failure may have impaired left ventricular systolic function, which is usually assessed on echocardiography by measuring the left ventricular ejection fraction. However, as many as 50% of patients with the syndrome may have preserved left ventricular ejection fraction (usually defined as >50%), and currently little evidence is available to guide management in these patients (box 1). It is important to distinguish between those with a low ejection fraction and those with a preserved ejection fraction because most of the research into treatment has been done on those with low ejection fraction. Many descriptive studies have shown that patients with diagnosed heart failure in the community are undertreated.[8]

How is heart failure diagnosed?

A patient with heart failure may present in several different ways. Table 3 describes the investigations available and assesses their usefulness.

In those who almost certainly have clinical heart failure

Patients who are acutely unwell are usually admitted to hospital urgently. They may have acute pulmonary oedema. A bedside clinical assessment is usually sufficient to make a diagnosis without the need for further investigations. An echocardiogram will help to guide treatment for those with heart failure and low ejection fraction.

Table 1 Key factors for the diagnosis of heart failure (with or without low ejection fraction)[4]

Diagnostic factor	Comment
Dyspnoea made worse with sometimes minimal exertion	Most common symptom of left sided heart failure; has a sensitivity of 87% (only symptom that has a sensitivity >80%); need to rule out chronic obstructive pulmonary disease and pneumonia, which may coexist
Fatigue	Common because of poor tissue perfusion
Presence of risk factors for cardiovascular disease, including old age, male sex, previous cardiovascular disease, diabetes or dyslipidaemia, hypertension, left ventricular ejection fraction hypertrophy	All are risk factors for cardiovascular disease and congestive heart failure
Previous myocardial infarction	Single best predictor of congestive heart failure; when present the likelihood of congestive heart failure is 21 times greater[5]
Neck vein distension*	Major Framingham† criteria for congestive heart failure*
Third heart sound (S3 gallop)	Major Framingham criteria for congestive heart failure, with a specificity of 99% (almost never seen in other conditions)
Cardiomegaly, dilation, or hypertrophy	Major Framingham criteria for congestive heart failure, with a specificity of 85% (uncommon in other conditions); can be assessed by chest radiography, electrocardiography, or echocardiography
Hepatojugular reflux	Major Framingham criteria for congestive heart failure
Lung crepitations*	Major Framingham criteria for congestive heart failure, with a specificity of 81% (uncommon in other conditions)
Ankle oedema	Minor Framingham criteria for heart failure; congestive heart failure is more likely in men with this and is given more prominence in the Health Technology Assessment[3]
Tachycardia >120 beats/min	A minor Framingham criterion for congestive heart failure
Hepatomegaly*	A minor Framingham criterion for congestive heart failure with a specificity of 97% (uncommon in other conditions)
Night cough	A minor Framingham criterion for congestive heart failure
Pleural effusion (less than one third maximum vital capacity)	A minor Framingham criterion for congestive heart failure
Thyroid enlargement	May point to thyroid disease

These signs are very specific but do not always occur (low sensitivity), which limits their usefulness.

†The Framingham study is a long term cohort study started in Framingham, Massachusetts, in 1948. Participants were seen every 2 years and checked for cardiovascular disease and risk factors. In 1971 their children were included in the study.[6]

Table 2 New York Heart Association classification of congestive heart failure and associated evidence based treatments[7]

Class	Symptoms	Treatment if left ventricular ejection fraction is low	Treatment if left ventricular ejection fraction is preserved
Class I (mild)	No limitation of physical activity; ordinary physical activity does not cause undue fatigue, palpitation, or dyspnoea (shortness of breath)	ACE inhibitor*; consider a β blocker†	
Class II (mild)	Slight limitation of physical activity; comfortable at rest, but ordinary physical activity results in fatigue, palpitation, or dyspnoea	ACE inhibitor; β blocker; candesartan§ (specialist advice needed if adding to an ACE inhibitor)	Candesartan (specialist advice needed)
Class III (moderate)	Marked limitation of physical activity; comfortable at rest, but less than ordinary activity causes fatigue, palpitation, or dyspnoea	ACE inhibitor; β blocker; candesartan (specialist advice needed if adding to an ACE inhibitor); spironolactone‡; digoxin	Candesartan (specialist advice needed)
Class IV (severe)	Cannot carry out any physical activity without discomfort; symptoms of cardiac insufficiency at rest; discomfort increases if any physical activity is undertaken	ACE inhibitor; carvedilol or bisoprolol as β blocker; spironolactone‡; digoxin	Candesartan (specialist advice needed)

**Any angiotensin converting enzyme inhibitor (ACE) inhibitor is recommended but not all have been evaluated in clinical trials.*

†Recommended β blockers are carvedilol, bisoprolol, nebivolol, and metoprolol succinate (not available in the UK).

‡Avoid giving an ACE inhibitor, angiotensin receptor blocker, and spironolactone together because of the risk of hypotension and hyperkalaemia.

§Uncertainty exists about angiotensin receptor blockers as a class because irbesartan is not effective whereas candesartan is.

Table 3 Investigations for the clinical congestive heart failure syndrome[4]

Test	Information added
Echocardiography	The gold standard test—confirms the diagnosis of heart failure and distinguishes heart failure with low ejection fraction from that with preserved ejection fraction
BNP or NT-pro BNP	When low or normal this test rules out congestive heart failure; both assays are accurate; better than electrocardiography for congestive heart failure[3]
Chest radiography	Will show cardiomegaly and pulmonary venous hypertension; when abnormalities are present very specific; useful for diagnosing respiratory causes of breathlessness
Electrocardiography	If normal this rules out congestive heart failure; useful for other diagnostic purposes such as irregular pulse and cardiac ischaemia; BNP test preferred if available[3]
Spirometry	Can diagnose respiratory causes of dyspnoea; does not rule out congestive heart failure because respiratory conditions can coexist with congestive heart failure
Full blood count	Anaemia may explain congestive heart failure
Thyroid function	Hyperthyroidism or hypothyroidism can be reversible causes of congestive heart failure
Renal function (eg, creatinine)	May explain overload if abnormal and needed for drug dosing
Blood glucose or glycosolated haemoglobin (HbA1c), lipids	Risk factors for cardiovascular disease that may need controlling
Liver function	Can be normal or raised; when raised may influence drug choice
Electrolytes	Of more interest once treatment has started

BNP=brain natriuretic peptide; NT-pro BNP=N-terminal pro-B-type brain natriuretic peptide.

BOX 1 THE TWO TYPES OF HEART FAILURE

Heart failure with low left ventricular ejection fraction
Left ventricular systolic dysfunction, commonly assessed using the left ventricular ejection fraction, refers to impaired left ventricular pump (contractile) function, usually termed heart failure with low ejection fraction. This is most commonly assessed by echocardiography. It is essential to determine left ventricular systolic function because most of the evidence on the life saving use of angiotensin converting enzyme inhibitor, β blockers, and aldosterone antagonists is based on studies with patients who have heart failure with low ejection fraction. Extensive evidence is available to guide management, including drugs and device based treatments (primary implantable cardiac defibrillators and biventricular pacing) in this group of patients.

Heart failure with preserved left ventricular ejection fraction
Around 50% of patients with heart failure will have preserved left ventricular ejection fraction when assessed using echocardiography. Although many will have left ventricular diastolic dysfunction this is difficult to assess accurately in clinical practice. Such patients have the clinical syndrome of congestive heart failure, with similar symptoms and signs as those who have heart failure with low ejection fraction. Echocardiography is still essential because it will help to define this group of patients, although techniques such as cardiac catheterisation may be needed to assess left ventricular diastolic dysfunction.

Table 4 Angiotensin converting enzyme (ACE) inhibitors and β blockers recommended for patients with heart failure and low ejection fraction*

Drug	Starting dose	Target dose	Comments
ACE inhibitors			
Captopril	6.25 mg TDS	50-100 TDS	Cough is a common adverse effect; monitor electrolytes and if creatinine increases >50% consider stopping; potassium can also rise
Cilazapril	0.5 mg OD	2.5 mg daily	As above
Enalapril	2.5 mg BD	10-20 mg daily	As above
Fosinopril	10 mg OD	40 mg OD	As above
Lisinopril[9]	2.5-5 mg	35 mg daily	As above
Perindopril	2 mg once daily	4 mg once daily	As above
Quinapril	2.5-5 mg OD	10-20 mg OD	As above
Ramipril	2.5 OD	5 mg BD or 10 mg OD	As above
β blockers			
Carvedilol†	3.125 mg BD	25-50 mg BD	Monitor all patients taking β blockers for bradycardia, atrial ventricular block, and bronchospasm
Bisoprolol	1.25 mg daily	10 mg daily	As above
Metoprolol succinate	23.75 mg daily	190 mg daily	Not to be used in New York Heart Association class IV disease
Nebivolol	1.25 mg daily	10 mg once daily	

*BD=twice daily; OD=once daily; TDS=three times daily.
†Carvedilol is preferred over metoprolol.[9]

BOX 2 DIFFERENTIAL DIAGNOSIS OF CLINICAL HEART FAILURE SYNDROME

Breathlessness
- Congestive heart failure
- Renal failure
- Depression, anxiety, or hyperventilation
- Anaemia
- Obesity
- Chronic obstructive pulmonary disease
- Pulmonary embolism
- Atrial fibrillation

Oedema
- Congestive heart failure
- Renal failure
- Depression (oedema as a result of inactivity)
- Drugs (calcium channel blockers and non-steroidal anti-inflammatory drugs)
- Benign ankle oedema
- Obesity
- Hypoalbuminaemia
- Pulmonary embolism
- Atrial fibrillation

In those with probable clinical heart failure

In patients with less acute symptoms who have a constellation of clinical symptoms and signs suggestive of heart failure the clinician might have a high degree of clinical certainty. Early treatment may be initiated and the patient referred for electrocardiography, chest radiography, and echocardiography. Although access to echocardiography may be delayed or restricted in some locations, refer as a priority for echocardiography patients who are at high risk of heart failure (if they have a history of myocardial infarction, basal lung crepitations, or are male and have swollen ankles).

In those in whom the diagnosis is very uncertain

In patients presenting in the community who have coexisting respiratory disease or are elderly, the diagnosis of heart failure is often difficult to make. Such a diagnosis can be improved by incorporating brain natriuretic peptide in clinical decision making pathways. The 2009 Health Technology Assessment group considers brain natriuretic peptide (measured using brain natriuretic peptide or N-terminal pro-B-type brain natriuretic peptide assays) better than electrocardiography for diagnosing congestive cardiac failure.[3] Low brain natriuretic peptide essentially rules out congestive heart failure as a cause of dyspnoea and guides investigation towards other causes, such as respiratory disease (see box 2 for differential diagnoses). All patients with confirmed congestive heart failure should undergo echocardiography to assess cardiac structure and function. Other tests discussed in table 3 can help establish a functional cause of heart failure or help guide drug treatments.

What treatments may be useful before results of diagnostic tests are available?

We suggest that when there is a strong clinical suspicion of congestive heart failure (with or without suggestive features on chest radiography and electrocardiography) but no access to echocardiography, patients should be given an angiotensin converting enzyme (ACE) inhibitor and a β blocker, titrated up to maximal doses (table 4). This means that patients with heart failure with low ejection fraction will be treated optimally and those with preserved ejection fraction will have their risk of cardiovascular disease lowered by virtue of a lower blood pressure. It is currently unclear if this approach would be beneficial or harmful but we would speculate that at least it would do no harm. For those with heart failure with preserved ejection fraction a change to candesartan could be considered once the diagnosis is confirmed. Although this approach is not ideal and extends beyond the current evidence, it is a pragmatic and reasonable approach to patient care in a resource poor environment because the adverse effects of ACE inhibitors and β blockers are not serious enough to limit their use.

How should a patient with heart failure be treated?[4 10]

Diuretics and assessment of fluid status

Consider treatment with diuretics in patients with heart failure who have dyspnoea or ankle or pulmonary oedema. These drugs should be given before or at the same time as ACE inhibitors, and both should precede the start of β blockers. We have no clear evidence that diuretics have a positive effect on mortality.[1] Diuretics are used on an individual basis to reduce fluid retention. Avoid overtreatment, which can lead to dehydration and renal dysfunction, particularly with loop diuretics.[4] Hypovolaemia can be assessed by measuring supine and standing blood pressures. A postural drop in blood pressure that causes light headedness or unconsciousness indicates hypovolaemia, particularly in elderly patients with heart failure.[1] Bumetanide, furosemide, and torasemide (loop diuretics) act at the loop of Henle, whereas thiazides, metolazone, and potassium sparing agents (such as spironolactone) act in the distal portion of the tubule.[1] The addition of a thiazide diuretic or a potassium sparing diuretic (or both) to loop diuretics can be useful if pulmonary or ankle oedema persists,[4] because the different classes of diuretic are thought to have an additive effect. It is essential to monitor electrolytes in the early phase of diuretic administration. The side effects of diuretics, such as frequent micturition, are unpleasant, especially for elderly patients, and in those with stable symptoms (ideally on maximum doses of ACE inhibitor and β blocker) consider lowering the dose of the loop diuretic, stepping down to a thiazide diuretic, or stopping diuretics completely.

Evidence based drug based treatment in heart failure with low ejection fraction

If the patient has limited fluid retention or is back to their baseline weight an ACE inhibitor can be started at a low dose. It is common practice to start the ACE inhibitor before the β blocker. Several high quality clinical trials have shown that treatment with ACE inhibitors and β blockers at the suggested maximum doses reduces mortality and decreases hospital admissions in people with heart failure. It is important to try to achieve the maximum dose because these benefits have not been confirmed at lower doses.[1 10 11] The dose of ACE inhibitor can be increased every two weeks until the maximum dose is achieved. Consider this approach in all patients except those who have low blood pressure (<100 systolic), are clinically hypotensive, or have terminal comorbidities.[12] Once the maximum dose is achieved add one of the recommended β blockers. If the patient has been assessed for intolerance you can start at a low dose and double it every two weeks.[12] Both drugs can be started even in patients with some degree of dyspnoea, although ideally fluid retention should be minimal by the time the β blocker is started. Tailor treatment to the patient's needs and comorbidities—for example, negotiate with patients about up-titration or considering cardioselective β blockers in those with chronic obstructive pulmonary disease.[13] One study suggested that patients can increase doses at home if they live with an adult who can call for help if any (rare) severe adverse reactions occur.[14] If this is not the case patients could be given the increased dose in the practice surgery and then wait until it is safe to go home. Most patients cope well with increasing doses of β blockers, but up-titration requires a conscious commitment on the part of the clinician to maintain the momentum. For most patients treatment can be managed by primary care clinicians and does not require the input of secondary care clinicians.

Aldosterone antagonists for patients with heart failure with low ejection fraction[15 16]

A systematic review of randomised trials in patients with heart failure with low ejection fraction found that in those categorised as New York Heart Association class III or IV an aldosterone antagonist such as spironolactone may be life saving.[14] Hyperkalaemia is a recognised adverse effect, especially when starting the drug, so patients need to be monitored. Doses of spironolactone higher than 25 mg daily should be used with caution. The combination of spironolactone and an ACE inhibitor can result in worsening renal function or hyperkalaemia (or both), which can occur many months after starting treatment, and may occur at the time of intercurrent illness such as diarrhoea and vomiting. Advise patients to stop the drug themselves if such an illness occurs.

Adding digoxin

If dyspnoea remains a problem despite the treatment recommended above, digoxin may be used even in patients who are in sinus rhythm. A Cochrane systematic review showed that digoxin reduces the combined end point of death and hospital admission in those with both heart failure with low ejection fraction and heart failure with preserved ejection fraction, but most studies have been done on patients who were not taking a β blocker.[17 18]

Drug based treatment for patients with heart failure and preserved ejection fraction[19]

One large randomised controlled trial published in 2003 found that the angiotensin receptor blocker candesartan may reduce readmissions in patients with heart failure and preserved ejection fraction.[20] In this trial about 20% of patients were already taking an ACE inhibitor and about 50% were taking a β blocker. Another randomised trial found that the angiotensin receptor blocker irbesartan made no difference to mortality or readmissions when used in patients with heart failure and preserved ejection fraction.[21] However, because evidence to guide the use of other drugs is limited and treatment is largely empirical, management is probably best guided by advice from secondary care. Heart failure with preserved ejection fraction is commonly associated with hypertension, so effective management of blood pressure is important. Atrial fibrillation can also contribute to the heart failure syndrome in those with a preserved ejection fraction, and effective management of heart rate and anticoagulation is important in patients with atrial fibrillation.[22]

Other drugs

Scottish Intercollegiate Guidelines Network (SIGN) guidelines state that hydralazine and isosorbide dinitrate are options for patients who are intolerant of ACE inhibitors or angiotensin receptor blockers but should not be considered first line except in African-Americans.[23] Statins to lower cholesterol reduced ischaemic heart events in the Heart Protection Study and could be considered for those with suspected ischaemic heart disease.[24] The usefulness of antiplatelet agents for those without evidence of ischaemic heart disease is unclear.[12]

Education and multidisciplinary interventions[25]

Education regarding their condition should be available for all patients with congestive heart failure.[12] Education should cover self management strategies (including recognition of

TIPS FOR NON-SPECIALISTS

- If heart failure is suspected but clinical uncertainty remains test for brain natriuretic peptide. A normal test result makes congestive heart failure unlikely. If the result is abnormal consider starting angiotensin converting enzyme inhibitor and β blocker while waiting for echocardiography
- Echocardiography is essential to determine whether the patient has impaired ejection fraction or preserved systolic function (usually assessed by left ventricular ejection fraction). It can also assess valve disease. Treatment for patients with heart failure and low ejection fraction has a clear evidence base, whereas treatment for those with preserved ejection fraction is less clear
- Ask patients to weigh themselves at the same time each day. If their weight goes up more than 2 kg in one to three days ask them to increase their loop diuretic and see their general practitioner. This is the simplest way for doctors and patients to assess fluid retention
- Consider giving all patients an angiotensin converting enzyme inhibitor. Once the maximum dose is achieved add a β blocker and increase to the maximum dose if possible. Try to do this for all patients with heart failure and in particular those with low ejection fraction. This can be done at home as long as another adult is present
- Use spironolactone and digoxin cautiously, perhaps with cardiological advice. It is essential to monitor serum potassium in patients taking spironolactone and other aldosterone antagonists. Extra care should be taken if creatinine is raised because most patients will be elderly and have poor renal function. Patients should be advised to stop the drugs if they become unwell, especially with vomiting and diarrhoea
- Once patients are stable on an angiotensin converting enzyme inhibitor and β blocker consider reducing the dose of their loop diuretic or stepping down to a thiazide and then cutting it out entirely if tolerated
- Patients with heart failure, low ejection fraction, and no complications can often be managed without cardiological advice. However, factors such as underlying cause of congestive heart failure or consideration of device based treatments (implantable cardiac defibrillator or biventricular pacing) may prompt early referral
- Consider referral for patients with heart failure caused by valvular disease, severe heart failure, symptomatic arrhythmia, women who are pregnant or planning a pregnancy, patients with renal failure with a creatinine concentration greater than 200 μmol/l, those with poorly controlled angina, and those not improving with guideline advised treatment

ADDITIONAL EDUCATIONAL RESOURCES

Resources for patients

- Patient UK (www.patient.co.uk/health/Heart-Failure.htm)—Good overview pamphlet
- British Cardiac Patients Association (www.bcpa.co.uk/)—Useful pamphlet on echocardiography

Resources for healthcare professionals

- National Institute for Health and Clinical Excellence. Chronic heart failure. 2003. http://guidance.nice.org.uk/CG5/Guidance/pdf/English
- Scottish Intercollegiate Guideline Network. Management of chronic heart failure. 2007. www.sign.ac.uk/pdf/sign95.pdf
- A Report of the American College of Cardiology Foundation/American Heart Association Task Force on Practice Management of Heart Failure in Adults; with the International Society for Heart and Lung Transplantation. The diagnosis and management of heart failure in adults. a focused update. *J Am Coll Cardiol* 2009;53:1343-82
- European Society of Cardiology, Heart Failure Association of the ESC, European Society of Intensive Care. ESC guidelines for the diagnosis and treatment of acute and chronic heart failure 2008. *Eur J Heart Failure* 2008;10:933-89

TOPICS AND QUESTIONS FOR FUTURE RESEARCH

- Further research is needed on the treatment of patients with heart failure and preserved ejection fraction, in particular new treatment targets
- Is a high dose of β blocker more effective than a low dose?
- How feasible and effective is treatment guided by brain natriuretic peptide test results for patients with heart failure in primary care?
- How can we improve attempts at maximal dosing of angiotensin converting enzyme inhibitors and β blockers in primary care?
- Does salt and fluid restriction improve survival?
- Does exercise improve survival in heart failure?

fluid retention with daily weight monitoring and a low salt diet) and use of drugs.[12] In our experience an action plan on what the patients should do in the case of worsening symptoms is useful. Multidisciplinary interventions such as structured nurse telephone contact with and without home visits are recommended by the SIGN group.[23] Randomised trials in which nurses could alter doses of diuretics reported reductions in combined end points of mortality and hospital readmission.[23] SIGN also reported improved adherence to drugs as a result of review by a pharmacist. A randomised trial of education and self management—which comprised clinical review at a hospital based heart failure clinic early after discharge, individual and group education sessions, a personal diary to record drugs and body weight, information booklets, and regular clinical follow-up alternating between the general practitioner and heart failure clinic—reported a reduction in hospital bed days and an improvement in quality of life.[26] However, most assessments of multidisciplinary interventions have been conducted in academic centres and the results may not generalise to smaller centres or community settings.

What non-drug based treatments are recommended?

Several non-drug treatments are available but most are not based on evidence from randomised trials. Approaches include sodium restriction, fluid restriction, daily weighing, avoiding alcohol and tobacco, and losing weight. Systematic reviews of exercise have shown benefits in terms of exercise tolerance and quality of life.[12]

Discussing end of life care

Heart failure has a poor prognosis but predicting the illness trajectory can be difficult.[6] A paper from 2004 showed that the death rate for those with systolic dysfunction is 11.2% in 12 months and 29.9% in 36 months.[27] Another cohort study from the same year found that β blockers improved prognosis so death rates may improve with increased use of such drugs.[28] It is advisable to discuss end of life wishes, living with uncertainty, and the concerns surrounding possible sudden death with all patients who are diagnosed with heart failure.[6] A qualitative study of 40 patients with heart failure showed that the palliative care values of a "good death" from cancer may not apply to elderly people with heart failure.[29] An author of a book criticising the "over-medication" of fragile elderly people suggests asking patients whether they would like quality or quantity (longer life) of life.[30]

When and to whom to refer?

Patients with heart failure may need referral for cardiological assessment at any stage of assessment and treatment. Use clinical judgment and referral criteria to decide about referral on an individual basis. We recommend a low threshold for referral in view of the malignant nature of the heart failure syndrome. Patients with heart failure associated with clinical signs of valvular disease and those with severe coexisting angina usually require urgent referral early on in the assessment phase. Patients with severe heart failure or those who are not improving despite appropriate evidence based treatment, those with symptomatic arrhythmias, women being treated for heart failure syndrome who are pregnant or planning a pregnancy, patients with renal failure with a creatinine concentration greater than 200 μmol/l, and those with poorly controlled angina should be referred.[1]

Patients with heart failure with low ejection fraction may be candidates for device based treatments, such as a primary implantable cardiac defibrillator or biventricular pacing, once standard medical treatment has been optimised. Local and national guidelines are usually available to guide appropriate selection of patients for such treatments.

Contributors: BA wrote the first draft. RD and VA commented on all drafts and supplied relevant references. RD provided the cardiology input. BA is guarantor.

Competing interests: BA is on the educational committee for Pharmac the New Zealand government purchasing agency for drugs. He was on the primary care advisory board for the Future forum from 2003 to 2008. This forum is funded by Astra Zeneca (UK). RD and VA have no competing interests.

Provenance and peer review: Commissioned; externally peer reviewed.

1 National Institute for Health and Clinical Excellence. Chronic heart failure. 2003. http://guidance.nice.org.uk/CG5/Guidance/pdf/English.
2 Ho KK, Anderson KM, Kannel WB, Grossman W, Levy D. Survival after the onset of congestive heart failure in Framingham Heart Study subjects. *Circulation* 1993;88:107-15.
3 Mant J, Doust J, Roalfe A, Barton P, Cowie MR, Glasziou P, et al. Systematic review and individual patient data meta-analysis of diagnosis of heart failure, with modelling of implications of different diagnostic strategies in primary care. *Health Technol Assess* 2009;13(32). www.hta.ac.uk/project/1509.asp.
4 Chronic congestive heart failure. *BMJ Best Practice* http://bestpractice.bmj.com/best-practice/monograph/61.html.
5 Chen YT, Vaccarino V, Williams CS, Butler J, Berkman LF, Krumholz HM. Risk factors for heart failure in the elderly: a prospective community-based study. *Am J Med* 1999;106:605-12.
6 Mckee PA, Castelli WP, McNamara PA, Kannel WB. The natural history of congestive heart failure: the Framingham study. *N Engl J Med* 1971;285:1441-6.
7 Heart Failure Society of America. The stages of heart failure—NYHA classification. www.abouthf.org/questions_stages.htm.
8 Calvert MJ, Shankar A, McManus RJ, Ryan R, Freemantle N. Evaluation of the management of heart failure in primary care. *Fam Pract* 2009;26:145-53.
9 Poole-Wilson PA, Swedberg K, Cleland JG, Di Lendarda A, Hanrath P, Komajda M, et al. A comparison of carvedilol and metoprolol on clinical outcomes in patients with chronic heart failure in the comet trial randomised controlled trial. *Lancet* 2003;362:7-13.
10 Massie BM, Armstrong PW, Cleland JG, Horowitz JD, Packer M, Poole-Wilson PA, et al. Toleration of high doses of angiotensin-converting enzyme inhibitors in patients with chronic heart failure: results from the ATLAS trial. The Assessment of Treatment with Lisinopril and Survival. *Arch Intern Med* 2001;161:165-71.
11 Konstam MA, Neaton JD, Dickstein K, Drexler H, Komajda M, Martinez FA, et al. Effects of high-dose versus low dose losartan on clinical outcomes in patients with heart failure (HEAAL study) a randomised, double blind trial. *Lancet* 2009;374:1840-8.
12 European Society of Cardiology, Heart Failure Association of the ESC, European Society of Intensive Care. ESC guidelines for the diagnosis and treatment of acute and chronic heart failure 2008: *Eur J Heart Failure* 2008;10:933-89.
13 Salpeter SR, Ormiston TM, Salpeter EE. Cardioselective beta-blockers for chronic obstructive pulmonary disease. *Cochrane Database Syst Rev* 2005;4:CD003566.
14 Wald DS, More RS, Martin M, Hughes L, Reid CJ. Can beta blockers be safely initiated at home in patients with heart failure. *Q J Med 2002* 2002;95:55-9.
15 Pitt B, Zannad F, Remme WJ, Cody R, Castaigne A, Perez A, et al. The effect of spironolactone on morbidity and mortality in patients with severe heart failure. randomized aldactone evaluation study investigators. *N Engl J Med* 1999;341:709-17.
16 Ezekowitz JA, McAlister FA. Aldosterone blockade and left ventricular dysfunction: a systematic review of randomized clinical trials. *Eur Heart J* 2009.30:469-7.
17 Meyer P, White M, Mujib A, Nozza T, Love I, Aban J, et al. Digoxin and reduction of heart failure hospitalization in chronic systolic and diastolic heart failure. *Am J Cardiol* 2008;102:1681-6.
18 Hood WB, Dans AL, Guyatt GH, Jaeschke R, McMurray JJ. Digitalis for treatment of congestive heart failure in patients in sinus rhythm. *Cochrane Database Syst Rev* 2004;2:CD002901.
19 Report of the American College of Cardiology Foundation/American Heart Association Task Force on Practice Management of Heart Failure in Adults; with the International Society for Heart and Lung Transplantation. The diagnosis and management of heart failure in adults. a focused update. *J Am Coll Cardiol* 2009;53:1343-82.
20 CHARM Investigators and Committees. Effects of candesartan in patients with chronic heart failure and preserved left-ventricular ejection fraction: the CHARM-Preserved Trial. *Lancet* 2003;362:777-81.
21 I-PRESERVE Investigators. Irbesartan in patients with heart failure and preserved ejection fraction. *N Engl J Med* 2008;359:2456-67.
22 Lafuente-Lafuente C, Mahe I, Extramiana F. Management of atrial fibrillation. *BMJ* 2010;339:b5216.
23 Scottish Intercollegiate Guideline Network. The management of chronic heart failure. 2007. www.sign.ac.uk/pdf/sign95.pdf.
24 Emberson JR, Ng LL, Armitage J, Bowman L, Parish S, Collins R, Heart Protection Study Collaborative Group. N-terminal pro-B-type natriuretic peptide, vascular disease risk, and cholesterol reduction among 20536 patients in the MRC/BHF heart protection study. *J Am Coll Cardiol* 2007;49:311-9.
25 McKelvie R. Heart failure. *Clin Evid* 2010; http://clinicalevidence.bmj.com/ceweb/conditions/cvd/0204/0204.jsp.
26 Doughty RN, Wright SP, Pearl A, Walsh HJ, Muncaster S, Whalley GA, et al. Randomized, controlled trial of integrated heart failure management: the Auckland Heart Failure Management Study. *Eur Heart J* 2002;23:139-46.
27 Brophy JM, Dagenais GR, McSherry F, Williford W, Yusuf S. A multivariate model for predicting mortality in patients with heart failure and systolic dysfunction. *Am J Med* 2004;116:300-4.
28 Koelling TM, Joseph S, Aaronson KD. Heart failure survival score continues to predict clinical outcomes in patients with heart failure receiving beta-blockers. *J Heart Lung Transplant* 2004;23:1414-22.
29 Gott M, Small N, Barnes S, Payne S, Seamark D. Older peoples views of a good death in heart failure. Implications for palliative care provision. *Soc Sci Med* 2008;67:1113-21.
30 Sloan J. A bitter pill: how the medical system is failing the elderly. Greystone Books, D & M Publishers, 2009.

Diagnosis and management of supraventricular tachycardia

Zachary I Whinnett, consultant cardiologist, S M Afzal Sohaib, British Heart Foundation clinical research training fellow and cardiology specialty registrar, D Wyn Davies, consultant cardiologist

[1]Waller Department of Cardiology, St Mary's Hospital, Imperial College Healthcare NHS Trust, London W2 1NY, UK

Correspondence to: D W Davies dwyndavies@aol.com

Cite this as: *BMJ* 2012;345:e7769

‹DOI› 10.1136/bmj.e7769
http://www.bmj.com/content/345/bmj.e7769

The term supraventricular tachycardia (SVT) encompasses many tachycardias in which atrial or atrioventricular nodal tissue are essential for sustaining the arrhythmia (box 1). In practice, however, the term SVT is generally used to refer to atrioventricular nodal re-entry tachycardia (AVNRT), atrioventricular re-entry tachycardia (AVRT), and atrial tachycardia[1]; in this review we follow that convention. We reviewed the literature to provide an up to date summary of our understanding of the mechanism for these arrhythmias, and we describe the approach to their diagnosis and management. Atrial fibrillation has been reviewed recently[2] so is not discussed in detail here. Much of the clinical evidence in this field is derived from observational and registry data, with a limited number of randomised control studies.

What is a supraventricular tachycardia?

SVTs are produced by disorders of impulse formation (causing generation of rapid electrical impulses from a small area) and/or disorders of impulse conduction, which result in re-entrant tachycardias, where tachycardia is produced because the electrical impulse repeatedly travels around a circuit. Re-entrant tachycardias typically require an extrasystole to initiate them. SVTs are among the few medical conditions that can be cured.

SOURCES AND SELECTION CRITERIA

As well as using our personal reference collections, we searched PubMed to identify peer reviewed original articles, meta-analyses, observational studies, and reviews, as well as searching Clinical Evidence (http://clinicalevidence.bmj.com) and the Cochrane Collaboration databases. We used the search terms supraventricular tachycardia, atrioventricular nodal re-entry tachycardia, atrioventricular re-entry tachycardia, atrial flutter, atrial tachycardia, Wolff-Parkinson-White syndrome.

We selected randomised controlled studies or meta-analyses when available; if none were available, we used observational studies and registry data.

SUMMARY POINTS

- Supraventricular tachycardia comprises a group of conditions in which atrial or atrioventricular nodal tissues are essential for sustaining the arrhythmia
- Common symptoms include palpitations, chest pain, anxiety, light headedness, pounding in the neck, shortness of breath, and uncommonly syncope
- They are produced either by disorders of impulse formation and/or disorders of impulse conduction
- For patients presenting with a regular narrow complex tachycardia, initial management is usually to slow atrioventricular node conduction, using either vagal manoeuvres or adenosine
- Drug treatment may reduce the frequency of symptoms, but complete suppression is uncommon
- Catheter ablation, a procedure done under local anaesthesia in the cardiac catheter laboratory, is usually curative

What are the different types of SVT?

AVNRT

AVNRT is caused by a re-entrant circuit involving the posterior and anterior inputs into the compact atrioventricular node.[3] A quarter of the population has two pathways that input into the compact atrioventricular node, one of which is a rapidly conducting pathway and the other a slower conducting pathway; these two pathways form the circuit for AVNRT (fig 1).

The extrasystole that triggers the tachycardia is critically timed so that the faster pathway is still refractory from the last sinus beat (that is, it is not yet ready to conduct an impulse because it is still recovering from depolarisation). The electrical impulse therefore propagates exclusively down the slow pathway, which has a shorter refractory period (that is, it takes less time to recover from depolarisation) and then returns up the fast pathway, which has by then recovered. The circuit for typical AVNRT is thus formed.

Less commonly, activation travels anterogradely down the fast pathway and returns up the slow pathway, forming atypical AVNRT. These different mechanisms result in very different appearances on the surface electrocardiogram (ECG). In the typical form, atrial and ventricular activation occur virtually simultaneously (because the impulse returns up the fast pathway at the same time as travelling down the His-Purkinje system), so the P waves are invisible in the QRS complexes (a pseudo-RSR' pattern in lead V1 often provides a clue to the presence of the P wave), whereas the delayed atrial activation via the slow pathway in atypical AVNRT produces inverted P waves typically in the middle of or late in the RR interval.

Typical AVNRT presents as a short RP tachycardia (the ECG during tachycardia has a RP interval shorter than PR interval) while atypical AVNRT produces a long RP tachycardia (RP interval longer than PR interval) (fig 2).

BOX 1 DIFFERENTIAL DIAGNOSIS OF A NARROW COMPLEX TACHYCARDIA

Common causes

- Sinus tachycardia
- Atrioventricular nodal re-entry tachycardia (AVNRT)
- Atrioventricular re-entry tachycardia (AVRT)
- Atrial tachycardia
- Atrial flutter
- Atrial fibrillation

Rare causes

- Inappropriate sinus tachycardia
- Sinus node re-entry
- Permanent junctional reciprocating tachycardia
- Non-paroxysmal junctional tachycardia
- Focal junctional tachycardia

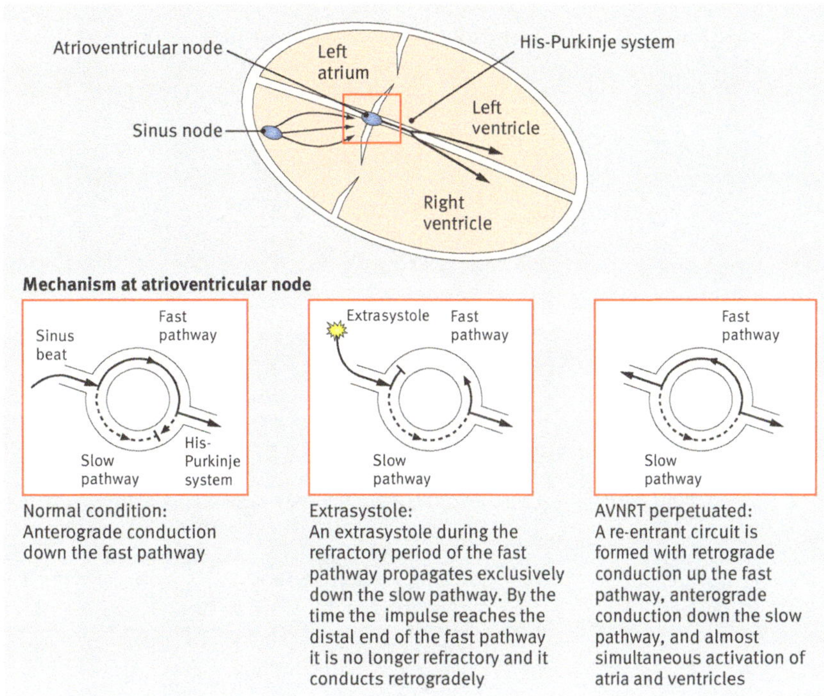

Fig 1 Mechanism for atrioventricular nodal re-entry tachycardia

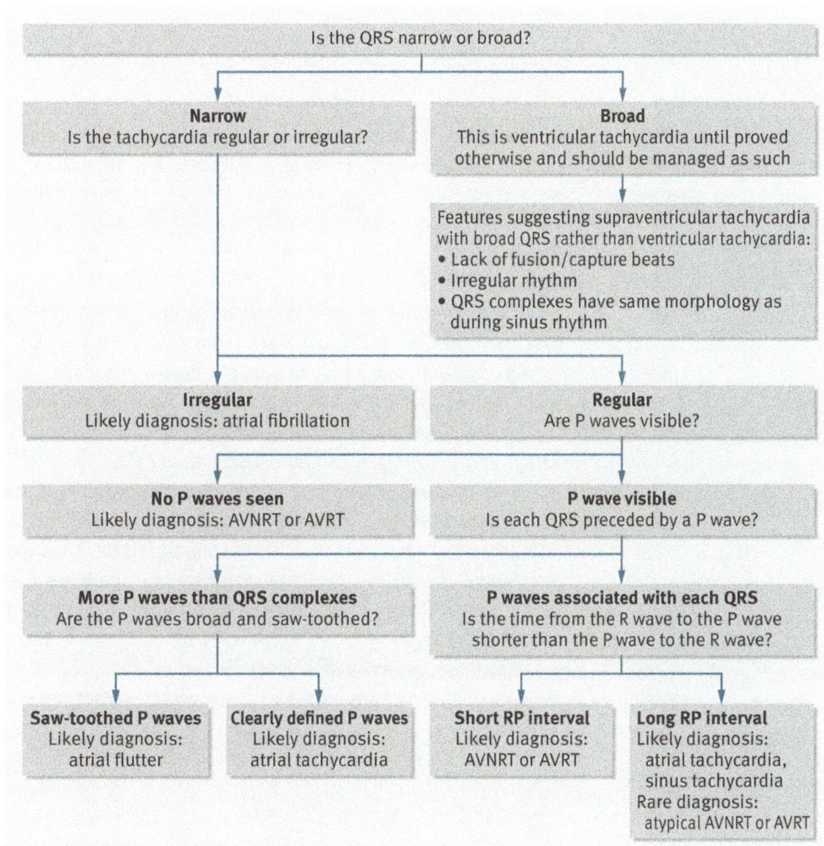

Fig 2 Interpretation of ECG showing tachycardia

AVRT (including Wolff-Parkinson-White syndrome)

AVRT is also a re-entrant tachycardia; it requires the presence of an accessory pathway, a small strand of myocardium that bridges the normal insulation between atria and ventricles (fig 3).

Some pathways can conduct impulses only from the ventricle to the atrium and are known as concealed accessory pathways. Others can conduct in both directions and usually produce pre-excitation of the ventricle because they conduct more rapidly than the atrioventricular node. This early ventricular activation shows on the 12 lead ECG as a delta wave at the start of the QRS (fig 3). The terminal portion of the QRS complex is narrow, reflecting the rapid conduction via the His-Purkinje system once the

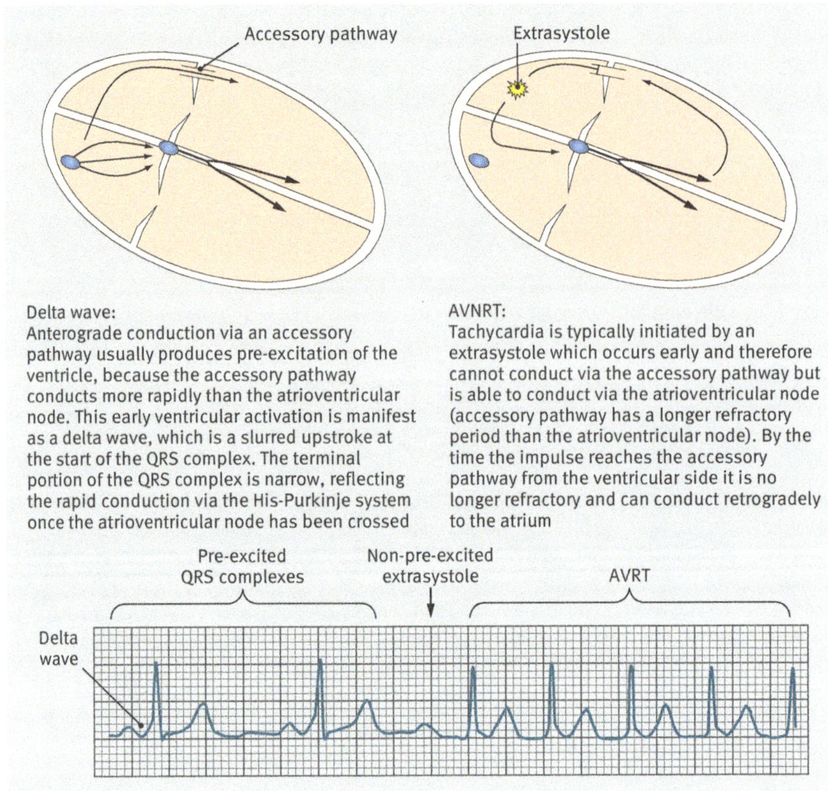

Fig 3 Mechanism for atrioventricular re-entry tachycardia

atrioventricular node has been crossed. The degree of pre-excitation varies depending on the time required to cross the atrioventricular node and the location of the accessory pathway.

The diagnosis of Wolff-Parkinson-White syndrome describes patients with a delta wave on the surface ECG who also experience palpitations.

AVRT is usually triggered by a critically timed atrial extrasystole that finds the accessory pathway refractory, therefore antegrade conduction occurs exclusively down the atrioventricular node. The accessory pathway is no longer refractory by the time the wave front reaches its ventricular insertion and it therefore conducts retrogradely to the atrium— the re-entrant circuit is thus formed (fig 3); this activation pattern is termed orthodromic AVRT, and produces a narrow complex tachycardia. Rarely, anterograde conduction travels down the accessory pathway returning to the atrium via the atrioventricular node, producing antidromic AVRT, which has broad QRS complexes that exaggerate the pattern of pre-excitation seen in sinus rhythm because ventricular activation occurs exclusively via the accessory pathway.

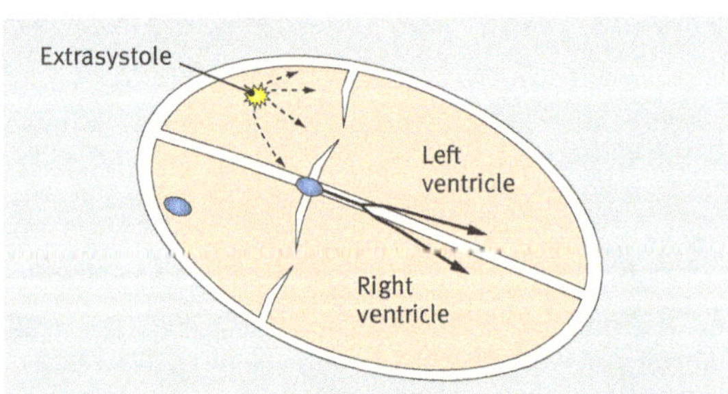

Fig 4 Mechanism for focal atrial tachycardia. Generation of rapid electrical impulses from a small localised area in the atria (in this example, the left atrium)

Atrial tachycardia

Atrial tachycardia may result from either abnormal impulse formation or a re-entrant mechanism. Atrial tachycardias are commonly classified according to whether they originate from a small localised area in the atrium (focal atrial tachycardia) or involve a larger re-entrant circuit (macro re-entry).

Focal atrial tachycardia

In focal atrial tachycardia there is generation of rapid electrical impulses from a small localised area in the atria (fig 4).

Multifocal atrial tachycardia

Multifocal atrial tachycardia is less common than focal atrial tachycardia and occurs most often in acutely unwell patients and those with pulmonary disease and/or digoxin toxicity. At least three different morphologies of P wave are usually present.[4]

Macro re-entrant atrial tachycardia

The re-entrant circuit involves a large area of the atrium. The commonest is "typical" atrial flutter where the re-entrant loop circles the right atrium (fig 5). Other re-entrant atrial tachycardias are seen in patients who have structural heart disease and in those who have had previous surgery (increasingly in those who have had catheter ablation procedures to treat atrial fibrillation).[5]

Who gets SVT?

People of all ages, either sex, and any ethnicity can develop SVT. In a large retrospective observational study in the United States the peak incidence of SVT presentation was in the middle decades of life (AVNRT at 48 (range 30-66) years; AVRT at 36 (18-64) years; and atrial fibrillation at 50 (31-69) years).[6]

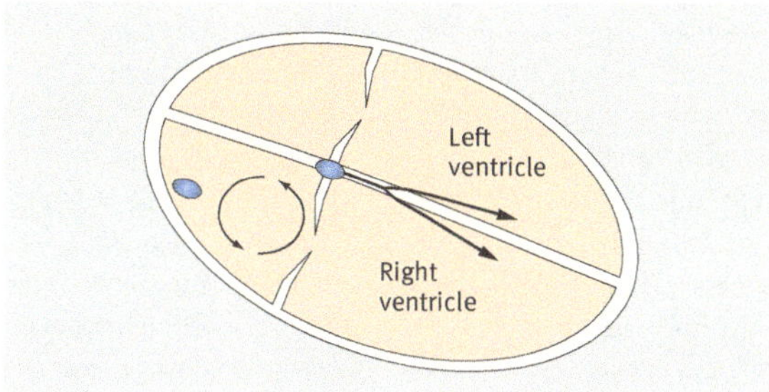

Fig 5 Mechanism for atrial flutter, an example of a macro re-entrant circuit. The electrical activation circles the right atrium

A higher proportion of AVNRT cases occur in women, and AVRT is more likely to affect men.[7] No sex difference was observed for atrial fibrillation.

SVTs usually manifest themselves as recurrent palpitations, can seriously impair quality of life,[8] and often prompt visits to primary care doctors and acute medical units. The incidence in a large cohort in the United States was found to be 35/100 000 patient years, with a prevalence of 0.2%.[9] An estimated prevalence for atrial fibrillation is 0.4% to 1% in the general population.[10]

How does SVT present?

Common symptoms include palpitations, chest pain, anxiety, lightheadedness, pounding in the neck, shortness of breath, and uncommonly syncope.[11]

Sudden onset and offset of palpitations is typical for a re-entrant arrhythmia, while for sinus tachycardia onset and offset is usually gradual. Patients with AVNRT or AVRT may be able to terminate palpitations with vagal manoeuvres such as the Valsalva manoeuvre, breath holding, or coughing.

Some patients can identify triggers such as caffeine or alcohol intake, which can initiate re-entrant tachycardia by increasing the frequency of extrasystoles.

In the absence of an acute episode the examination is usually normal. In a patient with tachycardia, prominent jugular venous A waves caused by atrial contraction against the closed tricuspid valve may be seen.[12]

What investigations are needed?

Electrocardiography

Attempts should always be made to capture the arrhythmia during an episode of palpitations. We recommend giving the patient a copy to ensure it is never lost and is easily available to health professionals. A rhythm strip should be recorded if 12 lead electrocardiography is not available, and every effort should be made to capture the termination of the tachycardia.

For patients with non-sustained episodes of palpitations, an ambulatory electrocardiograph or an event monitor can be useful in capturing an ECG during an episode.

Narrow complex tachycardia is most frequently seen (QRS <120 ms), but less commonly the QRS complexes are broad during tachycardia. Even though supraventricular tachycardias can present with broad QRS complexes, in the initial evaluation, a broad complex tachycardia should be treated as a ventricular tachycardia until proven otherwise.

A 12 lead ECG in sinus rhythm should also be recorded and carefully examined for the presence of a delta wave. In figure 2 we suggest how to analyse the 12 lead ECG during tachycardia.

Echocardiography

Echocardiography is an important investigation for patients presenting with palpitations. The presence of structural heart disease such as left ventricular impairment should prompt urgent referral and investigation. Left ventricular impairment is associated with an increased risk of sudden cardiac death,[13] and patients are less likely to tolerate tachycardia. Such patients should not be prescribed class 1 antiarrhythmic drugs, such as flecainide.[1]

Most patients with SVT have a structurally normal heart. In a series of 145 patients referred for ablation, only 4% had heart failure.[14] However, certain types of structural heart disease are associated with particular SVTs. Patients with Ebstein's anomaly (congenital displacement of the septal tricuspid valve leaflet into the right ventricle) have an increased frequency of right sided accessory pathways.[15] Incisional atrial tachycardia occurs as a result of re-entry around surgical scars and is a major source of morbidity in the growing population of survivors of congenital heart disease.[16]

What are the acute management options in SVT?

Non-drug treatment

Patients presenting with sustained tachycardia should be assessed for haemodynamic stability; rarely, the arrhythmia is so poorly tolerated that immediate electrical cardioversion is needed. With the important exception of pre-excited atrial fibrillation (in which case the ECG shows an irregular, broad complex tachycardia, with variation of the QRS morphology (fig 6)), the first line manoeuvre is usually to slow conduction through the atrioventricular node. This may either terminate the tachycardia if the mechanism is dependent on the atrioventricular node (AVNRT, AVRT) or provide diagnostic information in the case of atrial tachycardia (P wave morphology exposed and lack of dependence on the atrioventricular node to maintain the tachycardia). A continuous 12 lead ECG recording should be made during these manoeuvres (fig 7).

Atrioventricular node conduction can be slowed by vagal stimulation with carotid sinus massage or the Valsalva manoeuvre.

Pre-excited atrial fibrillation should be managed with electrical cardioversion, or by flecainide infusion if the tachycardia is haemodynamically well tolerated and the heart is normal.

Drug treatment

If vagal manoeuvres are unsuccessful in slowing atrioventricular conduction then, unless the patient is asthmatic, the ACC/AHA/ESC guidelines[1] recommend

---

BOX 2 WHICH PATIENTS SHOULD YOU REFER TO AN ELECTROPHYSIOLOGIST?

Urgent referral

Patients with:

- Syncope with palpitations on exertion
- Broad complex tachycardia
- Pre-excitation (delta wave) on a 12 lead ECG
- Structural heart disease
- Severe symptoms

Routine referral

Those with:

- Drug resistance or intolerance
- Preference not to take medication
- Diagnostic uncertainty

intravenous adenosine as first line medication. Adenosine is preferred owing to its rapid onset of action and short half life. In a randomised double blinded placebo trial in participants with SVT, tachycardia was terminated in 91% of those who received adenosine (at a dose of either 6 mg or 12 mg) and in 16% of those receiving placebo.[17] When administering adenosine, ensure that resuscitation equipment is available in case the rare complications of bronchospasm or ventricular fibrillation occur.

The effectiveness of intravenous verapamil seems similar to that of adenosine in terminating SVT. In a randomised controlled trial, intravenous verapamil (2.5-7.5 mg) resulted in termination of tachycardia in 91% of patients, compared with termination in 93% of those receiving adenosine (6 mg dose followed by a 12 mg dose if required).[17] A meta-analysis of eight trials with a total of 605 patients, found similarly high rates of termination with both adenosine and verapamil (91% *v* 90%), with slightly higher rates of minor adverse effects and lower rates of hypotension described with adenosine.[18] β blockers are a further option and are effective in lowering heart rate, but in a small randomised study intravenous esmolol converted only 6% of SVTs to sinus rhythm.[19] Amiodarone[20] and flecainide are further options. Acute administration of flecainide successfully restored sinus rhythm in 72% of patients with AVRT and 83% with AVNRT.[21]

Macro re-entrant atrial tachycardias are not usually responsive to antiarrhythmic drugs and usually require electrical cardioversion (or overdrive atrial pacing, where tachycardia is terminated by rapid pacing of the atrium using either an existing pacemaker or temporary pacing lead in the right atrium) to restore sinus rhythm. The ACC/AHA/ESC guidelines recommend that before cardioversion the same guidelines for thromboembolic prophylaxis are followed for atrial flutter as for atrial fibrillation (international normalised ratio 2-3, or arrhythmia duration <48 hours, or no evidence of atrial thrombus on transoesophageal echocardiography).[1]

What are the long term management options?

In general, improvement of quality of life is the major therapeutic goal for SVTs, and treatment strategies should be guided according to symptoms and patient preference. Patients troubled by recurrent symptomatic episodes should be offered treatment; options include medication or catheter ablation. Patients can be taught the Valsalva manoeuvre and some find this helpful in controlling their symptoms. This

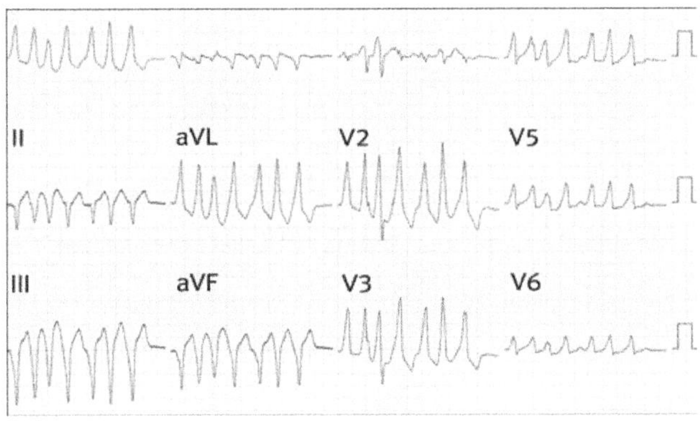

Fig 6 Pre-excited atrial fibrillation

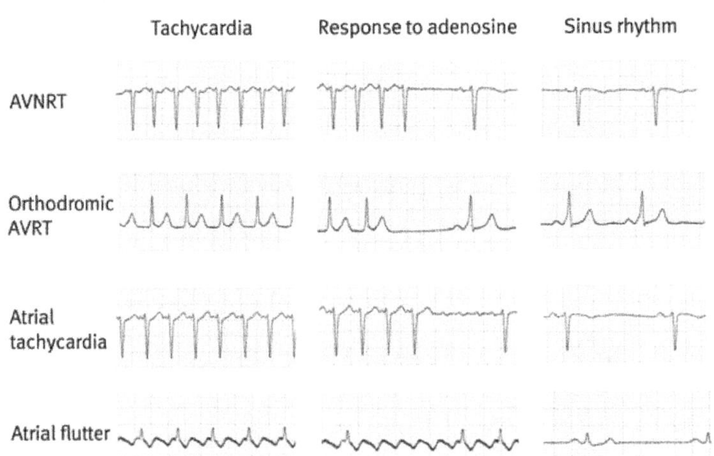

Fig 7 Typical electrocardiographic recordings for four common SVTs during tachycardia, administration of adenosine, and sinus rhythm. AVNRT: As atrial and ventricular activation occurs virtually simultaneously in typical AVNRT, the retrograde P waves are either hidden in the QRS complex or produce a pseudo r′ in V1. Tachycardia is usually terminated with adenosine. Orthodromic AVRT: During tachycardia ventricular activation occurs exclusively via the atrioventricular node and His-Purkinje system; tachycardia is therefore narrow complex. Typically, the RP interval is short; less commonly, if the accessory pathway conducts slowly, a long RP interval is observed. Adenosine usually terminates the tachycardia and in sinus rhythm a delta wave is commonly seen. Atrial tachycardia: Often the RP interval is long. Tachycardia is not dependent on the atrioventricular node so it usually continues even after the administration of adenosine (though adenosine may terminate focal atrial tachycardia). When atrioventricular conduction is blocked the underlying P waves can be clearly seen. Atrial flutter: The characteristic flutter waves are seen clearly after administration of adenosine, and tachycardia continues because it does not depend on the atrioventricular node.

can be described to the patient as simulating straining on the toilet, or trying to breathe out forcefully while keeping the mouth closed and nose pinched.

There have been no large scale randomised studies comparing these treatments. However, data from prospective non-randomised studies suggest that catheter ablation results in a greater reduction in symptoms and higher quality of life scores compared with medical treatment.[22 23]

Patients with pre-excitation (delta wave on ECG) warrant special consideration. Such patients are at risk of sudden cardiac death from ventricular fibrillation induced by rapidly conducted atrial fibrillation. The findings from a recent meta-analysis suggest that in patients who do not have palpitations, this risk seems to be relatively low (1.25 per 1000 person years, 95% confidence interval 0.57 to 2.19 per 1000 person years).[24] Symptoms of palpitations appear to be associated with an increased risk of ventricular fibrillation.[25]

We advise referring patients with pre-excitation to an electrophysiologist for further assessment. Patients with documented broad complex tachycardia (QRS duration >120 ms and heart rate >100 beats/min), even if they have only had a single episode, are also best referred early. Box 2 outlines which patients to refer to an electrophysiologist.

Drug treatment

In general drug treatment is reserved for minimising symptoms while awaiting catheter ablation or for long term management of patients who decline catheter ablation or in whom the procedure carries an unacceptably high risk. Drug treatment may be effective in reducing the frequency of symptoms but complete suppression is uncommon.[26]

A major limitation in evaluating antiarrhythmic agents for treatment of SVTs is the absence of large, multicentre, randomised, placebo controlled studies.

For AVNRT and AVRT without pre-excitation, agents to block atrioventricular node conduction are commonly used as first line medication, although only limited data are available on the long term efficacy of these medications. Data from a small, randomised, double blind trial, showed that verapamil, propranolol, and digoxin all reduced the frequency of symptoms, with all equally effective.[26]

For patients who do not respond to these drugs, alternatives include flecainide and sotalol.[27] Although only relatively small numbers of patients have been included in randomised studies of flecainide and sotalol, the available data suggest they can be effective in reducing symptoms. In one small placebo controlled study 79% of patients in the flecainide group and 15% in the placebo group did not experience symptoms, though the follow-up period was only eight weeks.[28] Proarrhythmia, including ventricular tachycardia, has been reported in 6% of patients.[29] Agents to slow atrioventricular node conduction are often co-administered, as flecainide may predispose to atrial flutter with 1:1 atrioventricular conduction.[29]

Flecainide is not recommended in patients with structural or ischaemic heart disease, in whom it is associated with an increased risk of sudden cardiac death.[30] Amiodarone is generally not recommended owing to the potential for serious adverse effects in patients with a benign condition. However, it may be used to treat atrial tachycardias resistant to other treatments, particularly in patients with structural heart disease and in elderly people.

Catheter ablation

Catheter ablation provides a definitive management option for SVT and is usually done under local anaesthesia as a day case. Catheters capable of recording electrical activation in the heart are inserted via the femoral vessels and manipulated under x ray guidance. Radiofrequency energy delivered via a catheter is used to create small localised areas of scar.

In AVNRT, the slow pathway is targeted with the aim of modifying conduction so that re-entrant tachycardia can no longer be sustained. Both acute and long term success rates for this procedure are high. In a large observational study acute success was achieved in 98% of cases.[31] A meta-analysis of 10 observational studies comprising 1204 patients reported a 4.3% recurrence rate.[32] Serious complications are uncommon, the most serious being atrioventricular block requiring pacemaker therapy (affecting 1% of patients in early series).[31 33 34]

AVRT is also amenable to catheter ablation. No randomised prospective studies have been conducted, but observational studies and registries have observed acute success rates of more than 95% and recurrence rates less than 5%.[33 35] Atrioventricular block is a risk in cases where the accessory pathway is close to the atrioventricular node and the His bundle; the use of cryothermal energy may reduce this risk.[36] Other complications are reported to occur in less than 2-3% of patients and include vascular injury, bleeding, venous thrombosis, pulmonary embolism, myocardial perforation, systemic embolism (in the case of a left sided accessory pathway), and rarely, death (0-0.2%).[33 34 35]

Focal atrial tachycardia can also be successfully treated with catheter ablation, although randomised control trials are lacking, and evidence is limited to small observational studies. Acute success rates of 85%[37 38] with recurrence rates of 8% have been reported.[39]

For re-entrant atrial tachycardias, radiofrequency ablation has high success rates and is often used as first line treatment.[5 40] Radiofrequency ablation is the treatment of choice for typical atrial flutter. This practice is supported by the findings from a medium sized randomised study which found that, compared with medical treatment, as first line treatment ablation produced higher rates of sinus rhythm (80% *v* 36%), fewer hospital admissions, and a lower occurrence of atrial fibrillation.[40]

After the procedure, most patients can return to their normal activities very quickly. We recommend they avoid heavy lifting for two weeks after the procedure. In the UK, the Driver and Vehicle Licensing Agency states that car drivers (group 1 entitlement) may not drive for two days after successful catheter ablation (vocational drivers (group 2) for two weeks afterwards) if the arrhythmia was not or did not have the potential to be incapacitating. If the arrhythmia was or had the potential to be incapacitating, the restriction is six weeks after successful ablation.[41]

Contributors: All authors contributed fully to all stages of the planning, researching, and preparation of the manuscript. DWD and ZIW are the guarantors.

Competing interests: All authors have completed the ICMJE uniform disclosure form at www.icmje.org/coi_disclosure.pdf (available on request from the corresponding author) and declare: SMAS is funded by the British Heart Foundation; no financial relationships with any organisations that might have an interest in the submitted work in the previous three years; no other relationships or activities that could appear to have influenced the submitted work.

Provenance and peer review: Commissioned; externally peer reviewed.

TIPS FOR NON-SPECIALISTS

- If a patient presents with tachycardia always record an ECG and give the patient a copy; this can be helpful for future management
- Broad complex tachycardia is ventricular tachycardia until proved otherwise
- For narrow complex tachycardia, the first step is usually to slow AV node conduction with either a Valsalva manoeuvre or adenosine. This provides diagnostic information and will usually terminate AVNRT and AVRT
- For patients with recurring symptoms, catheter ablation has high acute and long term success rates

ADDITIONAL EDUCATIONAL RESOURCES

For healthcare professionals

- The Resuscitation Council provides free algorithms for the acute management of tachycardia: www.resus.org.uk/pages/glalgos.htm
- ACC/AHA/ESC guidelines for the management of patients with supraventricular arrhythmias. 2003. www.escardio.org/guidelines-surveys/esc-guidelines/Pages/supraventricular-arrhythmias.aspx
- Fox DJ, Tischenko A, Krahn AD, Skanes AC, Gula LJ, Yee RK, et al. Supraventricular tachycardia: diagnosis and management. *Mayo Clin Proc* 2008;83:1400-11.
- Delacrétaz E. Clinical practice: supraventricular tachycardia. *N Engl J Med* 2006;354:1039-51.

For patients (free web based resources)

- Arrhythmia Alliance (www.heartrhythmcharity.org.uk)—The patient pages give information on the full range of rhythm disturbances and treatments available, and downloadable single sheet summaries for different arrhythmias
- British Heart Foundation (www.bhf.org.uk)—The "Heart Health" pages give information on different cardiac conditions and investigations including electrophysiology studies; telephone advice line (Heart Helpline) is also available.
- NHS Choices (www.nhs.uk/conditions/supraventricular-tachycardia)—Simple overview of supraventricular tachycardia
- Patient.co.uk website (www.patient.co.uk/health/Supraventricular-Tachycardia-(SVT).htm)—Brief overview of SVT in lay terms

QUESTIONS FOR FUTURE RESEARCH

- Uncertainty remains about the optimal management of patients with asymptomatic pre-excitation (delta wave on the ECG)—in particular, whether sufficiently sensitive risk stratification is possible or whether most patients should be managed with catheter ablation of their accessory pathway
- There is ongoing development of invasive and non-invasive methods for mapping complex arrhythmias, such as atrial tachycardias occurring after ablation for atrial fibrillation. These have the potential to help with diagnosis and to guide the catheter ablation procedure

1 Blomström-Lundqvist C, Scheinman MM, Aliot EM, Alpert JS, Calkins H, Camm AJ, et al. ACC/AHA/ESC guidelines for the management of patients with supraventricular arrhythmias—executive summary. A report of the American College of Cardiology/American Heart Association Task Force on practice guidelines and the European Society of Cardiology committee for practice guidelines (writing committee to develop guidelines for the management of patients with supraventricular arrhythmias) developed in collaboration with NASPE-Heart Rhythm Society. *J Am Coll Cardiol* 2003;42:1493-531.

2 Lafuente-Lafuente C, Mahé I, Extramiana F. Management of atrial fibrillation. *BMJ* 2009;339:b5216.

3 McGuire MA, Bourke JP, Robotin MC, Johnson DC, Meldrum-Hanna W, Nunn GR, et al. High resolution mapping of Koch's triangle using sixty electrodes in humans with atrioventricular junctional (AV nodal) reentrant tachycardia. *Circulation* 1993;88:2315-28.

4 Kastor JA. Multifocal atrial tachycardia. *N Engl J Med* 1990;322:1713-7.

5 Wasmer K, Mönnig G, Bittner A, Dechering D, Zellerhoff S, Milberg P, et al. Incidence, characteristics, and outcome of left atrial tachycardias after circumferential antral ablation of atrial fibrillation. *Heart Rhythm* 2012;9:1660-6.

6 Porter MJ, Morton JB, Denman R, Lin AC, Tierney S, Santucci PA, et al. Influence of age and gender on the mechanism of supraventricular tachycardia. *Heart Rhythm* 2004;1:393-6.

7 Tada H, Oral H, Greenstein R, Pelosi F Jr, Knight BP, Strickberger SA, et al. Analysis of age of onset of accessory pathway-mediated tachycardia in men and women. *Am J Cardiol* 2002;89:470-1.

8 Walfridsson U, Strömberg A, Janzon M, Walfridsson H. Wolff-Parkinson-White syndrome and atrioventricular nodal re-entry tachycardia in a Swedish population: consequences on health-related quality of life. *Pacing Clin Electrophysiol* 2009;32:1299-306.

9 Orejarena LA, Vidaillet H Jr, DeStefano F, Nordstrom DL, Vierkant RA, Smith PN, et al. Paroxysmal supraventricular tachycardia in the general population. *J Am Coll Cardiol* 1998;31:150-7.

10 Fuster V, Rydén LE, Cannom DS, Crijns HJ, Curtis AB, Ellenbogen KA, et al. 2011 ACCF/AHA/HRS focused updates incorporated into the ACC/AHA/ESC 2006 Guidelines for the management of patients with atrial fibrillation: a report of the American College of Cardiology Foundation/American Heart Association Task Force on Practice Guidelines developed in partnership with the European Society of Cardiology and in collaboration with the European Heart Rhythm Association and the Heart Rhythm Society. *J Am Coll Cardiol* 2011;57:e101-98.

11 Delacretaz E. Supraventricular tachycardia. *N Engl J Med* 2006;354:1039-51.

12 Gursoy S, Steurer G, Brugada J, Andries E, Brugada P. The hemodynamic mechanism of pounding in the neck in atrioventricular nodal reentrant tachycardia. *N Engl J Med* 1992;327:772-4.

13 Myerburg RJ, Kessler KM, Castellanos A. Sudden cardiac death: epidemiology, transient risk, and intervention assessment. *Ann Intern Med* 1993;119:1187-97.

14 Wood KA, Drew BJ, Scheinman MM. Frequency of disabling symptoms in supraventricular tachycardia *Am J Cardiol* 1997;79:145-9..

15 Ho S, Goltz D, McCarthy K, Cook A, Connell M, Smith A, et al. The atrioventricular junctions in Ebstein malformation. *Heart* 2000;83:444-9.

16 Walsh EP. Arrhythmias in patients with congenital heart disease. *Card Electrophysiol Rev* 2002;6:422-30.

17 DiMarco JP, Miles W, Akhtar M, Milstein S, Sharma AD, Platia E, et al. Adenosine for paroxysmal supraventricular tachycardia: dose ranging and comparison with verapamil: assessment in placebo-controlled, multicenter trials. *Ann Intern Med* 1990;113:104-10.

18 Delaney B, Loy J, Kelly AM. The relative efficacy of adenosine versus verapamil for the treatment of stable paroxysmal supraventricular tachycardia in adults: a meta-analysis. *Eur J Emerg Med* 2011;18:148-52.

19 Anderson S, Blanski L, Byrd RC, Das G, Engler R, Laddu A, et al. Comparison of the efficacy and safety of esmolol, a short-acting beta blocker, with placebo in the treatment of supraventricular tachyarrhythmias. *Am Heart J* 1986;111:42-8.

20 Holt P, Crick JC, Davies DW, Curry P. Intravenous amiodarone in the acute termination of supraventricular arrhythmias. *Int J Cardiol* 1985;8:67-79.

21 Hohnloser SH, Zabel M. Short- and long-term efficacy and safety of flecainide acetate for supraventricular arrhythmias. *Am J Cardiol* 1992;70:3-9A.

22 Bathina MN, Mickelsen S, Brooks C, Jaramillo J, Hepton T, Kusumoto FM. Radiofrequency catheter ablation versus medical therapy for initial treatment of supraventricular tachycardia and its impact on quality of life and healthcare costs. *Am J Cardiol* 1998;82:589-93.

23 Goldberg AS, Bathina MN, Mickelsen S, Nawman R, West G, Kusumoto FM. Long-term outcomes on quality-of-life and health care costs in patients with supraventricular tachycardia (radiofrequency catheter ablation versus medical therapy). *Am J Cardiol* 2002;1;89:1120-3.

24 Obeyesekere MN, Leong-Sit P, Massel D, Manlucu J, Modi S, Krahn AD, et al. Risk of arrhythmia and sudden death in patients with asymptomatic preexcitation: a meta-analysis. *Circulation* 2012;125:2308-15.

25 Klein GJ, Bashore TM, Sellers TD, Pritchett EL, Smith WM, Gallagher JJ. Ventricular-fibrillation in the Wolff-Parkinson-White Syndrome. *N Engl J Med* 1979;301:1080-5.

26 Winniford MD, Fulton KL, Hillis LD. Long-term therapy of paroxysmal supraventricular tachycardia: a randomized, double-blind comparison of digoxin, propranolol and verapamil. *Am J Cardiol* 1984;54:1138-9.

27 Kunze KP, Schlutter M, Kuck KH. Sotalol in patients with Wolff-Parkinson-White syndrome. *Circulation* 1987;75:1050-7.

28 Henthorn RW, Waldo AL, Anderson JL, Gilbert EM, Alpert BL, Bhandari AK, et al. Flecainide acetate prevents recurrence of symptomatic paroxysmal supraventricular tachycardia. *Circulation* 1991;83:119-125.

29 Benditt DG, Dunnigan A, Buetikofer J, Milstein S. Tachyarrhythmias. Flecainide acetate for long-term prevention of paroxysmal supraventricular. *Circulation* 1991;83:345-9.

30 Cardiac Arrhythmia Suppression Trial (CAST) Investigators. Preliminary report: effect of encainide and flecainide in a randomized trial of arrhythmia suppression after myocardial infarction. *N Engl J Med* 1989;321:406-12.

31 Feldman A, Voskoboinik A, Kumar S, Spence S, Morton JB, Kistler PM, et al. Predictors of acute and long-term success of slow pathway ablation for atrioventricular nodal reentrant tachycardia: a single center series of 1,419 consecutive patients. *Pacing Clin Electrophysiol* 2011;34:927-33.

32 Stern JD, Rolnitzky L, Goldberg JD, Chinitz LA, Holmes DS, Bernstein NE, et al. Meta-analysis to assess the appropriate endpoint for slow pathway ablation of atrioventricular nodal reentrant tachycardia. *Pacing Clin Electrophysiol* 2011;34:269-77.

33 Scheinman MM, Huang S. The 1998 NASPE prospective catheter ablation registry. *Pacing Clin Electrophysiol* 2000;23:1020-8.

34 Ganz LI, Friedman PL. Supraventricular tachycardia. *N Engl J Med* 1995;332:162-73.

35 Calkins H, Yong P, Miller JM, Olshansky B, Carlson M, Saul JP, et al. Catheter ablation of accessory pathways, atrioventricular nodal reentrant tachycardia, and the atrioventricular junction: final results of a prospective, multicenter clinical trial. The Atakr Multicenter Investigators Group. *Circulation* 1999;99:262-70.

36 Friedman PL, Dubuc M, Green MS, Jackman WM, Keane DT, Marinchak RA, et al. Catheter cryoablation of supraventricular tachycardia: results of the multicenter prospective "frosty" trial. *Heart Rhythm* 2004;1:129-38.
37 Kay GN, Epstein AE, Dailey SM, Plumb VJ. Role of radiofrequency ablation in the management of supraventricular arrhythmias: experience in 760 consecutive patients. *J Cardiovasc Electrophysiol* 1993;4:371-89.
38 Biviano AB, Bain W, Whang W, Leitner J, Dizon J, Hickey K, et al. Focal left atrial tachycardias not associated with prior catheter ablation for atrial fibrillation: clinical and electrophysiological characteristics. *Pacing Clin Electrophysiol* 2012;35:17-27.
39 Lesh MD, van Hare GF, Epstein LM, Fitzpatrick AP, Scheinman MM, Lee RJ, et al. Radiofrequency catheter ablation of atrial arrhythmias. Results and mechanisms. *Circulation* 1994;89:1074-89.
40 Natale A, Newby KH, Pisanó E, Leonelli F, Fanelli R, Potenza D, et al. Prospective randomized comparison of antiarrhythmic therapy versus first-line radiofrequency ablation in patients with atrial flutter. *J Am Coll Cardiol* 2000;35:1898-904.
41 Driver and Vehicle Licensing Agency (UK). For medical practitioners: at a glance guide to the current medical standards of fitness to drive. 2012. www.dft.gov.uk/dvla/medical/ataglance.aspx.

Related links

bmj.com

- All the latest BMJ Group articles on cardiovascular medicine

bmj.com/archive

Previous articles in this series

- Diagnosis and management of supraventricular tachycardia (2012;345:e7769)
- Generalized anxiety disorder: diagnosis and treatment (2012;345:e7500)
- Resistant hypertension (2012;345:e7473)
- Childhood constipation (2012;345:e7309)
- Preparing young travellers for low resource destinations (2012;345:e7179)

BMJ BPP UNIVERSITY SCHOOL OF HEALTH

Management of atrial fibrillation

Carmelo Lafuente-Lafuente, consultant, internal medicine[1], Isabelle Mahé, professor of therapeutics[2], Fabrice Extramiana, associate professor of cardiology[3]

[1]Service de Médecine A, Hôpital Lariboisière, Université Paris 7, Paris

[2]Service de Médecine Interne 5, Hôpital Louis Mourier, Université Paris 7, Paris

[3]Service de Cardiologie, Hôpital Lariboisière, Université Paris 7, Paris

Correspondence to: Dr C Lafuente-Lafuente, Service de Médecine A, Clinique Thérapeutique, Hôpital Lariboisière, Assistance Publique–Hôpitaux de Paris, Université Paris 7 Diderot, 2, rue Ambroise Paré, 75010 Paris, France c.lafuente@nodo3.net

Cite this as: *BMJ* 2009;339:b5216

‹DOI› 10.1136/bmj.b5216
http://www.bmj.com/content/339/bmj.b5216

Atrial fibrillation is the commonest sustained arrhythmia encountered in clinical practice. Its prevalence increases with age, rising from 0.7% in people aged 55-59 years to 18% in those older than 85 years.[1] Consequently, the public health burden associated with atrial fibrillation is increasing.[w1] The therapeutics of atrial fibrillation is evolving. In recent years, publication of several randomised controlled trials and meta-analyses have improved our understanding of the advantages and inconveniences of rate and rhythm control strategies, and effective, new non-pharmacological treatments have been introduced. New antiarrhythmic and anticoagulant drugs are expected in the near future.

Clinical manifestations of atrial fibrillation: what is important to know?

Atrial fibrillation is characterised by a chaotic electrical activity in the atria that induces an irregular and usually rapid contraction of the ventricles (figure 1). Patients may be asymptomatic; may have mild symptoms, such as palpitations, weariness, and reduced effort capacity; or may present with syncope, heart failure, or angina. Many of the presenting symptoms, as well as their intensity, are related to the degree of associated tachycardia. Aside from tachycardia, the major complication of atrial fibrillation is systemic embolism, usually cerebral.

Atrial fibrillation may be self limiting (paroxysmal, which may recur) or sustained (termed "persistent" if lasting more than seven days). "Permanent" atrial fibrillation refers to persistent atrial fibrillation in which cardioversion has failed or restoration of sinus rhythm is no longer considered possible (table 1). An individual can have different types of atrial fibrillation over time—for example, it can evolve from paroxysmal to persistent.

In most cases, atrial fibrillation is associated with hypertension, coronary disease, heart failure, valvular diseases, or cardiomyopathies that result in a dysfunctional heart muscle. Correct recognition and treatment of underlying conditions is essential.

How should we investigate a patient presenting with atrial fibrillation?

Diagnosis of atrial fibrillation requires electrocardiographic documentation. In patients with suspected symptoms but in sinus rhythm at the time of consultation, ambulatory electrocardiography (a 24 hour monitor or an event recorder) may be needed. History taking and physical examination are important for defining whether the atrial fibrillation is paroxysmal or persistent and which symptoms it produces, and for enabling detection of possible causes and precipitating factors, as well as any underlying heart disease (table 2).

US and UK guidelines recommend transthoracic echocardiography in all patients with atrial fibrillation to identify underlying heart disease and to assess signs associated with increased risk of recurrence and embolism (dilated atria, presence of thrombus).[2 3] The US guidelines also recommend measurement of serum electrolytes, blood count, and renal, hepatic, and thyroid function in all patients at least once. Sometimes referral will be needed for specialised investigations, such as transoesophageal echocardiography in patients in whom a cardioversion without previous anticoagulation is being considered, electrophysiological study in patients with wide QRS complex tachycardia, or exercise testing when ischaemia is suspected (table 2).

What are the general principles of the treatment?

Managing acutely unwell patients

Current guidelines for atrial fibrillation agree in several aspects.[2 3 w2] Patients presenting with rapid atrial fibrillation and acute symptoms (hypotension, syncope, chest pain, dyspnoea, heart failure, or neurological symptoms) require urgent control of their heart rate and possibly emergency cardioversion, in a hospital setting.

It is usual to admit to hospital any patient with symptomatic atrial fibrillation of recent onset, even if stable, to expedite investigation and treatment. Some experts advocate trying early restoration of sinus rhythm in these patients to prevent further atrial remodelling and reduce the risk of persistence and recurrence of the arrhythmia.[w3] However, this approach has not been tested in randomised trials.

SOURCES AND SELECTION CRITERIA

We searched the Cochrane database of systematic reviews, *Clinical Evidence*, and the US National Guideline Clearinghouse up to 20 September 2009. We also used personal databases (www.nodo3.net/) and reference collections. We selected well conducted systematic reviews, meta-analyses, and large randomised controlled trials. When no study of those types was available, we considered small randomised controlled trials and cohort studies

SUMMARY POINTS

- Atrial fibrillation is common and highly variable in its clinical presentation and evolution; it causes substantial morbidity and mortality, including impaired quality of life, heart failure, systemic emboli, and stroke
- The first priority is to control heart rate (if tachycardia is present) and provide adequate antithrombotic treatment for preventing complications of embolism
- Patients with moderate to high risk of stroke require warfarin long term for preventing emboli; aspirin is adequate in patients with low risk of stroke
- When a patient should but cannot take warfarin, aspirin plus clopidogrel can be an intermediate option
- For long term treatment of atrial fibrillation, rate control matches rhythm control in terms of mortality and major cardiovascular events but has fewer adverse events related to the treatment and fewer hospital admissions
- Consider referring for rhythm control younger patients with lone atrial fibrillation, patients with symptomatic atrial fibrillation, and patients with atrial fibrillation secondary to a corrected precipitant
- If antiarrhythmic drugs fail to maintain sinus rhythm, percutaneous catheter ablation is an alternative for rhythm control

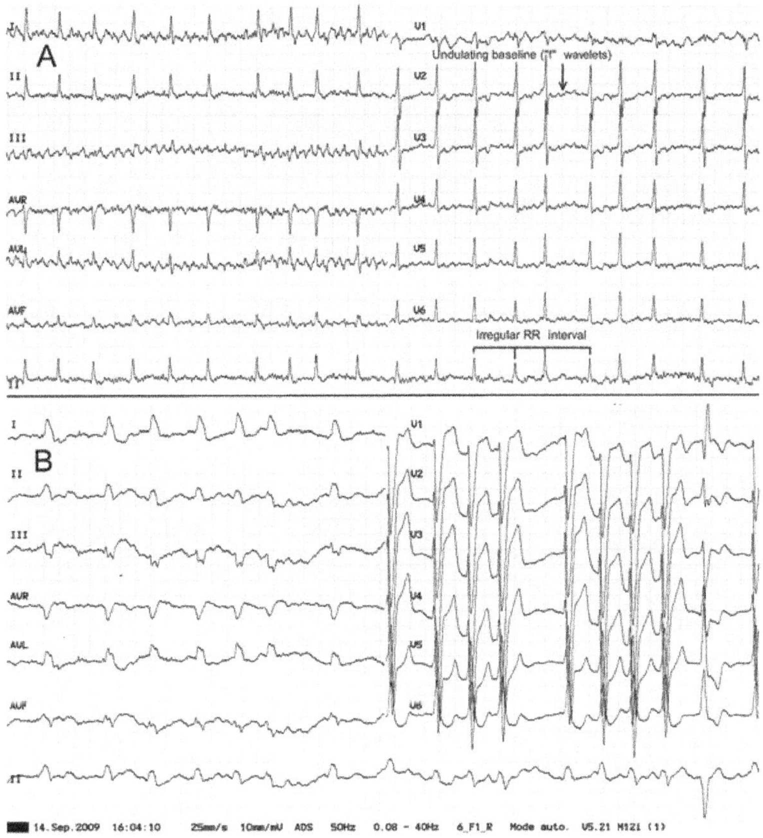

Fig 1 Top panel (A): Typical electrocardiogram of patient with atrial fibrillation. Bottom panel (B): Atrial fibrillation in patient with concomitant left bundle branch block causing enlarged and abnormal QRS complexes

Table 1 Classification of atrial fibrillation*

Type	Definition	Recurrence
Recent onset or first detected	First diagnosed episode (sometimes an incidental diagnosis and precise duration is not known)	May or may not recur
Paroxysmal	Terminates spontaneously in <7 days	Tends to recur
Persistent	Sustained beyond 7 days; rarely terminates spontaneously	Often recurs
Permanent	Cardioversion has failed or restoration of sinus rhythm is no longer considered possible	Established

**Adapted from joint guidelines from the American College of Cardiology, American Heart Association, and European Society of Cardiology.*[2]

Managing patients who are stable at presentation

For patients who are haemodynamically stable and have few or tolerable symptoms the initial management is to slow down the heart rate to the normal range and provide adequate treatment to prevent emboli. Subsequent long term management will focus on rate control or rhythm control. Additionally, adequate treatment of cardiovascular risk factors, especially of hypertension, and avoiding hypokalaemia when using diuretics, can contribute to reduce recurrences of atrial fibrillation.

Which drugs should be used to control heart rate?

Table 3 lists the most common drugs used for controlling heart rate. A systematic review of randomised trials found that first generation calcium channel blockers, β blockers, digoxin, or a combination of these drugs are more effective than placebo in slowing tachycardia associated with atrial fibrillation.[4] Digoxin seemed less effective at controlling heart rate during exercise than β blockers or diltiazem (mean difference 15 to 30 beats/min higher with digoxin). In the AFFIRM trial,[5] a large randomised trial that studied rate versus rhythm control, β blockers were the most effective drugs for slowing heart rate, but frequent treatment changes or combination with other drugs were often needed to achieve adequate rate control.

A randomised trial found that intravenous diltiazem was better than intravenous digoxin (90% versus 74% of patients were well controlled at 24 hours) for rapid rate control of acute, symptomatic, uncomplicated atrial fibrillation.[w4] In patients with decompensated heart failure, current US guidelines recommend intravenous administration of digoxin or amiodarone to slow heart rate, and avoidance of acute use of calcium channel blockers or acute large doses of β blockers as both are negative inotropes.[2]

How do we choose an antithrombotic treatment?

Full anticoagulation is warranted whenever pharmacological or electrical cardioversion is considered, for at least three weeks before and four weeks after the procedure, except when atrial fibrillation has existed for less than 48 hours.[2] If pharmacological or electrical cardioversion is not considered, then a systematic assessment of embolic and haemorrhagic risk in each patient with atrial fibrillation should guide the choice of antithrombotic treatment.[2] [w5] Several scores have been developed to help in this assessment. A large cohort study found that the CHADS-2 tool was the best of three schemes for estimating the risk of stroke in patients with

Table 2 Investigations in patients with atrial fibrillation

Investigation	Purpose
Basic evaluation (history)	
Presence of symptoms, type, intensity	To assess clinical impact
Date of onset or discovery, frequency, duration	To characterise as paroxysmal or persistent
Antecedents, cardiac and non-cardiac diseases, cardiovascular risk factors, alcohol and drugs intake	To look for possible causes, precipitating factors, and possible underlying heart disease
Any previous treatment and response	To plan future treatment
Basic evaluation (physical examination)	
Blood pressure	To rule out hypertension
Heart rate	To establish degree of tachycardia
Heart murmurs, signs of heart failure	To consider probability of heart disease
Enlarged or nodular thyroid	To consider lung and thyroid diseases (possible causes of atrial fibrillation)
Signs of respiratory disease	
Basic evaluation (other)	
Transthoracic echocardiography	To identify heart disease: valvular disease, left ventricle size, hypertrophy, and function
	To establish precise risk of recurrence and of embolism: atrial size, presence of thrombus in left atria (low sensibility)
Blood tests: electrolytes, thyroid function	To identify possible causes or precipitating factors
Blood tests: blood count, renal and hepatic function	To adequately establish dose of drugs and follow side effects
Additional testing	
24 hour electrocardiographic monitoring or event recorder	To diagnose the type of arrhythmia if unknown, and to assess adequacy of rate control
Six-minute walk test	To assess adequacy of rate control
Exercise testing	To evaluate ischaemia if suspected, reproduce exercise induced atrial fibrillation, assess adequacy of rate control
Transoesophageal echocardiography	To identify thrombus in left atrium (high sensibility) and guide cardioversion accordingly
Electrophysiological study	To clarify the mechanism of wide QRS complex tachycardia (accessory pathway?) and to study further any patient considered for ablation of atrial fibrillation, of atrioventricular node, or of other supraventricular arrhythmias
Chest radiography	To identify lung diseases if suggested by clinical findings

**Adapted from joint guidelines from the American College of Cardiology, American Heart Association, and European Society of Cardiology.*[2]

Table 3 Drugs commonly used to control heart rate in atrial fibrillation

Drug	Dose range	Use in heart failure	Major and common side effects
β blockers			
Atenolol	25-100 mg daily	Negative inotropes. Avoid in acute decompensated heart failure. Recommended in chronic, stable systolic heart failure	Hypotension, bradycardia, atrioventricular block, heart failure, bronchospasm, impotence, asthenia, depression
Bisoprolol	2.5-10 mg daily		
Metoprolol	Intravenously 2.5-5 mg (up to three doses) or orally 25-200 mg every 12 hours		
Any other β blocker at appropriate doses			
Calcium channel blockers			
Diltiazem	Intravenously 0.25 mg/kg ororally 120-360 mg daily, in two to three doses	Negative inotropes. Use caution in decompensated heart failure	Hypotension, bradycardia, atrioventricular block, heart failure
Verapamil	120-360 mg daily in two to three doses		
Digoxin	Intravenously 0.25 mg every two hours, up to 1-1.5 mg, or orally 0.125-0.5 mg daily	Positive inotrope. Improves symptoms of heart failure	Bradycardia; intoxication (nausea, abdominal pain, vision changes, confusion, various arrhythmias)

BOX 1 SCORING SYSTEM FOR ESTIMATING RISK OF STROKE PATIENTS WITH ATRIAL FIBRILLATION NOT ASSOCIATED WITH VALVULAR DISEASE*

Risk factors

- Age >75 years—1 point
- Hypertension—1 point
- Diabetes mellitus—1 point
- Congestive heart failure—1 point
- History of stroke or transient ischaemic attack—2 points

Annual risk of stroke (based on points accrued)

- 0 points—1.9%
- 1 point—2.8%
- 2 points—4.0%
- 3 points—5.9%
- 4 points—8.5%
- 5 points—12.5%
- 6 points—18.2%

**Using the CHADS-2 tool*[6]

BOX 2 SCORING SYSTEM FOR ESTIMATING RISK OF MAJOR BLEEDING RELATED TO WARFARIN*

Risk factors

- Age >65 years—1 point
- History of stroke—1 point
- History of gastrointestinal bleeding—1 point
- Any, or several combined, of the following—1 point:
  - Diabetes mellitus
  - Recent myocardial infarction
  - Packed cell volume <30%
  - Creatinine >1.5 mg/l

Annual risk of stroke (based on points accrued)

- Low risk (0 points)—0.8%
- Intermediate risk (1 to 2 points)—2.5%
- High risk (3 to 4 points)—10.6%

**Using the bleeding risk index*[8]

atrial fibrillation not associated with valvular disease (box 1).[6] Echographic demonstration of intra-auricular thrombus or an enlarged left atrium also indicate increased risk of emboli.[7] A score for predicting the risk of bleeding in outpatients treated with warfarin has also been developed (box 2).[8]

Which patients should receive aspirin?

Systematic reviews of randomised trials show that aspirin reduces the risk of stroke by about 22-36%.[9 10] According to guidelines, aspirin is adequate for *(a)* patients at low risk of stroke (those aged under 75 years with no prior thromboembolism and no additional risk factor such as hypertension, diabetes, or heart failure) and *(b)* when warfarin is contraindicated.[2 3 11]

Which patients should receive warfarin?

In well conducted systematic reviews warfarin reduced rate of stroke by 65-68% compared with placebo and 32-47% compared with aspirin, at the expense of increasing haemorrhages (2.5 to 5 major bleedings per 100 patient years, compared with one to two major bleedings in aspirin treated patients).[9 10 12] Guidelines strongly recommend warfarin for patients with atrial fibrillation and moderate to high risk of stroke, such as those with *(a)* mitral stenosis or prosthetic heart valve, *(b)* a history of prior ischaemic stroke or systemic embolism, or *(c)* two or more thromboembolic risk factors (box 2).[2 3 11]

In patients with an intermediate to low risk of stroke (no previous stroke and only one risk factor), either aspirin or warfarin is reasonable. A patient's individual characteristics and preferences should be considered. It is important to *(a)* explain clearly to patients that their disease carries a risk of embolism and stroke and that they need to take a treatment continuously to reduce this risk and *(b)* describe the relative advantages and inconveniences of aspirin and warfarin (especially the needs of regular monitoring and dose adaptations). A semiquantitative ("low, moderate, or high") or quantitative ("x cases in every 100 persons every year") estimate of patients' individual risks may be given. A large randomised trial[13] and a cohort study[w5] have found that elderly patients obtain greater net benefit from warfarin despite their higher haemorrhagic risk.

What about paroxysmal atrial fibrillation?

Cohort studies have found that thromboembolic risk in recurrent paroxysmal atrial fibrillation is closely similar to persistent or permanent atrial fibrillation.[w6] Current guidelines recommend using the same criteria to select antithrombotic treatment irrespective of the pattern of atrial fibrillation.[2 3] Anticoagulation is commonly stopped some weeks after cardioversion, but in a retrospective analysis of data from a large randomised trial this approach was associated with increased incidence of stroke.[w7]

Are there alternatives to aspirin or warfarin for preventing thromboembolic events?

Two large randomised trials, the ACTIVE trials, have studied outcomes in patients treated with aspirin plus clopidogrel. In one of them, aspirin plus clopidogrel proved inferior to warfarin in preventing embolism.[w8] The other found that in patients with atrial fibrillation who were considered unsuitable for warfarin, aspirin and clopidogrel combined reduced stroke and major cardiovascular events further than aspirin alone (relative risk 0.89).[14] However, the combination increased major bleeding by a similar magnitude.

Which long term treatment strategy: rate or rhythm control?

In rate control, in which the aim of treatment is to slow the heart rate and prevent emboli, atrial fibrillation is tolerated. In rhythm control, the objective is to restore and maintain sinus rhythm. To restore sinus rhythm, pharmacological or electrical cardioversion can be used, always after adequate anticoagulation. Pharmacological cardioversion can be tried with antiarrhythmic drugs, administered intravenously or orally; patients receive the treatment usually as inpatients but sometimes as outpatients. In electrical cardioversion, a low voltage electric current, synchronised with the R wave, is delivered through pads placed appropriately on the chest and back. The shock is painful, so it requires sedation or anaesthesia. After cardioversion, atrial fibrillation often recurs (70-85% of patients at one year[15]), so most patients need treatment with antiarrhythmic drugs to stay in sinus rhythm.

Several good quality randomised trials,[16 17 w9] pooled in meta-analysis,[18 19] have compared rate and rhythm control in a variety of patients with atrial fibrillation. No study found any difference between the strategies in terms of mortality, major cardiovascular events, or stroke. Rate control was better for some secondary outcomes: it produced fewer side effects and fewer admissions to hospital. Regardless of whether patients received rate control or rhythm control, those who were in sinus rhythm reported better scores for quality of life. However, when the results were analysed on the basis of intention to treat, quality of life scores did not differ for rate control and rhythm control.[w10 w11]

On the basis of these findings, many specialists consider rate control to be the default strategy for most patients with atrial fibrillation.[w2] However, these result are averaged over a wide range of patients, and many patients in the studies had persistent atrial fibrillation and were aged over 65 years. Other specialists believe that rhythm control might provide better outcomes or quality of life in some subgroups of patients.

Which patients should be referred for rhythm control?

Current guidelines recommend considering rhythm control in patients with *(a)* lone atrial fibrillation, especially younger patients; *(b)* symptomatic atrial fibrillation, such as frequent symptomatic paroxysmal atrial fibrillation or symptoms despite rate control; or *(c)* atrial fibrillation secondary to a corrected precipitant.[3] In addition, patients who should but cannot take warfarin might reduce their risk of stroke if sinus rhythm is restored. Nevertheless, rhythm control in those subgroups has not yet been proved in controlled trials to be better than rate control.

Rhythm control has also been recommended for patients with heart failure. However, a recent large randomised trial in patients with systolic heart failure found no difference between rate and rhythm control for any outcome, including worsening heart failure.[17]

Which antiarrhythmic drugs are used to maintain sinus rhythm?

Two meta-analyses and a systematic review[15 20 21] have found that several class I and III antiarrhythmics (table 4) are effective in reducing recurrences of atrial fibrillation, but all of them cause adverse effects, many have a proarrhythmic

Table 4 Antiarrhythmic drugs commonly used to maintain sinus rhythm*

Drug	Maintenance dose	Use in heart failure	Major and common side effects
Class IA			
Quinidine, disopyramide	Not applicable	Avoid (owing to increased mortality)	Avoid (owing to increased mortality)
Class IC			
Flecainide	50-200 mg every 12 hours	No (negative inotropes); risk of increasing mortality in patients with structural heart disease	Heart failure, gastrointestinal and neurological side effects, blurred vision, proarrhythmia
Propafenone	150-300 mg every 8 hours		Gastrointestinal, dizziness, proarrhythmia
Class III			
Sotalol	80-160 mg every 12 hours	No (negative inotrope)	Hypotension, bradycardia, heart failure, neurological side effects , proarrhythmia
Dofetilide†	125-500 micrograms every 12 hours; monitor QTc interval; start in inpatient setting	Possible	Headache, dizziness, nausea, bradycardia, proarrhythmia
Amiodarone‡	100-200 mg daily	Yes	Bradycardia, atrioventricular block. Thyroid, dermatological, pulmonary, corneal, and liver toxicities

**Antiarrhythmic drugs should be withdrawn in any patients presenting with a long QT interval, new or increasing QRS widening, pronounced bradycardia, or unexplained syncope. β blockers might have a modest effect in preventing recurrences of atrial fibrillation, according to some randomised controlled trials.*[w27 w28]

†Not available in Europe.

‡Not approved by the US Food and Drug Administration for this indication.

activity (that is, they may induce or aggravate arrhythmias), and none improve survival. Furthermore, class IA drugs were associated with increased mortality.

Amiodarone does not increase mortality, can be given to patients with heart failure, and seems to be more effective than other drugs in maintaining sinus rhythm. Unfortunately, amiodarone causes frequent and varied adverse effects, which can be severe.[22 w12] Overall, the benefit to risk ratio of antiarrhythmic drugs is low and they should be prescribed by experienced specialists.

Are there other alternatives for rhythm control?

Patients with infrequent paroxysmal atrial fibrillation may receive no treatment between episodes. If their atrial fibrillation recurs they may have repeated electrical or pharmacological cardioversion, sometimes following a "pill in the pocket" approach (that is, patients who have been given flecainide or propafenone in hospital to reduce paroxysmal atrial fibrillation, and tolerate them well, can be prescribed a single, oral loading dose of flecainide or propafenone for them to take outside hospital if they experience sudden and persistent heart palpitations). A prospective non-controlled trial found that this approach was effective and safe in patients with no underlying heart disease.[23]

Which non-pharmacological treatments can be used for atrial fibrillation?

Atrioventricular nodal catheter ablation with permanent ventricular pacing is used as a palliative approach for controlling ventricular rate in patients with symptomatic atrial fibrillation refractory to medical treatment. A meta-analysis of randomised and non-randomised studies showed that this technique is highly effective and significantly improves quality of life.[24] The main limitations are a small risk of sudden death during the few months after ablation and lifelong dependency on a pacemaker.

Non-pharmacological interventions aiming to "cure" atrial fibrillation have been tried, initially using open surgery.[w13] A more successful approach has been the development of closed chest endocardial ablation, after the discovery that in many patients atrial fibrillation is triggered and/or perpetuated by extrasystoles originating in the pulmonary veins.[25] Briefly, catheters are introduced into the left atrium after a transeptal puncture, and atrial tissue is selectively destroyed (by radiofrequency or cryoenergy) to electrically isolate pulmonary veins. In experienced centres, the success rates are above 70% at one year for paroxysmal atrial fibrillation. In persistent atrial fibrillation, pulmonary vein isolation alone is not sufficient to achieve acceptable success rates, and atrial substrate modification (discrete ablation and/or linear ablations) is usually necessary. Redoing procedures is required in 9-20% of patients. The rate of related major complications of ablation is below 5%.[w14] The advances obtained with endocardial catheter ablation have also led to the development of off-pump, epicardial surgical ablation, following the same principles.

Which patients should be referred for catheter ablation?

Catheter ablation for patients with atrial fibrillation has become widely used only recently and has not yet been tested in large randomised studies with a mortality end point. However, several well conducted randomised trials and systematic reviews have shown that, in both paroxysmal and persistent atrial fibrillation, catheter ablation is better than antiarrhythmic drugs at preventing recurrences of atrial fibrillation.[26 27 w14-w17] According to recent guidelines, prevention of recurrence of atrial fibrillation by ablation is justified only when atrial fibrillation is associated with disabling symptoms, and its use depends on the type of atrial fibrillation.[2]

In patients with paroxysmal symptomatic atrial fibrillation, catheter ablation may be considered after failure of a first line antiarrhythmic drug. Hence, in patients with a structurally normal heart, ablation is an alternative to amiodarone if a class IC antiarrhythmic fails. When amiodarone is the first line treatment because class IC drugs are contraindicated, ablation can be considered if amiodarone fails.

The guidelines are less clear for patients with persistent atrial fibrillation. In such patients, catheter ablation can be considered for "severely symptomatic recurrent atrial fibrillation after failure of greater than or equal to one antiarrhythmic drug plus rate control."[2] This recommendation is not based on strong evidence but is supported by small case series and randomised studies showing that restoration of sinus rhythm by catheter ablation may be associated with a significant improvement in left ventricular ejection fraction in patients with either heart failure induced by tachycardia or pre-existing heart failure.[28 w18]

Can we expect any new treatments for atrial fibrillation?

New antiarrhythmic drugs are being developed. In a randomised trial, vernakalant, a new atrial selective agent, was effective for rapid cardioversion of recent onset atrial fibrillation.[w19] In several randomised trials, dronedarone, a derivative of amiodarone, was more effective than placebo in maintaining sinus rhythm and reducing admission to hospital[29 w20] but increased mortality in patients with heart failure.[w21] The results from a study comparing dronedarone with amiodarone are expected soon.

New oral anticoagulant drugs not requiring blood tests for monitoring are being developed. In a recent large randomised trial, dabigatran, a direct thrombin inhibitor, was as good as warfarin for the primary end point of stroke or systemic embolism and was associated with comparable or lower rates of major haemorrhage.[30]

A randomised trial has shown that percutaneous occlusion of left atrial appendage is as good as warfarin in preventing stroke in patients with atrial fibrillation.[w22] The best indications for such devices remain to be determined.

TOPICS FOR FUTURE RESEARCH

- Understand the mechanism of atrial remodelling (the changes in atrial substrate that usually precede the development of atrial fibrillation and are accentuated by its persistence) and find effective treatments for preventing or reducing it
- Clarify the utility of angiotensin converting enzyme inhibitors and angiotensin II receptor blockers to prevent atrial fibrillation or reduce recurrences. Results of randomised trials and one meta-analysis have been contradictory[w23-w26]
- Compare new oral anticoagulants (dabigatran, rivaroxaban, factor VIIa/tissue factor inhibitors, tecarfarin) with warfarin, the current treatment of choice
- Establish the indications of percutaneous occlusion of left atrial appendage for preventing emboli
- Define the role of new antiarrhythmic drugs (dronedarone, vernakalant) in the management of atrial fibrillation
- Determine the best treatment for elderly patients
- Evaluate the effect of percutaneous catheter ablation of atrial fibrillation on mortality

TIPS FOR NON-SPECIALISTS

- Patients with tachycardia plus syncope, chest pain, dyspnoea, or acute neurological symptoms should be sent immediately to hospital for urgent treatment
- Use β blockers, diltiazem, or digoxin (if heart failure is present), or a combination of these drugs at standard doses to slow heart rate in atrial fibrillation if tachycardia is present

ADDITIONAL EDUCATIONAL RESOURCES

For healthcare professionals

- National Institute for Health and Clinical Excellence. Atrial fibrillation. Clinical guideline CG36. www.nice.org.uk/Guidance/CG36
- ACC/AHA/ESC 2006 guidelines for the management of patients with atrial fibrillation. (Executive summary: http://circ.ahajournals.org/cgi/content/full/114/7/700; full guidelines: http://content.onlinejacc.org/cgi/reprint/48/4/e149.pdf; pocket guidelines: www.acc.org/qualityandscience/clinical/pdfs/AF_PocketGuide.pdf)
- NHS Clinical Knowledge Summaries—source of evidence based information and practical "know how" about common conditions managed in primary care; provides answers to questions that arise in the consultation, with links to answers outlining the evidence (www.cks.nhs.uk/atrial_fibrillation)

For patients

- Shea JB, Sears SF. A patient's guide to living with atrial fibrillation. *Circulation.* 2008;117:e340-43. http://circ.ahajournals.org/cgi/content/full/117/20/e340
- Medline Plus. www.nlm.nih.gov/medlineplus/atrialfibrillation.html
- NHS Clinical Knowledge Summaries (patient information leaflet, atrial fibrillation). www.cks.nhs.uk/patient_information_leaflet/Atrial_fibrillation (Free access)
- Wikipedia. http://en.wikipedia.org/wiki/Atrial_fibrillation

Contributors: CL-L coordinated the review and wrote the introduction and the sections on rate control, rhythm control, and antiarrhythmic drugs. IM wrote about anticoagulants and the choice of antithrombotic treatment. FE wrote about non-pharmacological treatments, ablation, and percutaneous procedures. All the authors revised the draft and approved the complete final version. CL-L is the guarantor.

Competing interests: None declared.

Provenance and peer review: Commissioned; externally peer reviewed.

1 Heeringa J, van der Kuip DA, Hofman A, Kors JA, van Herpen G, Stricker BH, et al. Prevalence, incidence and lifetime risk of atrial fibrillation: the Rotterdam study. *Eur Heart J* 2006;27:949-53.
2 Fuster V, Ryden LE, Cannom DS, Crijns HJ, Curtis AB, Ellenbogen KA, et al. ACC/AHA/ESC 2006 guidelines for the management of patients with atrial fibrillation. *Circulation* 2006;114:e257-354.
3 National Institute for Health and Clinical Excellence (NICE). Atrial fibrillation. (Clinical guideline CG36.) 2006. www.nice.org.uk/Guidance/CG36.
4 Segal JB, McNamara RL, Miller MR, Kim N, Goodman SN, Powe NR, et al. The evidence regarding the drugs used for ventricular rate control. *J Fam Pract* 2000;49(1):47-59.
5 AFFIRM Investigators. The atrial fibrillation follow-up investigation of rhythm management (AFFIRM) study: approaches to control rate in atrial fibrillation. *J Am Coll Cardiol* 2004;43:1201-8.
6 Gage BF, Waterman AD, Shannon W, Boechler M, Rich MW, Radford MJ. Validation of clinical classification schemes for predicting stroke: results from the National Registry of Atrial Fibrillation. *JAMA* 2001;285:2864-70.
7 Atrial Fibrillation Investigators. Echographic predictors of stroke in patients with atrial fibrillation: a prospective study of 1066 patients from three clinical trials. *Arch Intern Med* 1998;158:1316-20.
8 Aspinall SL, DeSanzo BE, Trilli LE, Good CB. Bleeding risk index in an anticoagulation clinic assessment by indication and implications for care. *J Gen Intern Med* 2005;20:1008-13.
9 Cooper NJ, Sutton AJ, Lu G, Khunti K. Mixed comparison of stroke prevention treatments in individuals with nonrheumatic atrial fibrillation. *Arch Intern Med* 2006;166:1269-75.
10 Hart RG, Pearce LA, Aguilar MI. Meta-analysis: antithrombotic therapy to prevent stroke in patients who have nonvalvular atrial fibrillation. *Ann Intern Med* 2007;146:857-67.
11 Singer DE, Dalen JE, Fang MC, Go AS, Halperin JL, Lip GJH, et al. Antithrombotic therapy in atrial fibrillation: American College of Chest Physicians evidence-based clinical practice guidelines (8th edition). *Chest* 2008;133:S546-92.
12 Aguilar MI, Hart R, Pearce LA. Oral anticoagulants versus antiplatelet therapy for preventing stroke in patients with non-valvular atrial fibrillation and no history of stroke or transient ischemic attacks. *Cochrane Database Syst Rev* 2007;(3):CD006186.
13 BAFTA investigators, Midland Research Practices Network (MidReC); Mant J, Hobbs FD, Fletcher K, Roalfe A, et al. Warfarin versus aspirin for stroke prevention in an elderly community population with atrial fibrillation (the Birmingham atrial fibrillation treatment of the aged study, BAFTA): a randomised controlled trial. *Lancet* 2007;370:493-503.
14 ACTIVE Investigators; Connolly SJ, Pogue J, Hart RG, Hohnloser SH, Pfeffer M, et al. Effect of clopidogrel added to aspirin in patients with atrial fibrillation. *N Engl J Med* 2009;360:2066-78.
15 Lafuente-Lafuente C, Mouly S, Longas-Tejero MA, Bergmann JF. Antiarrhythmics for maintaining sinus rhythm after cardioversion of atrial fibrillation. *Cochrane Database Syst Rev* 2007;(4):CD005049.
16 Atrial Fibrillation Follow-up Investigation of Rhythm Management (AFFIRM) Investigators; Wyse DG, Waldo AL, DiMarco JP, Domanski MJ, Rosenberg Y, et al. A comparison of rate control and rhythm control in patients with atrial fibrillation (the AFFIRM STUDY). *N Engl J Med* 2002;347:1825-33.
17 Atrial Fibrillation and Congestive Heart Failure (AF-CHF) Investigators; Roy D, Talajic M, Nattel S, Wyse DG, Dorian P, et al. Rhythm control versus rate control for atrial fibrillation and heart failure. *N Engl J Med* 2008;358:2667-77.
18 De Denus S, Sanoski CA, Carlsson J, Opolski G, Spinler SA. Rate vs rhythm control in patients with atrial fibrillation: a meta-analysis. *Arch Intern Med* 2005;165:258-62.
19 Testa L, Biondi-Zoccai GG, Russo AD, Bellocci F, Andreotti F, Crea F. Rate-control vs rhythm-control in patients with atrial fibrillation: a meta-analysis. *Eur Heart J* 2005;26:2000-6.
20 Miller MR, McNamara RL, Segal JB, Kim N, Robinson KA, Goodman SN, et al. Efficacy of agents for pharmacologic conversion of atrial fibrillation and subsequent maintenance of sinus rhythm: a meta-analysis of clinical trials. *J Fam Pract* 2000;49:1033-46.
21 Nichol G, McAlister F, Pham B, Laupacis A, Shea B, Green M, et al. Meta-analysis of randomised controlled trials of the effectiveness of antiarrhythmic agents at promoting sinus rhythm in patients with atrial fibrillation. *Heart* 2002;87:535-43.
22 Doyle JF, Ho KM. Benefits and risks of long-term amiodarone therapy for persistent atrial fibrillation: a meta-analysis. *Mayo Clin Proc* 2009;84:234-42.
23 Alboni P, Botto GL, Baldi N, Luzi M, Russo V, Gianfranchi L, et al. Outpatient treatment of recent-onset atrial fibrillation with the "pill-in-the-pocket" approach. *N Engl J Med* 2004;351:2384-91.

24 Wood MA, Brown-Mahoney C, Kay GN, Ellenbogen KA. Clinical outcomes after ablation and pacing therapy for atrial fibrillation: a meta-analysis. *Circulation* 2000;101:1138-44.

25 Haïssaguerre M, Jaïs P, Shah DC, Takahashi A, Hocini M, Quiniou G, et al. Spontaneous initiation of atrial fibrillation by ectopic beats originating in the pulmonary veins. *N Engl J Med* 1998;339:659-66.

26 Noheria A, Kumar A, Wylie Jr, Josephson ME. Catheter ablation vs antiarrhythmic drug therapy for atrial fibrillation: a systematic review. *Arch Intern Med* 2008;168:581-6.

27 Jaïs P, Cauchemez B, Macle L, Daoud E, Khairy P, Subbiah R, et al. Catheter ablation versus antiarrhythmic drugs for atrial fibrillation: the A4 study. *Circulation* 2008;118:2498-505.

28 PABA-CHF Investigators; Khan MN, Jaïs P, Cummings J, di Biase L, Sanders P, et al. Pulmonary-vein isolation for atrial fibrillation in patients with heart failure. *N Engl J Med* 2008;359:1778-85.

29 ATHENA Investigators; Hohnloser SH, Crijns HJ, van Eickels M, Gaudin C, Page RL, et al. Effect of dronedarone on cardiovascular events in atrial fibrillation. *N Engl J Med* 2009;360:668-78.

30 RE-LY Steering Committee and Investigators; Connolly SJ, Ezekowitz MD, Yusuf S, Eikelboom J, Oldgren J, et al. Dabigatran versus warfarin in patients with atrial fibrillation. *N Engl J Med* 2009;361:1139-51.

BMJ BPP UNIVERSITY SCHOOL OF HEALTH

Anticoagulation in atrial fibrillation

Benjamin A Steinberg, postdoctoral fellow[1 2], Jonathan P Piccini, assistant professor of medicine[1 2]

[1]Electrophysiology Section, Duke Clinical Research Institute, Duke University Medical Center, Durham, NC 27715, USA

[2]Duke Clinical Research Institute, Durham, NC, USA

Correspondence to: B A Steinberg benjamin.steinberg@duke.edu

Cite this as: *BMJ* 2014;348:g2116

‹DOI› 10.1136/bmj.g2116
http://www.bmj.com/content/348/bmj.g2116

Atrial fibrillation increases the risk of stroke, which is a leading cause of death and disability worldwide. The use of oral anticoagulation in patients with atrial fibrillation at moderate or high risk of stroke, estimated by established criteria, improves outcomes. However, to ensure that the benefits exceed the risks of bleeding, appropriate patient selection is essential. Vitamin K antagonism has been the mainstay of treatment; however, newer drugs with novel mechanisms are also available. These novel oral anticoagulants (direct thrombin inhibitors and factor Xa inhibitors) obviate many of warfarin's shortcomings, and they have demonstrated safety and efficacy in large randomized trials of patients with non-valvular atrial fibrillation. However, the management of patients taking warfarin or novel agents remains a clinical challenge. There are several important considerations when selecting anticoagulant therapy for patients with atrial fibrillation. This review will discuss the rationale for anticoagulation in patients with atrial fibrillation; risk stratification for treatment; available agents; the appropriate implementation of these agents; and additional, specific clinical considerations for treatment.

Introduction

Atrial fibrillation is the most common disturbance of cardiac rhythm in adults, and its prevalence is increasing.[1] Patients with this condition have a significantly increased risk of stroke, and thromboembolic events are a major source of morbidity and mortality.[2 3 4 5] Strokes caused by atrial fibrillation affect a larger part of the brain and are therefore more likely to be fatal or leave patients bedridden than non-cardioembolic strokes.[6 7 8] The use of long term oral anticoagulation reduces the risk of stroke or systemic embolism in patients with atrial fibrillation.[9 10] However, the use of these drugs can be challenging because they significantly increase the risk of bleeding, which can be fatal.[11] The appropriate selection of patients for treatment represents an important clinical dilemma. In this review, we will discuss the background and rationale for long term anticoagulation in patients with atrial fibrillation; appropriate risk stratification for such patients; and the selection and management of oral anticoagulants, including emerging treatments.

SOURCES AND SELECTION CRITERIA

We based this review on a comprehensive literature review and prioritized well conducted studies of high impact and clinical relevance to the topic. Data sources included PubMed, as well as reference lists from included articles. Searches were limited to English language results. Our search terms included atrial fibrillation, prevalence, incidence, stroke, bleeding, and names of individual anticoagulants (such as warfarin, dabigatran, and rivaroxaban). We included MeSH terms, where applicable. In addition, we searched the clinicaltrials.gov database for ongoing trials of novel agents. Most clinical data on novel oral anticoagulants were derived from large randomized clinical trials and retrospective analyses of such trials. The data were supplemented with expert interpretation of the results and summary of the cumulative data.

SUMMARY POINTS

- Stroke is a major cause of morbidity and mortality in patients with atrial fibrillation
- Oral systemic anticoagulation provides significant clinical benefit by reducing stroke or systemic embolism in patients with atrial fibrillation at moderate or high risk
- Although warfarin has been the agent of choice in the past, several newly available oral anticoagulants (direct thrombin and factor Xa inhibitors) have shown superior safety and efficacy in clinical trials
- Although novel oral anticoagulants are a major advance over warfarin, attention to dosing, potential interactions, and adherence are important
- Management of bleeding in patients receiving oral systemic anticoagulation is an ongoing challenge to providers

Epidemiology

The prevalence of atrial fibrillation in the United States has been projected to increase 2.5-fold during the first half of the 21st century.[1] This trend was confirmed in a recent review of worldwide rates of atrial fibrillation in the past 20 years.[12] Cohort studies in North America and Europe show the high burden of disease, which translates into a lifetime risk of about one in four.[13 14 15] Recently the incidence of atrial fibrillation has been shown to vary by race.[16] Nevertheless, the association between atrial fibrillation and adverse events, including all cause mortality and stroke, has been well described. The most recent data suggest that atrial fibrillation related mortality is about 1.6 per 100000, a twofold increase over the past 20 years.[3 11 12 17]

Background and rationale for anticoagulation in atrial fibrillation

The association between atrial fibrillation and stroke was first described in analyses from the Framingham Heart Study cohorts.[4 5 17 18] The earliest study detailed a fivefold increased risk of stroke in patients with non-rheumatic atrial fibrillation, and a 17-fold increase in patients whose atrial fibrillation was rheumatic in origin.[4] Subsequent studies have tried to elucidate the causal pathway between atrial fibrillation and stroke. Many patients with atrial fibrillation also have traditional risk factors for atherosclerotic cerebrovascular disease, and some ischemic events have been attributed to carotid stenoses.[19] However, the most often cited link is the high prevalence of left atrial appendage thrombus in patients with atrial fibrillation. This is attributed mainly to relative stasis of flow in the fibrillating atrium,[20] although in vitro studies have also shown a relative hypercoagulable state in patients with atrial fibrillation.[21 22] Nevertheless, cardiac thromboembolism causes most atrial fibrillation related strokes, so patients are also at increased risk of non-central nervous system systemic embolism.

The association between atrial fibrillation and stroke led to the pursuit of treatments that could reduce this risk. Several randomized trials established the efficacy of antithrombotic drugs for preventing stroke in patients with atrial fibrillation, with both antiplatelet agents and oral anticoagulants showing benefit. Concurrently, risk factors were identified that could stratify patients with atrial fibrillation on the basis of stroke risk, as a way to pinpoint those patients most likely to benefit from anticoagulation despite the increased risks of bleeding.

Risk stratification for stroke, bleeding, and net clinical benefit

The risk of stroke conveyed by atrial fibrillation is not uniform; event rates vary across populations and subgroups. The first observation, in the Framingham cohort, was the pronounced increase in risk for patients with rheumatic heart disease and atrial fibrillation.[4] This association, predominantly related to rheumatic mitral stenosis, has led to the discrete characterization of "valvular atrial fibrillation." Further risk stratification in these patients is not helpful—their risk is very high irrespective of additional risk factors. In contrast, for patients with non-valvular atrial fibrillation, additional risk stratification can yield better resolution of estimated event rates and identify patients at higher versus lower risk.

Stroke risk scores

The most widely used algorithm for estimation of stroke risk in patients with non-valvular atrial fibrillation has been the CHADS2 score.[23] It assigns 1 point to each of congestive heart failure, hypertension, age over 75 years, and diabetes mellitus; and 2 points for a history of stroke or transient ischemic attack. The score was developed from risk factors identified in clinical trials and was subsequently measured and validated in 1733 patients in the national registry of atrial fibrillation, a combined dataset of Medicare patients participating in a quality improvement initiative. The score robustly identifies patients at significantly increased risk of stroke and has been validated repeatedly in other cohorts.[24]

However, in an effort to improve risk stratification in seemingly low risk patients, the CHADS2 score was expanded to incorporate additional risk factors.[25] The CHA2DS2-VASc score further stratified age (1 point for age 65-74 years, 2 points for age ≥75 years) and added 1 point each for female sex and the presence of vascular disease (coronary, peripheral, or aortic plaque on imaging). The CHA2DS2-VASc score was tested and validated in 1084 Euro Heart Survey patients with non-valvular atrial fibrillation who were not taking oral anticoagulation. It showed improved resolution of patients at the lowest scores—no patients with a CHA2DS2-VASc score of 0 had events during follow-up and the adjusted rate of stroke was 0.7% for patients with a score of 1 (fig 1).

However, the CHADS2 and CHA2DS2-VASc scores have limitations. Although they have been validated across many different cohorts of thousands of patients, the discriminatory power of the scores is limited (c statistics range 0.5-0.6). This may be partly because of the relatively narrow cohorts from which they were derived.[24 28] In addition, although the CHA2DS2-VASc score improved discrimination at the lower end of the risk spectrum, stratification remains challenging—confidence intervals for the rate of stroke in patients with a CHA2DS2-VASc score of 1 range from 0% to 3.4%.[25] Thus, guidelines committees have modified the CHA2DS2-VASc score further, downplaying the risk conveyed by a CHA2DS2-VASc score of only 1 when the single point comes from female sex.[29] This is because studies have yielded conflicting estimates on the risk conveyed by female sex. In summary, risk factors can vary in the severity of risk they convey; and the same risk factor may not be equivalent across populations.[24 28 30]

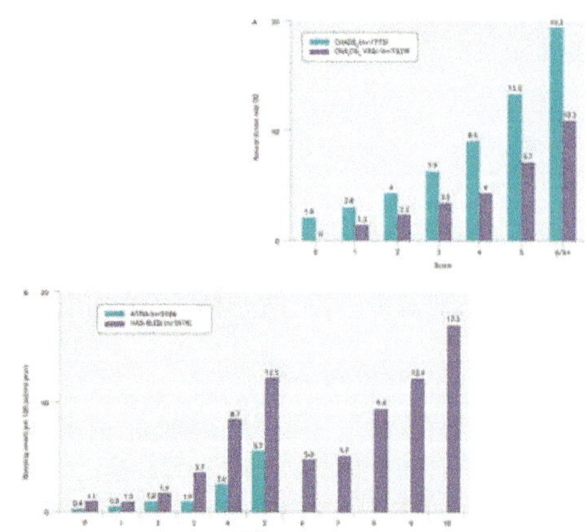

Fig 1 Event rates, according to scores on the various risk stratification algorithms, for (A) stroke and (B) bleeding[23 25 26 27]

Bleeding scores

Because the risk of stroke needs to be balanced against the risk of bleeding, several scoring algorithms have been developed to identify patients at highest risk of bleeding in the setting of oral anticoagulation. The most commonly cited algorithms are the ATRIA, HAS-BLED, and HEMORR2HAGES scores.[26 27 31] Each combines several potential markers for future bleeding and has performed relatively well in large derivation and validation cohorts.

However, in clinical practice not all data points from these scores are readily available or calculable, and no robust prospective studies have shown any benefit for withholding anticoagulation on the basis of a high bleeding score. Furthermore, large observational datasets have failed to identify a group of patients whose risk of intracranial hemorrhage from anticoagulation outweighs the risk of stroke from withholding anticoagulation.[32]

Thus, it is difficult to identify patients with atrial fibrillation whose bleeding risk represents a true contraindication to antithrombotic therapy, and the decision is largely up to the subjective judgment of the individual provider (see box). Guidelines cite bleeding scores as potential tools to reduce the subjectivity involved in the decision but emphasize that these scores should not be the sole basis for a patient being excluded from treatment.[33] Although stroke and bleeding risk factors overlap (for example, advanced age), current evidence suggests net clinical benefit for all but those with the highest risk of bleeding.[32]

Available agents

Warfarin

Vitamin K antagonists have been the mainstay of oral anticoagulation for nearly half a century, particularly for patients with atrial fibrillation. Several randomized clinical trials showed that warfarin was significantly better than placebo and antiplatelet agents (aspirin) for the prevention of stroke in patients with atrial fibrillation. The most important of these were the SPAF-I, SPAF-II, SPINAF, and AFASAK trials.[34 35 36 37] In a meta-analysis of these and other randomized trials, warfarin reduced stroke in untreated patients at intermediate risk from 4.3% to 1.1% (1.4% for aspirin), and in high risk patients from 12% to 4% (10% for aspirin).[38] An updated meta-analysis of 29 trials across comparators confirmed these findings; dose adjusted warfarin was associated with a 64% (95% confidence interval 49% to 74%) relative risk reduction for stroke compared with placebo and a 39% (22% to 52%) relative risk reduction compared with antiplatelet drugs.[10]

SCORES FOR RISK STRATIFICATION IN ATRIAL FIBRILLATION

Stroke risk scores

- CHADS2[23]
- Congestive heart failure (1 point)
- Hypertension (1 point)
- Age ≥75 years (1 point)
- Diabetes (1 point)
- Stroke or transient ischemic attack (2 points)
- CHA2DS2-VASc[25]
- Congestive heart failure (1 point)
- Hypertension (1 point)
- Age ≥75 (2 points)
- Diabetes (1 point)
- Stroke or transient ischemic attack (2 points)
- Vascular disease (1 point)
- Age 65-74 (1 point)
- Sex category (1 point for female)

Bleeding risk scores

- ATRIA[27]
- Anemia (3 points)
- Severe renal disease (3 points)
- Age ≥75 (2 points)
- Previous bleeding (1 point)
- Hypertension (1 point)
- HAS-BLED[26]
- Hypertension (1 point)
- Abnormal liver or renal function (1 point each)
- Stroke (1 point)
- Bleeding (1 point)
- Labile international normalized ratio (1 point)
- Elderly: >65 years (1 point)
- Drugs or alcohol (1 point each)

Warfarin was also compared with newer antiplatelet regimens, including the combination of aspirin and clopidogrel in the ACTIVE W trial.[39] Warfarin was significantly better than dual antiplatelet therapy for the prevention of stroke, without a significant increased risk of bleeding. In fact, in patients who had previously taken warfarin, the risk of bleeding was numerically higher in the dual antiplatelet group. Therefore, despite the development of highly potent oral antiplatelet agents, warfarin remained the standard for stroke prevention in patients with atrial fibrillation through the turn of the century.

Subsequent analyses of the bleeding risk associated with warfarin have shown minimal additional risk in patients treated in the community, outside the setting of well conducted clinical trials. An observational study of 11 526 outpatients with non-valvular atrial fibrillation found a significant benefit of warfarin for the prevention of stroke or systemic embolism (51% reduction compared with no treatment or aspirin, 95% confidence interval 39% to 60%).[9] Furthermore, although warfarin use was associated with a small but significant increased risk of intracranial hemorrhage (0.46 *v* 0.23 events/100 person years; adjusted hazard 1.97, 1.24 to 3.13), it was associated with lower all cause mortality (0.69, 0.61 to 0.77).

Dabigatran

In 2010, the direct thrombin inhibitor dabigatran etexilate became the first alternative to vitamin K antagonism approved for the prevention of stroke or systemic embolism in patients with non-valvular atrial fibrillation. The RE-LY (Randomized Evaluation of Long-Term Anticoagulation Therapy) trial, a prospective open label randomized trial compared dose adjusted warfarin to dabigatran at 150 mg twice daily or 110 mg twice daily in 18 113 patients with non-valvular atrial fibrillation.[40] The primary endpoint of stroke or systemic embolism was similar between warfarin and dabigatran 110 mg (relative risk 0.91 for dabigatran 110 mg; P<0.001 for non-inferiority) and lower in patients receiving dabigatran 150 mg (0.66; P<0.001). Rates of major bleeding were lowest in the 110 mg dabigatran group (2.71%) and equivalent between warfarin (3.36%) and dabigatran 150 mg (3.11%; P=0.31 for warfarin *v* dabigatran 150 mg), whereas intracranial hemorrhage was highest in the warfarin group (0.31 for dabigatran 110 mg, 0.4 for dabigatran 150 mg; P<0.001 for both comparisons with warfarin). Risk of gastrointestinal bleeding was significantly higher in patients receiving both doses of dabigatran compared with warfarin (1.50 for dabigatran 150 mg, 1.36 for dabigatran 110 mg; P<0.001 and P=0.007, respectively). Largely on the basis of this trial, dabigatran was approved in the US at doses of 150 mg and 75 mg (for patients with creatinine clearance 15-30 mL/min/1.73 m^2) and in the European Union at doses of 110 and 150 mg (dose based on clinical judgment).[41 42]

Several additional analyses have provided further data on the use of dabigatran. Firstly, the efficacy of the 150 mg dose and the safety of the 110 mg dose were both consistent with the overall trial across the spectrum of warfarin management quality (as assessed by time in therapeutic range).[43] An in-depth review of intracerebral haemorrhage events in the RE-LY trial found a similar spectrum of severity of bleeding between warfarin and dabigatran.[44] Patients in this trial who needed an invasive procedure had equivalent rates of periprocedural bleeding events (after carefully scripted discontinuation and restart of their anticoagulant),[45] although this has not been a consistent finding across procedures and anticoagulation indications.[46]

In an observational extension of the RE-LY trial, the RELY-ABLE (Long-term Multicenter Extension of Dabigatran Treatment in Patients with Atrial Fibrillation) trial demonstrated efficacy of dabigatran up to 28 months beyond the original RE-LY follow-up period, with a consistent lower risk of bleeding in patients taking 110 mg (*v* 150 mg).[47]

Of note, the primary results of the RE-LY trial suggested a potential signal for increased risk of myocardial ischemic events. A subsequent meta-analysis of dabigatran trials across disease states confirmed such an association,[48] although a mechanism has yet to be confirmed. To date, observational "real world" cohort studies of dabigatran users have demonstrated safety and effectiveness consistent with the RE-LY trial, without a signal for increased risk of myocardial events or higher than expected bleeding.[49 50 51] Further investigation of this potential signal for myocardial events is warranted.

Rivaroxaban

In 2011, rivaroxaban became the first oral factor Xa inhibitor approved for the prevention of stroke in patients with non-valvular atrial fibrillation. The ROCKET AF (Rivaroxaban Once Daily Oral Direct Factor Xa Inhibition Compared with Vitamin K Antagonism for Prevention of Stroke and Embolism) trial is a double blind double dummy trial, which randomized 14 246 patients with non-valvular atrial fibrillation to dose adjusted warfarin (international normalized ratio (INR) 2-3) or rivaroxaban, 20 mg daily (15 mg for creatinine clearance 30-49 mL/min/1.73 m²).[52] This trial enrolled a population with a moderate to high risk of stroke (mean CHADS2 score 3.5; 55% had previous stroke or transient ischemic attack). In the intention to treat analysis, rivaroxaban was non-inferior to warfarin for the endpoint of stroke or systemic embolism (1.7% for rivaroxaban v 2.2% for warfarin; P<0.001 for non-inferiority).[53] Overall major and clinically relevant non-major bleeding was similar between rivaroxaban and warfarin (14.9 v 14.5 events/100 patient years; P=0.44), although rates of intracerebral hemorrhage were significantly lower with rivaroxaban (hazard ratio 0.67; P=0.02). In contrast, gastrointestinal bleeding was significantly more common in the rivaroxaban group (3.15% v 2.16%; P<0.001). The treatment effects were consistent in patients with renal impairment treated with the 15 mg dose.[54]

When interpreting the ROCKET AF data, it should be noted that the time in therapeutic range (a well known marker of anticoagulation quality[55 56 57]) in those randomized to warfarin was lower than in other randomized trials of anticoagulation therapy (mean 55% of the time). However, the treatment effects of rivaroxaban were consistent over the spectrum of low and high time in therapeutic range.[58] Secondly, the number of strokes in the rivaroxaban group increased after mandatory discontinuation of rivaroxaban at the end of the trial. This increase in stroke events was attributed to the delayed therapeutic effect of transitioning to open label warfarin (median 13 days to therapeutic INR when transitioning from rivaroxaban v 3 days in the warfarin arm).[59 60] On the basis of these and other data, careful attention to the transition from a short acting anticoagulant to warfarin is warranted, regardless of the agent(s) used.[61]

An additional randomized trial of rivaroxaban was performed separately in Japan, the J-ROCKET AF trial.[62] This was done for two reasons—firstly, pharmacokinetic data suggested that Japanese patients required lower dosing to achieve target drug concentrations; and, secondly, anticoagulation goals are generally lower in Japanese practice. The investigators randomized 1280 patients to rivaroxaban 15 mg daily or dose adjusted warfarin (INR goals 2-3 for patients <70 years, 1.6-2.6 for age >70 years). Rivaroxaban was non-inferior for the efficacy endpoint of stroke or systemic embolism (hazard ratio 0.49 for rivaroxaban, 0.24 to 1.00), and the safety endpoint of major bleeding or non-major clinically relevant bleeding (1.11 for rivaroxaban; P<0.001 for non-inferiority). Finally, rivaroxaban is the only once daily dosed novel anticoagulant available for stroke prevention in patients with atrial fibrillation.[63]

Apixaban

In 2012, apixaban became the second factor Xa inhibitor to be approved for patients with non-valvular atrial fibrillation. It was shown to be safe and effective in two large phase III trials of patients with non-valvular atrial fibrillation: the AVERROES (Apixaban Versus Acetylsalicylic Acid (ASA) to Prevent Stroke in Atrial Fibrillation Patients Who Have Failed or Are Unsuitable for Vitamin K Antagonist Treatment) trial and the ARISTOTLE (Apixaban for Reduction in Stroke and Other Thromboembolic Events in Atrial Fibrillation) trial.

In the AVERROES trial, 5599 patients with non-valvular atrial fibrillation, who were deemed by their physician not to be candidates for warfarin (40% had previously taken warfarin), were blindly randomized to daily aspirin or twice daily apixaban (5 mg).[64] Reasons for not using warfarin included: difficulty with performing INR testing (43%); inability to maintain appropriate INR therapeutic range (42%); only moderate risk for stroke (CHADS2 score 1, 21%); and refusal to take warfarin (37%; sole reason in 15%). The trial was stopped prematurely, and at one year follow-up the primary outcome of stroke or systemic embolism significantly favored apixaban (1.6% v 3.7%; P<0.001). Rates of bleeding were low, but statistically equivalent between the two groups (hazard ratio for apixaban 1.13, 0.74 to 1.75; P=0.57), including gastrointestinal bleeding (0.86, 0.40 to 1.86; P=0.71).

In the ARISTOTLE trial, 18 201 patients with non-valvular atrial fibrillation were blindly randomized to dose adjusted warfarin (INR 2-3) or apixaban 5 mg twice daily.[65] Patients with at least two of three select risk factors (age ≥80 years, weight ≤60 kg, and serum creatinine ≥1.5 mg/dL; 1 mg/dL=88.4 μmol/L) received 2.5 mg twice daily. After a median follow-up of 1.8 years, apixaban was superior for the reduction of stroke or systemic embolism (hazard ratio for apixaban 0.79; P=0.01 for superiority). Major bleeding occurred in 2.13% of patients taking apixaban each year versus 3.09% in those taking warfarin (P<0.001); gastrointestinal bleeding was equivalent between the groups (0.89, 0.70 to 1.15; P=0.37). Furthermore, the ARISTOTLE trial was the only study of an approved novel anticoagulant to show significantly lower rates of all cause mortality in the novel anticoagulant group (3.52% v 3.94%; P=0.047); however, a non-significant trend has been consistent in trials of other novel agents. Additional analyses of ARISTOTLE have shown consistently positive results across different types of atrial fibrillation (paroxysmal v persistent),[66] degrees of warfarin anticoagulation control (time in therapeutic range),[67] and stroke and bleeding risk score groups.[68]

Emerging treatments

In addition to the approved agents above, several anticoagulants are at various stages of development. The most advanced is edoxaban, another oral factor Xa inhibitor. The ENGAGE AF-TIMI 48 (Effective Anticoagulation with Factor Xa Next Generation in Atrial Fibrillation–Thrombolysis in Myocardial Infarction) trial is a randomized double blind double dummy trial that compared two different once daily doses (30 mg and 60 mg) to dose adjusted warfarin.[69] A total of 21 105 patients with moderate to high risk non-valvular atrial fibrillation were randomized, and the trial mandated a dose reduction (by half) for patients with any of the following: creatinine clearance 30-50 mL/min; weight ≤60 kg; or concomitant use of verapamil, quinidine, or dronedarone. Rates of stroke or systemic embolism were similar to those of warfarin for edoxaban 30 mg (hazard ratio 1.07; P=0.005 for non-inferiority) and 60 mg (0.79; P<0.001 for non-inferiority), with an increased risk of ischemic stroke in the low dose edoxaban group compared with warfarin (1.77; P<0.001). Compared with warfarin, rates of major bleeding were lower for both doses (30 mg edoxaban 0.47, 60 mg edoxaban 0.80; P<0.001 for both), and mortality was lower for low dose edoxaban (0.87; P=0.006), with a similar trend for high dose edoxaban (0.92; P=0.08).

Other novel oral anticoagulants are at earlier stages of development, including the factor Xa inhibitors betrixaban and darexaban,[70 71] and the direct thrombin inhibitor AZD0837.[72] Interventional treatments for stroke prevention are also emerging, including left atrial appendage closure devices.[73 74 75 76 77]

Comparative pharmacology and choosing an agent

Warfarin has relatively non-specific anticoagulant properties, inhibiting the production of factors II, VII, IX, and X. Although this mechanism leads to its notorious long time to onset and offset, warfarin has robust therapeutic effectiveness across many disease states.[78 79] Furthermore, this pharmacodynamic profile is relatively forgiving of missed doses or poor adherence—the anticoagulant effect persists for days after the last warfarin dose. In addition, clearance of warfarin is not affected by renal function, so it can be used in patients across the spectrum of kidney disease.

For these reasons, warfarin remains the preferred anticoagulant for several specific patient groups. Firstly, patients with concomitant valve disease, including valve replacement or valvular atrial fibrillation (current or previous mitral stenosis), should be treated only with warfarin. Current data do not support the use of any of the novel anticoagulants in these patients. The only randomized trial of dabigatran in mechanical valves to date was halted prematurely owing to an increased risk of thrombosis and bleeding in patients assigned to dabigatran (*v* warfarin).[46]

Secondly, patients with the most severe renal dysfunction (estimate glomerular filtration rate <30 mL/min/1.73 m^2) were not included in randomized trials of novel anticoagulants, so these agents should be avoided in such patients. Lastly, providers may choose to use warfarin in patients for whom the ability to readily and objectively monitor the extent of anticoagulation is paramount (for example, for adherence or safety reasons). However, in the remaining patients with atrial fibrillation, the choice of anticoagulant for stroke prevention can be tailored to individual needs and may include new drugs. Regardless of the ultimate choice, the selection of anticoagulant should always be patient centered—no single approach is optimal for all patients, and the subtleties of each patient's characteristics and preferences should be considered.

The novel anticoagulants (dabigatran, rivaroxaban, apixaban, and edoxaban) have been shown collectively to be safer (for avoiding intracerebral hemorrhage) and more effective than warfarin,[80] leading some guidelines to recommend them preferentially.[33] However, these drugs have much shorter time to onset and offset compared with warfarin, and each exhibits some level of renal clearance (table). In addition, none of these agents can be easily monitored using readily available commercial assays for anticoagulation. However, there are additional drug specific considerations when selecting among them. Although some characteristics may favor one agent over another, no prospective randomized head to head comparisons have been made, so any conclusions about comparative safety and effectiveness are putative and remain inadequately tested. Indirect comparisons of these agents have been performed, but caution is needed when interpreting the results.[86 87] Characteristics of individual patients or drugs that may favor one agent over another are therefore subject to provider judgment.

Competing risks

All anticoagulants increase the risk of bleeding. However, apixaban is the only agent to demonstrate safety and efficacy in a randomized trial of patients thought to be suboptimal candidates for warfarin (the AVERROES trial).[64] In these patients, apixaban showed greater efficacy and equivalent safety compared with aspirin. Furthermore, the ARISTOTLE trial showed similar results with a reduced dosing regimen of apixaban in patients at particular risk of bleeding (based on age, weight, and serum creatinine, as noted above).[65] Thus, in patients considered at higher risk of bleeding and those who are not candidates for vitamin K antagonism, apixaban may have several advantages, particularly with respect to bleeding.

By contrast, for patients at particular risk of ischemic stroke, dabigatran may be the most suitable novel anticoagulant. Although apixaban and rivaroxaban prevented more strokes than warfarin through a reduction in the number of hemorrhagic events, dabigatran was the only one of the three drugs that also significantly reduced non-hemorrhagic stroke events (as seen in the RE-LY trial).[40] However, patients at high risk of non-hemorrhagic stroke may also be at high risk of acute coronary syndromes, and these risks must be balanced. Because of the observed association between dabigatran and increased risk of myocardial infarction, some investigators advocate that dabigatran should be avoided in patients with, or at risk of, coronary artery disease.[48] It is important to note though, that the association between dabigatran and acute coronary events stems from retrospective analyses of randomized

Pharmacologic properties of approved anticoagulants available for prevention of thromboembolism in atrial fibrillation*

	Drug			
Property	**Warfarin**	**Dabigatran**	**Rivaroxaban**	**Apixaban**
Mechanism	Vitamin K antagonist	Direct thrombin inhibitor	Factor Xa inhibitor	Factor Xa inhibitor
Dosing†	Variable (dose adjusted on the basis of international normalised ratio)	150 mg; 110 mg bid (Europe only); 75 mg bid for creatinine clearance‡ 15-30 (US only), not recommended if <15	20 mg daily; 15 mg daily for creatinine clearance‡ 15-50, not recommended if <15	5 mg bid; 2.5 mg bid for patients with >2 of the following: creatinine ≥133 µmol/L, age .80 years, or weight ≤60 kg; creatinine clearance‡ <15: no data available
Oral bioavailability	100%	3-7%	60%	58%
Time to effect (h)	72-96	1-2	2-4	3-4
Half life (h)	~40	12-17	5-9	8-15
Notable drug interactions	Numerous	Strong P-glycoprotein inducers		
		Strong P-glycoprotein inhibitors with concomitant kidney dysfunction	Strong P-glycoprotein inhibitors; strong cytochrome P450 inducers and inhibitors	

*As detailed in their regulatory approval packages (may differ from clinical trials protocols).[41 63 81-85]

†Patients with creatinine clearance <30 mL/min/1.73 m^2 were not included in any of the clinical trials of novel oral anticoagulants.

‡Creatinine clearance measured in mL/min/1.73 m^2.

Abbreviation: bid=twice daily.

trials, and subsequent observational data have been conflicting.[49,50,51]

Other populations

Patients with chronic kidney disease represent a challenging population for the prescription and management of anticoagulation. Chronic kidney disease increases the risks of both stroke and bleeding,[27,88] and patients with advanced disease are often under-represented in clinical trials. Each of the novel anticoagulant trials excluded patients with the most severe renal dysfunction, although both the ROCKET AF and ARISTOTLE trials tested reduced dosing of the drugs that they were testing.

In the ROCKET AF trial, the dose of rivaroxaban was reduced to 15 mg daily in patients with creatinine clearance of 30-49 mL/min/1.73 m^2 (and received regulatory approval down to 15 mL/min/1.73 m^2).[53,63] In the ARISTOTLE trial, the dose of apixaban was reduced to 2.5 mg twice daily for patients with two or more of the following: age ≥80 years, body weight ≤60 kg, or serum creatinine ≥133 µmol/L.[65] Although the use of serum creatinine as a measure of renal function has limitations, it does provide supporting data for the use of apixaban in such patients.

For dabigatran, pharmacokinetic studies were used to identify the preferred, renally adjusted dose in the US (75 mg), as is common practice for the Food and Drug Administration.[89] Thus, although some dose adjustment for renal impairment is available for each of the novel anticoagulants, the evidence base for such recommendations varies, and this should be taken into account for patients with marginal kidney function.

Although as a group novel agents have fewer drug-drug and food-drug interactions than warfarin, there are specific, major interactions to be aware of. Antifungal agents almost all have major interactions with novel anticoagulants, as do HIV protease inhibitors and rifampin (US) and rifampicin (UK) (although fewer data are available). In addition, both rivaroxaban and apixaban interact with drugs that are strong inhibitors or inducers of cytochrome P450 3A4. More specific interactions include those between dabigatran and verapamil, quinidine, amiodarone, and dronedarone. However, data on interactions with rivaroxaban or apixaban are more limited,[81] and many drugs have yet to be rigorously tested for interactions with these newer anticoagulants. The requirement for long term concomitant treatment with an interacting agent may guide the choice of anticoagulant in certain patients (table 1).

Additional considerations

Overall, the novel oral anticoagulants are well tolerated with few common side effects; however, dyspepsia is a problem in about 10% of patients receiving dabigatran and is relieved by a change of drug.[40] Thus, it may be best to avoid dabigatran in patients with known dyspepsia, reflux, or gastrointestinal motility disease. Apixaban is the only approved novel anticoagulant that is not associated with an increased risk of gastrointestinal bleeding. Adherence can be a challenge for patients managing anticoagulation. In those patients who find it difficult to manage multiple daily dosages or monitoring, rivaroxaban is the only once daily alternative to warfarin currently available. Lastly, in regions lacking a single payer healthcare system, cost may influence the decision of which, if any, novel anticoagulant to use. To date, cost effectiveness data have favored novel anticoagulants (mostly because they do not need to be monitored),[90] and as more become available they may become more affordable.

Patients stable on warfarin

The management of patients who are stable on warfarin is a challenge for clinicians. The decision to switch a stable patient (with adequate time in therapeutic range) to a new drug should be individually tailored; however, there are several considerations. Most importantly, clinical data to date show that novel oral anticoagulants are more efficacious and safe than dose adjusted warfarin (fig 2). Furthermore, stability on warfarin is highly variable—many patients may tolerate the drug but their time in therapeutic range is insufficient to confer a clinical benefit.[43,55,58,67]

Providers should consider exactly how well controlled the INR is in these patients because novel drugs may be more beneficial in patients with poor control on warfarin.[55]

Nevertheless, switching has additional implications for the individual patient, who may be accustomed to warfarin and reluctant to fix "what isn't broke." For some, an agent that does not require repeated blood draws or dietary restrictions will be appealing. However, all patients should be advised about the availability of these new

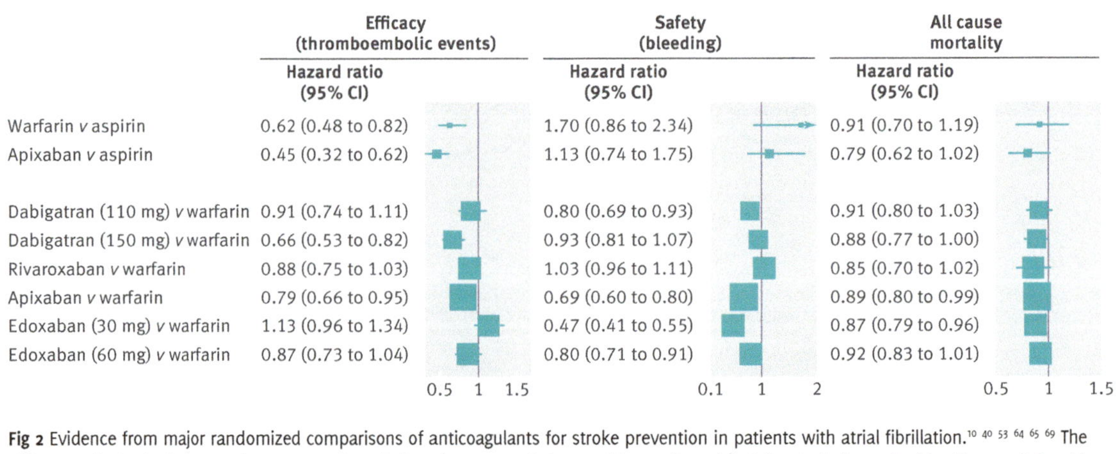

Fig 2 Evidence from major randomized comparisons of anticoagulants for stroke prevention in patients with atrial fibrillation.[10,40,53,64,65,69] The efficacy endpoint includes stroke or systemic embolism (except warfarin *v* aspirin, stroke only). Safety includes major bleeding, as defined by the trial (except warfarin *v* aspirin, extracranial bleeding only). Estimates for warfarin versus aspirin are approximate conversions from risk reduction to relative risk (hazard). ROCKET AF (Rivaroxaban Once Daily Oral Direct Factor Xa Inhibition Compared with Vitamin K Antagonism for Prevention of Stroke and Embolism trial) efficacy includes intention to treat analysis; safety and mortality include the on treatment population. ENGAGE AF-TIMI 48 (Effective Anticoagulation with Factor Xa Next Generation in Atrial Fibrillation-Thrombolysis in Myocardial Infarction 48 trial) efficacy includes intention to treat analysis. CI=confidence interval

drugs, their risks, and their benefits and should be offered these alternatives where clinically appropriate. Patients' engagement and subsequent adherence are paramount to the effective implementation of these newer treatments.

Adherence, planned interruptions, and transitions between drugs

Adherence to oral anticoagulation, particularly vitamin K antagonists, is a major problem. Vitamin K antagonists have myriad drug-drug and drug-food interactions that can dramatically modify the pharmacologic effect, so regular blood sampling and monitoring are required. However, novel oral anticoagulants do not require monitoring and interact with fewer foods and drugs. Yet because commercial assays specific to their activity are not widely available, adherence cannot be easily and objectively measured. Generic coagulation assays (such as prothrombin time and partial thromboplastin time) can be evaluated in patients taking these drugs, but they are not drug or dose specific.[63 91]

Management of planned and unplanned interruptions in chronic anticoagulation can be difficult. Data suggest a low risk of thrombotic events in patients who stop treatment for a short time (≤5 days),[92] and trials have failed to show a benefit of bridging anticoagulation therapy with shorter acting drugs (a larger, more conclusive trial is ongoing).[93] However, US guidelines call for a tailored approach because subgroups of patients seem to be at serious risk of short term thromboembolic events in the absence of anticoagulation.[78] They recommend bridging in patients at high risk of thromboembolic events, such as those who previously experienced an event while not receiving anticoagulation. The guidelines also state that bridging may be considered in those at moderate risk, such as patients with an increased CHADS2 score but no high risk features.[94] Nonetheless, there may be risks to starting and stopping multiple anticoagulants with varying degrees of overlap.

The bridging paradigm is less applicable to novel anticoagulants. Unlike warfarin, which takes a long time to reach maximum effect and has a long half life, newer agents exert systemic anticoagulation within hours—a similar pharmacodynamic profile to agents used for bridging (such as low molecular weight heparins). Thus, there is probably little benefit in substituting a low molecular weight heparin for one of the novel agents. Furthermore, early use of a novel anticoagulant may put patients at risk in the postoperative period—whereas warfarin can be started shortly after surgery with little effect on hemostasis for several days, newer anticoagulants could precipitate bleeding acutely within hours. This is why labels contain warnings against restarting these drug soon after certain types of invasive procedures (for example, neurosurgery and spinal procedures).[41 84 95]

Retrospective analyses of currently available randomized trials show favorable outcomes in patients taking novel anticoagulants who undergo invasive procedures when managed carefully. In 4591 patients in the RE-LY trial who underwent an invasive procedure, rates of major bleeding from a week before the procedure to 30 days after were similar across treatment groups (3.8% for dabigatran 110 mg, 5.1% for dabigatran 150 mg, and 4.6% for warfarin; P>0.05 for each two way comparison).[45] Of note, in this open label trial patients receiving dabigatran stopped the agent a median of 49 (35-85) hours before the procedure, compared with 114 (87-144) hours for patients treated with warfarin (P<0.001). Similar analyses from the ROCKET AF and ARISTOTLE trials are forthcoming, and preliminary results have consistently yielded favorable findings.[61 96]

Management of bleeding events

The management of bleeding in the setting of systemic anticoagulation is an ongoing clinical challenge. In patients receiving warfarin, providers have long experience with reversing the agent using blood products (acutely and temporarily) or replacing vitamin K (gradually and permanently). However, the clinical evidence to support these approaches is not robust. Although they can improve laboratory markers of systemic anticoagulation (INR), their impact on durable clinical outcomes has not been firmly established.[97] Nevertheless, the availability of, and experience with, such reversal strategies serve as a comfort to many clinicians, particularly interventional and surgical specialists.

By contrast, none of the novel oral anticoagulants (direct thrombin inhibitors or factor Xa inhibitors) has an effective reversal strategy that is supported by prospective data. Several approaches have been tested, including recombinant hemostatic factor concentrates and developmental small molecules.[91 95 98] However, studies are limited by their observational nature, small sample size, and lack of long term durable outcomes. None of these compounds is commercially available for this indication. Although more robust trials are planned, the limited data to date do not show increased morbidity or mortality in patients receiving novel oral anticoagulants who experience bleeding events compared with those taking warfarin.

The most recent large analysis of bleeding in patients receiving a novel anticoagulant included a combined population of more than 1000 patients with bleeding events from five phase III clinical trials of dabigatran versus warfarin.[99] It found that patients receiving dabigatran required more red blood cell transfusions, although they had lower rates of plasma transfusion and shorter stays in intensive care. Mortality at 30 days was lower in patients receiving dabigatran who experienced bleeding (9.1% *v* 13.0%; adjusted odds ratio 0.66; P=0.051). These data are limited because they are confined to the well controlled randomized trial population. Although rates of bleeding in several large observational analyses of dabigatran have not been higher than for warfarin,[50] conclusions regarding the outcomes in these patients remain tentative. Furthermore, similar data are not yet available for the factor Xa inhibitors.

Therefore, although guidelines include the reversal of vitamin K antagonists in patients who are bleeding,[78] recommendations for patients taking novel oral anticoagulants are mostly limited to supportive care (including volume resuscitation, hemodynamic support, and primary intervention).[33] The administration of plasma is unlikely to be useful in patients without a primary coagulopathy. Factor concentrates have attracted much attention but remain untested, and they carry a serious risk of thrombotic complications (stroke) that counterbalances their antihemorrhagic properties.[98]

Summary

Thromboembolism is the major source of morbidity and mortality in patients with atrial fibrillation. Oral anticoagulation is beneficial in patients at risk for stroke. However, safe and effective implementation of oral anticoagulation requires appropriate risk stratification. Additional research is needed on stratifying the risk of

GUIDELINES

Anticoagulation is universally recommended for patients with valvular atrial fibrillation or those with mechanical heart valves (who do not have a contraindication).[27 100] The most recent US guidelines for patients with non-valvular atrial fibrillation recommend stroke prophylaxis with oral anticoagulation for patients with a CHADS2 score of 2 or more and state that prophylaxis is reasonable for patients with a CHADS2 score of 1. In female patients with coronary artery disease or age 65-74 (CHA2DS2-VASc components), the guidelines suggest that anticoagulation is considered and weighed against its risks.[100] However, an update to these guidelines is expected imminently. The most recent European guidelines for patients with non-valvular atrial fibrillation recommend no treatment for patients with a CHA2DS2-VASc score of 0; oral anticoagulation with warfarin or a novel anticoagulant (preferred) is recommended for those with a CHA2DS2-VASc score of 2 or more. In patients with a CHA2DS2-VASc score of 1, oral anticoagulation therapy should be considered and weighed against the risks (except for women under 65 years of age, in whom it is reasonable to withhold treatment). Lastly, in patients who decline oral anticoagulation, dual antiplatelet therapy with aspirin and clopidogrel is a reasonable alternative.[33]

RESEARCH QUESTIONS

- What is the benefit of oral anticoagulation for stroke prevention in patients with atrial fibrillation at low to moderate risk of stroke?
- What role should formal assessment of bleeding risk play in the treatment decision?
- What is the comparative effectiveness of the novel oral anticoagulants in patients with atrial fibrillation being treated in the community?
- What is the optimal management of bleeding in patients receiving oral anticoagulation?

bleeding in these patients. Novel oral anticoagulants represent an important breakthrough in medical treatment and are generally more effective than warfarin, but the agent and dose must be chosen carefully. Although these agents may reduce the most serious intracranial bleeding, management of hemorrhage in patients taking anticoagulants remains a challenge and further development of reversal strategies is a priority.

Contributors: BAS performed the literature searches and compiled source documents. BAS and JPP jointly interpreted the data and drafted and revised the manuscript. Both authors approve the final version of the manuscript and are guarantors. The authors certify that the manuscript represents their own work and are solely responsible for its content.

Competing interests: We have read and understood the BMJ Group policy on declaration of interests and declare the following interests: JPP discloses institutional research grant support from Janssen Scientific, GE Healthcare, ARCA pharmaceuticals, and ResMed; and consulting relationships with Johnson & Johnson, Pfizer/BMS, Medtronic, and Spectranetics. BAS was funded by NIH T-32 training grant #5 T32 HL 7101-38.

Provenance and peer review: Commissioned; externally peer reviewed.

1 Go AS, Hylek EM, Phillips KA, Chang Y, Henault LE, Selby JV, et al. Prevalence of diagnosed atrial fibrillation in adults: national implications for rhythm management and stroke prevention: the AnTicoagulation and Risk Factors in Atrial Fibrillation (ATRIA) study. *JAMA* 2001;285:2370-5.
2 Conen D, Chae CU, Glynn RJ, Tedrow UB, Everett BM, Buring JE, et al. Risk of death and cardiovascular events in initially healthy women with new-onset atrial fibrillation. *JAMA* 2011;305:2080-7.
3 Benjamin EJ, Wolf PA, D'Agostino RB, Silbershatz H, Kannel WB, Levy D. Impact of atrial fibrillation on the risk of death: the Framingham Heart Study. *Circulation* 1998;98:946-52.
4 Wolf PA, Dawber TR, Thomas HE Jr, Kannel WB. Epidemiologic assessment of chronic atrial fibrillation and risk of stroke: the Framingham study. *Neurology* 1978;28:973-7.
5 Wolf PA, Abbott RD, Kannel WB. Atrial fibrillation: a major contributor to stroke in the elderly. The Framingham Study. *Arch Intern Med* 1987;147:1561-4.
6 Lin HJ, Wolf PA, Kelly-Hayes M, Beiser AS, Kase CS, Benjamin EJ, et al. Stroke severity in atrial fibrillation. The Framingham Study. *Stroke* 1996;27:1760-4.
7 Tu HT, Campbell BC, Christensen S, Collins M, De Silva DA, Butcher KS, et al. Pathophysiological determinants of worse stroke outcome in atrial fibrillation. *Cerebrovasc Dis* 2010;30:389-95.
8 McGrath ER, Kapral MK, Fang J, Eikelboom JW, O'Conghaile A, Canavan M, et al. Association of atrial fibrillation with mortality and disability after ischemic stroke. *Neurology* 2013;81:825-32.
9 Go AS, Hylek EM, Chang Y, Phillips KA, Henault LE, Capra AM, et al. Anticoagulation therapy for stroke prevention in atrial fibrillation: how well do randomized trials translate into clinical practice? *JAMA* 2003;290:2685-92.
10 Hart RG, Pearce LA, Aguilar MI. Meta-analysis: antithrombotic therapy to prevent stroke in patients who have nonvalvular atrial fibrillation. *Ann Intern Med* 2007;146:857-67.
11 Fang MC, Go AS, Chang Y, Borowsky LH, Pomernacki NK, Udaltsova N, et al. Thirty-day mortality after ischemic stroke and intracranial hemorrhage in patients with atrial fibrillation on and off anticoagulants. *Stroke* 2012;43:1795-9.
12 Chugh SS, Havmoeller R, Narayanan K, Singh D, Rienstra M, Benjamin EJ, et al. Worldwide epidemiology of atrial fibrillation: a global burden of disease 2010 study. *Circulation* 2014;129:837-47.
13 Lloyd-Jones DM. Lifetime risk for development of atrial fibrillation: the Framingham Heart Study. *Circulation* 2004;110:1042-46.
14 Piccini JP, Hammill BG, Sinner MF, Jensen PN, Hernandez AF, Heckbert SR, et al. Incidence and prevalence of atrial fibrillation and associated mortality among Medicare beneficiaries, 1993-2007. *Circ Cardiovasc Qual Outcomes* 2012;5:85-93.
15 Stewart S, Hart CL, Hole DJ, McMurray JJ. Population prevalence, incidence, and predictors of atrial fibrillation in the Renfrew/Paisley study. *Heart* 2001;86:516-21.
16 Dewland TA, Olgin JE, Vittinghoff E, Marcus GM. Incident atrial fibrillation among Asians, Hispanics, blacks, and whites. *Circulation* 2013;128:2470-7.
17 Brand FN, Abbott RD, Kannel WB, Wolf PA. Characteristics and prognosis of lone atrial fibrillation. 30-year follow-up in the Framingham study. *JAMA* 1985;254:3449-53.
18 Wolf PA, Abbott RD, Kannel WB. Atrial fibrillation as an independent risk factor for stroke: the Framingham Study. *Stroke* 1991;22:983-8.
19 Anderson DC, Kappelle LJ, Eliasziw M, Babikian VL, Pearce LA, Barnett HJ. Occurrence of hemispheric and retinal ischemia in atrial fibrillation compared with carotid stenosis. *Stroke* 2002;33:1963-7.
20 Transesophageal echocardiographic correlates of thromboembolism in high-risk patients with nonvalvular atrial fibrillation. The stroke prevention in atrial fibrillation investigators committee on echocardiography. *Ann Intern Med* 1998;128:639-47.
21 Uno M, Tsuji H, Sawada S, Toyoda T, Nakagawa M. Fibrinopeptide A (FPA) levels in atrial fibrillation and the effects of heparin administration. *Jpn Circ J* 1988;52:9-12.
22 Mitusch R, Siemens HJ, Garbe M, Wagner T, Sheikhzadeh A, Diederich KW. Detection of a hypercoagulable state in nonvalvular atrial fibrillation and the effect of anticoagulant therapy. *Thromb Haemost* 1996;75:219-23.
23 Gage BF, Waterman AD, Shannon W, Boechler M, Rich MW, Radford MJ. Validation of clinical classification schemes for predicting stroke: results from the national registry of atrial fibrillation. *JAMA* 2001;285:2864-70.
24 Olesen JB, Lip GY, Hansen ML, Hansen PR, Tolstrup JS, Lindhardsen J, et al. Validation of risk stratification schemes for predicting stroke and thromboembolism in patients with atrial fibrillation: nationwide cohort study. *BMJ* 2011;342:d124.
25 Lip GY, Nieuwlaat R, Pisters R, Lane DA, Crijns HJ. Refining clinical risk stratification for predicting stroke and thromboembolism in atrial fibrillation using a novel risk factor-based approach: the Euro Heart Survey on atrial fibrillation. *Chest* 2010;137:263-72.
26 Pisters R, Lane DA, Nieuwlaat R, de Vos CB, Crijns HJ, Lip GY. A novel user-friendly score (HAS-BLED) to assess 1-year risk of major bleeding in patients with atrial fibrillation: the Euro Heart Survey. *Chest* 2010;138:1093-100.
27 Fang MC, Go AS, Chang Y, Borowsky LH, Pomernacki NK, Udaltsova N, et al. A new risk scheme to predict warfarin-associated hemorrhage: the ATRIA (Anticoagulation and Risk Factors in Atrial Fibrillation) Study. *J Am Coll Cardiol* 2011;58:395-401.
28 Friberg L, Rosenqvist M, Lip GY. Evaluation of risk stratification schemes for ischaemic stroke and bleeding in 182 678 patients with atrial fibrillation: the Swedish atrial fibrillation cohort study. *Eur Heart J* 2012;33:1500-10.
29 Camm AJ, Kirchhof P, Lip GY, Schotten U, Savelieva I, Ernst S, et al. Guidelines for the management of atrial fibrillation: the task force for the management of atrial fibrillation of the European Society of Cardiology (ESC). *Eur Heart J* 2010;31:2369-429.
30 Keogh C, Wallace E, Dillon C, Dimitrov BD, Fahey T. Validation of the CHADS2 clinical prediction rule to predict ischaemic stroke. A systematic review and meta-analysis. *Thromb Haemost* 2011;106:528-38.
31 Gage BF, Yan Y, Milligan PE, Waterman AD, Culverhouse R, Rich MW, et al. Clinical classification schemes for predicting hemorrhage: results from the national registry of atrial fibrillation (NRAF). *Am Heart J* 2006;151:713-9.
32 Friberg L, Rosenqvist M, Lip GY. Net clinical benefit of warfarin in patients with atrial fibrillation: a report from the Swedish atrial fibrillation cohort study. *Circulation* 2012;125:2298-307.
33 Camm AJ, Lip GY, De Caterina R, Savelieva I, Atar D, Hohnloser SH, et al. 2012 focused update of the ESC guidelines for the management of atrial fibrillation: an update of the 2010 ESC guidelines for the management of atrial fibrillation. Developed with the special contribution of the European Heart Rhythm Association. *Eur Heart J* 2012;33:2719-47.
34 Warfarin versus aspirin for prevention of thromboembolism in atrial fibrillation: Stroke Prevention in Atrial Fibrillation II Study. *Lancet* 1994;343:687-91.

35 Design of a multicenter randomized trial for the Stroke Prevention in Atrial Fibrillation Study. The Stroke Prevention in Atrial Fibrillation Investigators. *Stroke* 1990;21:538-45.
36 Ezekowitz MD, Bridgers SL, James KE, Carliner NH, Colling CL, Gornick CC, et al. Warfarin in the prevention of stroke associated with nonrheumatic atrial fibrillation. Veterans Affairs Stroke Prevention in Nonrheumatic Atrial Fibrillation Investigators. *N Engl J Med* 1992;327:1406-12.
37 Petersen P, Boysen G, Godtfredsen J, Andersen ED, Andersen B. Placebo-controlled, randomised trial of warfarin and aspirin for prevention of thromboembolic complications in chronic atrial fibrillation. The Copenhagen AFASAK study. *Lancet* 1989;1:175-9.
38 Ezekowitz MD, Levine JA. Preventing stroke in patients with atrial fibrillation. *JAMA* 1999;281:1830-5.
39 Connolly S, Pogue J, Hart R, Pfeffer M, Hohnloser S, Chrolavicius S, et al. Clopidogrel plus aspirin versus oral anticoagulation for atrial fibrillation in the Atrial fibrillation Clopidogrel Trial with Irbesartan for prevention of Vascular Events (ACTIVE W): a randomised controlled trial. *Lancet* 2006;367:1903-12.
40 Connolly SJ, Ezekowitz MD, Yusuf S, Eikelboom J, Oldgren J, Parekh A, et al. Dabigatran versus warfarin in patients with atrial fibrillation. *N Engl J Med* 2009;361:1139-51.
41 Boehringer-Ingelheim. Dabigatran prescribing information. Secondary dabigatran prescribing information 2010. http://bidocs.boehringer-ingelheim.com/BIWebAccess/ViewServlet.ser?docBase=renetnt&folderPath=/Prescribing%20Information/PIs/Pradaxa/Pradaxa.pdf.
42 Boehringer-Ingelheim. Dabigatran prescribing information for stroke prevention in atrial fibrillation in the United Kingdom. 2013. www.pradaxa.co.uk/downloads/pi-spaf.pdf.
43 Wallentin L, Yusuf S, Ezekowitz MD, Alings M, Flather M, Franzosi MG, et al. Efficacy and safety of dabigatran compared with warfarin at different levels of international normalised ratio control for stroke prevention in atrial fibrillation: an analysis of the RE-LY trial. *Lancet* 2010;376:975-83.
44 Hart RG, Diener HC, Yang S, Connolly SJ, Wallentin L, Reilly PA, et al. Intracranial hemorrhage in atrial fibrillation patients during anticoagulation with warfarin or dabigatran: the RE-LY trial. *Stroke* 2012;43:1511-7.
45 Healey JS, Eikelboom J, Douketis J, Wallentin L, Oldgren J, Yang S, et al. Peri-procedural bleeding and thromboembolic events with dabigatran compared to warfarin: results from the RE-LY randomized trial. *Circulation* 2012;126:343-8.
46 Eikelboom JW, Connolly SJ, Brueckmann M, Granger CB, Kappetein AP, Mack MJ, et al. Dabigatran versus warfarin in patients with mechanical heart valves. *N Engl J Med* 2013;369:1206-14.
47 Connolly SJ, Wallentin L, Ezekowitz MD, Eikelboom J, Oldgren J, Reilly PA, et al. The long-term multicenter observational study of dabigatran treatment in patients with atrial fibrillation (RELY-ABLE) study. *Circulation* 2013;128:237-43.
48 Uchino K, Hernandez AV. Dabigatran association with higher risk of acute coronary events: meta-analysis of noninferiority randomized controlled trials. *Arch Intern Med* 2012;172:397-402.
49 Larsen TB, Rasmussen LH, Skjoth F, Due KM, Callreus T, Rosenzweig M, et al. Efficacy and safety of dabigatran etexilate and warfarin in "real-world" patients with atrial fibrillation: a prospective nationwide cohort study. *J Am Coll Cardiol* 2013;61:2264-73.
50 Southworth MR, Reichman ME, Unger EF. Dabigatran and postmarketing reports of bleeding. *N Engl J Med* 2013;368:1272-4.
51 Sorensen R, Gislason G, Torp-Pedersen C, Olesen JB, Fosbol EL, Hvidtfeldt MW, et al. Dabigatran use in Danish atrial fibrillation patients in 2011: a nationwide study. *BMJ Open* 2013;3:2758.
52 ROCKET AF Study Investigators. Rivaroxaban-Once daily, oral, direct factor Xa inhibition Compared with vitamin K antagonism for prevention of stroke and Embolism Trial in Atrial Fibrillation: rationale and design of the ROCKET AF study. *Am Heart J* 2010;159:340-47.
53 Patel MR, Mahaffey KW, Garg J, Pan G, Singer DE, Hacke W, et al. Rivaroxaban versus warfarin in nonvalvular atrial fibrillation. *N Engl J Med* 2011;365:883-91.
54 Fox KA, Piccini JP, Wojdyla D, Becker RC, Halperin JL, Nessel CC, et al. Prevention of stroke and systemic embolism with rivaroxaban compared with warfarin in patients with non-valvular atrial fibrillation and moderate renal impairment. *Eur Heart J* 2011;32:2387-94.
55 Connolly SJ, Pogue J, Eikelboom J, Flaker G, Commerford P, Franzosi MG, et al. Benefit of oral anticoagulant over antiplatelet therapy in atrial fibrillation depends on the quality of international normalized ratio control achieved by centers and countries as measured by time in therapeutic range. *Circulation* 2008;118:2029-37.
56 Morgan CL, McEwan P, Tukiendorf A, Robinson PA, Clemens A, Plumb JM. Warfarin treatment in patients with atrial fibrillation: observing outcomes associated with varying levels of INR control. *Thromb Res* 2009;124:37-41.
57 Rosendaal FR, Cannegieter SC, van der Meer FJ, Briet E. A method to determine the optimal intensity of oral anticoagulant therapy. *Thromb Haemost* 1993;69:236-9.
58 Food and Drug Administration. FDA draft briefing document for the cardiovascular and renal drugs advisory committee (CRDAC): rivaroxaban for the prevention of stroke and systemic embolism in patients with non-valvular atrial fibrillation. 2011. www.fda.gov/downloads/AdvisoryCommittees/CommitteesMeetingMaterials/drugs/CardiovascularandRenalDrugsAdvisoryCommittee/ucm270796.pdf.
59 Patel MR, Hellkamp AS, Lokhnygina Y, Piccini JP, Zhang Z, Mohanty S, et al. Outcomes of discontinuing rivaroxaban compared with warfarin in patients with nonvalvular atrial fibrillation: analysis from the ROCKET AF trial (Rivaroxaban Once-Daily, Oral, Direct Factor Xa Inhibition Compared With Vitamin K Antagonism for Prevention of Stroke and Embolism Trial in Atrial Fibrillation). *J Am Coll Cardiol* 2013;61:651-8.
60 Mahaffey KW, Hellkamp AS, Patel MR, Hannan KL, Schwabe K, Nessel CC, et al. End of study transition from study drug to open-label vitamin K antagonist therapy: the ROCKET AF experience. *Circ Cardiovasc Qual Outcomes* 2013;6:470-8.
61 Lopes RD, Garcia DA, Wojdyla D, Dorian P, Alexander JH, Wallentin L, et al. Use of apixaban and warfarin in patients undergoing invasive procedures: insights from ARISTOTLE. *Eur Heart J* 2013;34(suppl 1): doi:10.1093/eurheartj/eht307.P535.
62 Hori M, Matsumoto M, Tanahashi N, Momomura S, Uchiyama S, Goto S, et al. Rivaroxaban vs. warfarin in Japanese patients with atrial fibrillation—the J-ROCKET AF study. *Circ J* 2012;76:2104-11.
63 Pharmaceuticals J. Rivaroxaban prescribing information. Secondary rivaroxaban prescribing information 2011. www.xareltohcp.com/sites/default/files/pdf/xarelto_0.pdf#zoom=100.
64 Connolly SJ, Eikelboom J, Joyner C, Diener HC, Hart R, Golitsyn S, et al. Apixaban in patients with atrial fibrillation. *N Engl J Med* 2011;364:806-17.
65 Granger CB, Alexander JH, McMurray JJ, Lopes RD, Hylek EM, Hanna M, et al. Apixaban versus warfarin in patients with atrial fibrillation. *N Engl J Med* 2011;365:981-92.
66 Al-Khatib SM, Thomas L, Wallentin L, Lopes RD, Gersh B, Garcia D, et al. Outcomes of apixaban vs warfarin by type and duration of atrial fibrillation: results from the ARISTOTLE trial. *Eur Heart J* 2013;34:2464-71.
67 Wallentin L, Lopes RD, Hanna M, Thomas L, Hellkamp A, Nepal S, et al. Efficacy and safety of apixaban compared with warfarin at different levels of predicted international normalized ratio control for stroke prevention in atrial fibrillation. *Circulation* 2013;127:2166-76.
68 Lopes RD, Al-Khatib SM, Wallentin L, Yang H, Ansell J, Bahit MC, et al. Efficacy and safety of apixaban compared with warfarin according to patient risk of stroke and of bleeding in atrial fibrillation: a secondary analysis of a randomised controlled trial. *Lancet* 2012;380:1749-58.
69 Giugliano RP, Ruff CT, Braunwald E, Murphy SA, Wiviott SD, Halperin JL, et al. Edoxaban versus warfarin in patients with atrial fibrillation. *N Engl J Med* 2013;369:2093-104.
70 Hashimoto T, Suzuki K, Kihara Y, Iwatsubo T, Miyashita A, Heeringa M, et al. Absorption, metabolism and excretion of darexaban (YM150), a new direct factor Xa inhibitor in humans. *Xenobiotica* 2013;43:534-47.
71 Connolly SJ, Eikelboom J, Dorian P, Hohnloser SH, Gretler DD, Sinha U, et al. Betrixaban compared with warfarin in patients with atrial fibrillation: results of a phase 2, randomized, dose-ranging study (Explore-Xa). *Eur Heart J* 2013;34:1498-505.
72 Johansson S, Cullberg M, Eriksson UG, et al. Single-dose pharmacokinetics, pharmacodynamics and safety of AZD0837, a novel oral direct thrombin inhibitor, in young healthy male subjects. *Int J Clin Pharmacol Ther* 2011;49:258-67.
73 Bartus K, Han FT, Bednarek J, Elg M, Duner K, Jensen E, et al. Percutaneous left atrial appendage suture ligation using the LARIAT device in patients with atrial fibrillation: initial clinical experience. *J Am Coll Cardiol* 2013;62:108-18.
74 Bartus K, Bednarek J, Myc J, Myc J, Kapelak B, Sadowski J, et al. Feasibility of closed-chest ligation of the left atrial appendage in humans. *Heart Rhythm* 2011;8:188-93.
75 Reddy VY, Doshi SK, Sievert H, Buchbinder M, Neuzil P, Huber K, et al. Percutaneous left atrial appendage closure for stroke prophylaxis in patients with atrial fibrillation: 2.3-year follow-up of the PROTECT AF (Watchman Left Atrial Appendage System for Embolic Protection in Patients with Atrial Fibrillation) trial. *Circulation* 2013;127:720-9.
76 Reddy VY, Holmes D, Doshi SK, , Neuzil P, Kar S. Safety of percutaneous left atrial appendage closure: results from the Watchman Left Atrial Appendage System for Embolic Protection in Patients with AF (PROTECT AF) clinical trial and the continued access registry. *Circulation* 2011;123:417-24.
77 Landmesser U, Holmes DR Jr. Left atrial appendage closure: a percutaneous transcatheter approach for stroke prevention in atrial fibrillation. *Eur Heart J* 2012;33:698-704.
78 Guyatt GH, Akl EA, Crowther M, Gutterman DD, Schuunemann HJ; American College of Chest Physicians Antithrombotic Therapy and Prevention of Thrombosis Panel. Executive summary: antithrombotic therapy and prevention of thrombosis (9th ed). American College of Chest Physicians evidence-based clinical practice guidelines. *Chest* 2012;141(suppl 2):7S-47S.
79 Singer DE, Albers GW, Dalen JE, Fang MC, Go AS, Halperin JL, et al. Antithrombotic therapy in atrial fibrillation: American College of Chest Physicians evidence-based clinical practice guidelines (8th ed). *Chest* 2008;133(suppl 6):546S-92S.
80 Ruff CT, Giugliano RP, Braunwald E, Hoffman EB, Deenadayalu N, Ezekowitz MD, et al. Comparison of the efficacy and safety of new oral anticoagulants with warfarin in patients with atrial fibrillation: a meta-analysis of randomised trials. *Lancet* 2013; published 4 Dec.
81 Heidbuchel H, Verhamme P, Alings M, Antz M, Hacke W, Oldgren J, et al. European Heart Rhythm Association practical guide on the use of new oral anticoagulants in patients with non-valvular atrial fibrillation. *Europace* 2013;15:625-5.

82 Squibb B-M. Apixaban prescribing information. Secondary apixaban prescribing information 2012. http://packageinserts.bms.com/pi/pi_eliquis.pdf.

83 Perzborn E, Roehrig S, Straub A, Kubitza D, Misselwitz F. The discovery and development of rivaroxaban, an oral, direct factor Xa inhibitor. *Nat Rev Drug Discov* 2011;10:61-75.

84 Eriksson BI, Quinlan DJ, Weitz JI. Comparative pharmacodynamics and pharmacokinetics of oral direct thrombin and factor xa inhibitors in development. *Clin Pharmacokinet* 2009;48:1-22.

85 Pinto DJ, Orwat MJ, Koch S, Rossi KA, Alexander RS, Smallwood A, et al. Discovery of 1-(4-methoxyphenyl)-7-oxo-6-(4-(2-oxopiperidin-1-yl) phenyl)-4,5,6,7-tetrahydro-1H -pyrazolo[3,4-c]pyridine-3-carboxamide (apixaban, BMS-562247), a highly potent, selective, efficacious, and orally bioavailable inhibitor of blood coagulation factor Xa. *J Med Chem* 2007;50:5339-56.

86 Lip GY, Larsen TB, Skjoth F, Rasmussen LH. Indirect comparisons of new oral anticoagulant drugs for efficacy and safety when used for stroke prevention in atrial fibrillation. *J Am Coll Cardiol* 2012;60:738-46.

87 Dogliotti A, Paolasso E, Giugliano RP. Current and new oral antithrombotics in non-valvular atrial fibrillation: a network meta-analysis of 79 808 patients. *Heart* 2013; published online 5 Sep.

88 Piccini JP, Stevens SR, Chang Y, Singer DE, Lokhnygina Y, Go AS, et al. Renal dysfunction as a predictor of stroke and systemic embolism in patients with nonvalvular atrial fibrillation: validation of the R(2) CHADS(2) index in the ROCKET AF (Rivaroxaban Once-daily, oral, direct factor Xa inhibition Compared with vitamin K antagonism for prevention of stroke and Embolism Trial in Atrial Fibrillation) and ATRIA (AnTicoagulation and Risk factors In Atrial fibrillation) study cohorts. *Circulation* 2013;127:224-32.

89 Beasley BN, Unger EF, Temple R. Anticoagulant options—why the FDA approved a higher but not a lower dose of dabigatran. *N Engl J Med* 2011;364:1788-90.

90 Limone BL, Baker WL, Kluger J, Coleman CI. Novel anticoagulants for stroke prevention in atrial fibrillation: a systematic review of cost-effectiveness models. *PLoS One* 2013;8:e62183.

91 Eerenberg ES, Kamphuisen PW, Sijpkens MK, Meijers JC, Buller HR, Levi M. Reversal of rivaroxaban and dabigatran by prothrombin complex concentrate: a randomized, placebo-controlled, crossover study in healthy subjects. *Circulation* 2011;124:1573-9.

92 Garcia DA, Regan S, Henault LE, Upadhyay A, Baker J, Othman M, et al. Risk of thromboembolism with short-term interruption of warfarin therapy. *Arch Intern Med* 2008;168:63-9.

93 Wysokinski WE, McBane RD, Daniels PR, Litin SC, Hodge DO, Dowling NF, et al. Periprocedural anticoagulation management of patients with nonvalvular atrial fibrillation. *Mayo Clin Proc* 2008;83:639-45.

94 Douketis JD, Spyropoulos AC, Spencer FA, Mayr M, Jaffer AK, Eckman MH, et al. Perioperative management of antithrombotic therapy: antithrombotic therapy and prevention of thrombosis (9th ed). American College of Chest Physicians evidence-based clinical practice guidelines. *Chest* 2012;141(suppl 2):e326S-50S.

95 Marlu R, Hodaj E, Paris A, Albaladejo P, Crackowski JL, Pernod G. Effect of non-specific reversal agents on anticoagulant activity of dabigatran and rivaroxaban: a randomised crossover ex vivo study in healthy volunteers. *Thromb Haemost* 2012;108:217-24.

96 Sherwood MW, Douketis JD, Patel MR, Piccini JP, Hellkamp AS, Lokhnygina Y, et al. Outcomes of temporary interruption of rivaroxaban compared with warfarin in patients with nonvalvular atrial fibrillation: results from ROCKET AF. *Circulation* 2014; published online 19 Feb.

97 Bauer KA. Reversal of antithrombotic agents. *Am J Hematol* 2012;87(suppl 1):S119-26.

98 Lu G, DeGuzman FR, Hollenbach SJ, Karbarz MJ, Abe K, Lee G, et al. A specific antidote for reversal of anticoagulation by direct and indirect inhibitors of coagulation factor Xa. *Nat Med* 2013;19:446-51.

99 Majeed A, Hwang HG, Connolly SJ, Eikelboom JW, Ezekowitz MD, Wallentin L, et al. Management and outcomes of major bleeding during treatment with dabigatran or warfarin. *Circulation* 2013;128:2325-32.

100 Fuster V, Ryden LE, Cannom DS, Crijns HJ, Curtis AB, Ellenbogen KA, et al. 2011 ACCF/AHA/HRS focused updates incorporated into the ACC/AHA/ESC 2006 guidelines for the management of patients with atrial fibrillation: a report of the American College of Cardiology Foundation/American Heart Association task force on practice guidelines. *Circulation* 2011;123:e269-367.

Catheter ablation for atrial fibrillation

Steven A Lubitz, clinical cardiology fellow[1], Avi Fischer, assistant professor of medicine[1], Valentin Fuster, professor of medicine[1]

[1]Zena and Michael A Wiener Cardiovascular Institute, Marie-Josee and Henry R Kravis Center for Cardiovascular Health, Mount Sinai School of Medicine, Box 1030, New York, NY 10029, USA

Correspondence to: S A Lubitz steven.lubitz@mssm.edu

Cite this as: BMJ 2008;336:819-26

‹DOI› 10.1136/bmj.39513.555150.BE
http://www.bmj.com/content/336/7648/819

Atrial fibrillation is the most common arrhythmia in clinical practice and is associated with significant morbidity and mortality.[1] Catheter ablation is increasingly being used to treat atrial fibrillation, although it is not suitable for all patients.[2] Referring doctors must confront challenges such as the appropriate selection of patients for ablation and proper management of patients after the procedure, and must be familiar with the expected outcomes. Many unanswered questions exist surrounding the appropriate application of this technique.

This review summarises current ablative techniques and emphasises the appropriate application and limitations of catheter ablation on the basis of recent clinical trials and guidelines.

What is catheter ablation of atrial fibrillation?

After the transvenous insertion of catheters into the right atrium, the left atrium is accessed (in the absence of an atrial septal defect or patent foramen ovale) by trans-septal puncture. Catheter positioning, as well as the anatomy of the pulmonary veins and left atrium, are confirmed by fluoroscopy, pulmonary venography, three dimensional electroanatomical mapping, intracardiac echocardiography, computed tomography, remote guidance using magnetic resonance imaging, or combinations of these techniques. Through the application of thermal energy—most commonly by radiofrequency or cryothermy—injury is induced to the myocardium. Ablation can be done in atrial fibrillation or sinus rhythm.

SOURCES AND SELECTION CRITERIA

We searched all entries in PubMed through September 2007 with the medical subject headings "atrial fibrillation", "catheter ablation", and "anti-arrhythmia agents". We reviewed the reference lists of retrieved articles to identify any additional relevant articles for inclusion. Whenever available, we chose randomised controlled trials and meta-analyses over prospective cohort studies. When these were not available, we cited retrospective studies. We included other references if judged relevant for the purposes of discussion. Thus this work is not an exhaustive review but represents an overview of current clinical and technical aspects pertaining to catheter ablation of atrial fibrillation.

SUMMARY POINTS

- Atrial fibrillation is the most common arrhythmia in clinical practice
- Common triggers are ectopic pulmonary venous foci which conduct to the left atrium
- Catheter ablation techniques usually involve radiofrequency energy to electrically isolate the pulmonary veins from the left atrium
- Ablation may be more successful in patients with paroxysmal atrial fibrillation rather than persistent atrial fibrillation
- Atrial fibrillation ablation seems more successful than medical rhythm control therapy in carefully selected patients
- Ablation is indicated in patients requiring rhythm control and who have failed with at least one antiarrhythmic drug
- Long term data on the safety and efficacy of atrial fibrillation ablation are limited

How have catheter ablation techniques evolved?

The underlying factors contributing to atrial fibrillation are complex and multifactorial (fig 1). Current catheter ablation techniques target susceptible atrial substrate, electrical triggers, and autonomic tone, factors that are considered to be important for the initiation and maintenance of atrial fibrillation (box 1). Structural and electrical properties of the atria, such as fibrosis of the atrial myocardium, electromechanical remodelling, and genetic mutations affecting ion channels and gap junction proteins, are critical factors in the genesis of atrial fibrillation. Initial success with attempts to stop atrial fibrillation by creating linear incisions in the atria, as in the surgical Cox-Maze procedure, and replication of these lesions with radiofrequency catheter ablation, supported the concept of susceptible atrial substrate, although the contribution of pulmonary vein isolation was probably overlooked with these early techniques.

Ectopic pulmonary vein foci that communicate with the left atrium through muscular sleeves[3] (figs 2 and 3) were later discovered to trigger atrial fibrillation in most patients,[4] leading to targeted ablation within the pulmonary veins. As a result of pulmonary vein stenosis often associated with this procedure, techniques emerged that attempted to isolate the left atrium from the pulmonary veins. Predominant approaches included segmental ostial ablation at sites where pulmonary vein signals were detected,[5] and anatomically guided circumferential pulmonary vein ablation encircling individual or ipsilateral pairs of pulmonary veins (fig 4).[6]

Recently, ablation of ganglionated plexi innervating the pulmonary veins and left atrium has emerged with recognition that autonomic tone contributes to the genesis of atrial fibrillation.[7 8] Additionally, targeting complex fractionated electrograms—signals with rapid deflections and short cycle lengths corresponding to areas of wavebreak, vagal innervation, slow conduction, or re-entry—has become increasingly successful.[9 10]

The evolution of ablation techniques was illustrated in a survey of centres carrying out atrial fibrillation ablation worldwide between 1995 and 2002.[2] In 1995, isolation of pulmonary veins was not reported by any of the centres. Between 1998 and 1999, after elucidation of the role of pulmonary vein triggers in the genesis of atrial fibrillation,[4] selective ablation of triggers represented the preferred technique in about 46% of cases. By 2002, pulmonary vein isolation represented 80% of all atrial fibrillation ablation techniques. During the surveyed dates the frequency of the procedure grew from 18 procedures in 1995 to 5450 in 2002.

The multitude of ablation approaches is testimony to the multifactorial causes of atrial fibrillation. Despite the mechanistic rationale that justifies each specific ablative technique, approaches have overlapping effects. For example, during pulmonary vein isolation—the most widely used technique—ablation lines may encompass critical portions of the left atrium. Thus the technique may have

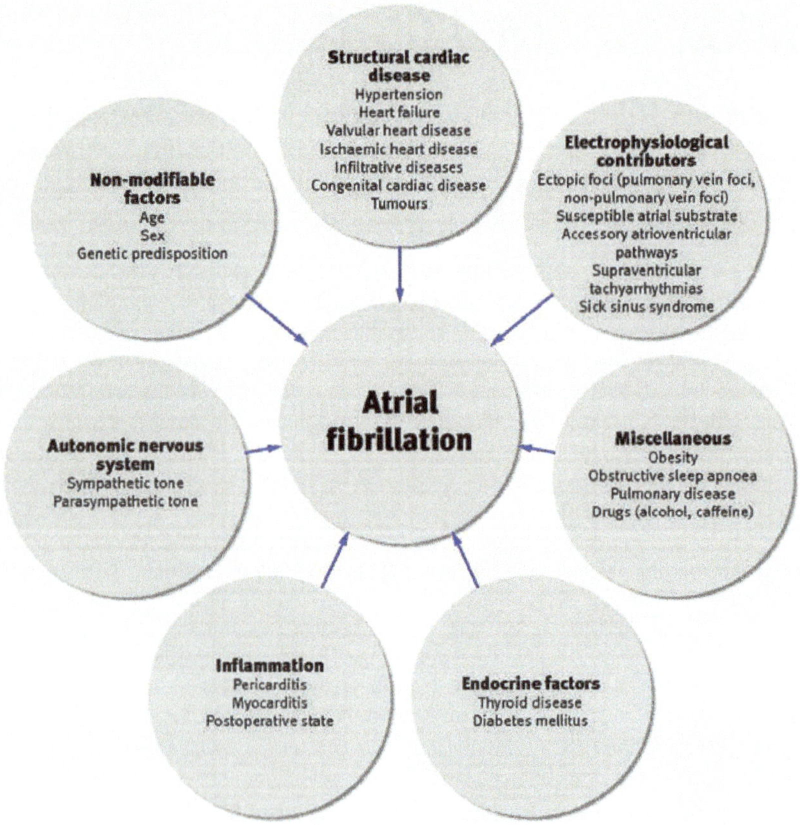

Fig 1 Factors contributing to development of atrial fibrillation. Clinical factors predisposing patients to atrial fibrillation are complex and may be inter-related. *These conditions may result in structural changes such as left atrial enlargement or stretch, myocardial hypertrophy, or left ventricular systolic dysfunction

BOX 1: TARGETS OF CURRENT ABLATION TECHNIQUES

- Electrical triggers (pulmonary vein foci, non-pulmonary vein foci, supraventricular tachyarrhythmias, accessory pathways)
- Susceptible atrial substrate (caused by, for example, fibrosis, hypertrophy, mutations of ion or gap junctions, electromechanical remodelling from previous atrial fibrillation*)
- Autonomic innervation

*Cellular electrical and structural remodelling occur as a result of previous atrial fibrillation, predisposing to subsequent episodes of atrial fibrillation

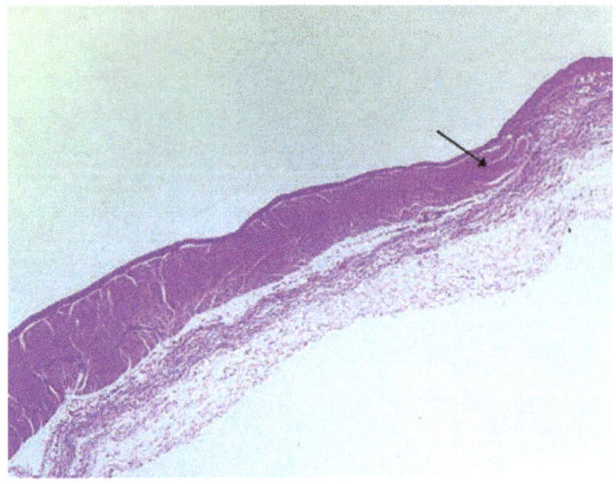

Fig 3 Muscular sleeves extending into pulmonary vein. Specimen from pulmonary vein showing muscular sleeves (arrowhead) extending from left atrium into pulmonary vein. Haematoxylin and eosin, ×2 magnification

substrate modification effects beyond the explicit intention of merely disrupting signal transmission from pulmonary veins to the left atrium.

How successful is ablation for atrial fibrillation?

The primary end point in most trials of ablation is recurrent atrial fibrillation or atrial arrhythmias in the absence of antiarrhythmic drugs, excluding early and often transient tachyarrhythmias that occur in up to half of patients within the first three months.[11 12 13] These are thought to result from recovered pulmonary vein conduction or proarrhythmic effects of ablation itself and are often treated with cardioversion, antiarrhythmic drugs, and repeat ablation.

Initial reports described success rates between 22% and 85%, with better results observed for patients with paroxysmal (self terminating and lasting less than seven days) rather than persistent (not self terminating) or permanent atrial fibrillation (terminating attempts failed or were not attempted). Randomised trials comparing pulmonary vein isolation in symptomatic patients, most with paroxysmal disease, reported success rates ranging from 31% to 88%, with no clearly superior strategy (table 1).[14 15 16 17 18] Long term results are limited by follow-up of generally no more than one year in most trials. Outcomes may have been influenced by the different patient

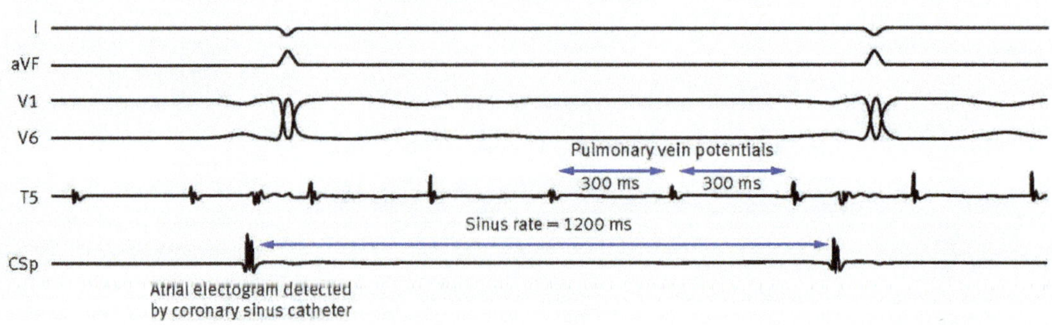

Fig 2 Intracardiac electrogram (recorded at a paper speed of 100 mm/s) from a patient with paroxysmal atrial fibrillation undergoing pulmonary vein isolation. Patient is in sinus rhythm at 50 bpm (cycle length=1200 ms), seen on surface electrograms (I, aVF, V1, V6). An intracardiac atrial electrogram is detected at the same cycle length by a catheter in the coronary sinus, preceding the surface electrogram deflection. A circular lasso catheter in the left upper pulmonary vein (T5) records pulmonary vein potentials occurring at a cycle length of 300 ms and dissociated from sinus activity. Other measurement points from lasso catheter were removed for simplicity

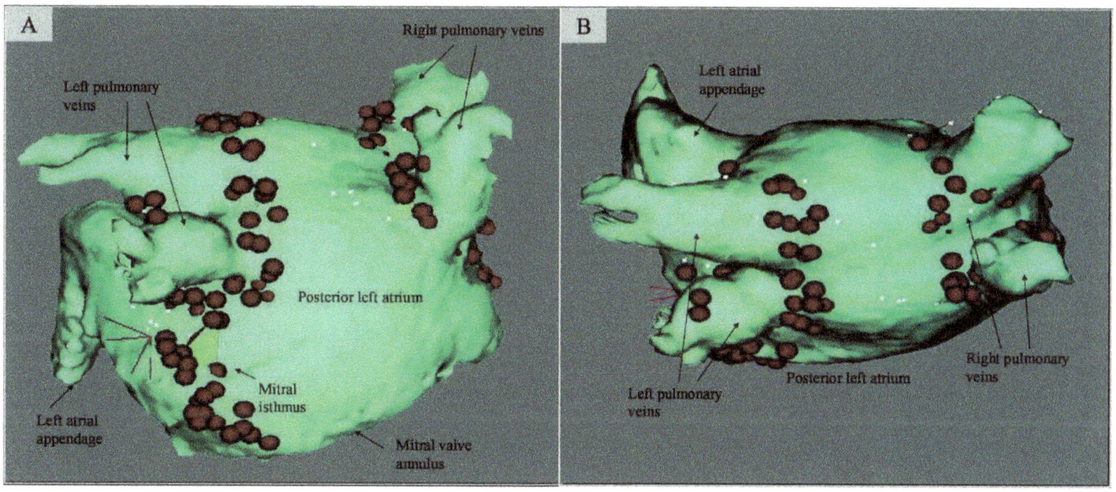

Fig 4 Electroanatomical map of left atrium in patient with persistent atrial fibrillation undergoing pulmonary vein isolation. Computed tomogram before ablation procedure is merged with three dimensional electroanatomical map of left atrium created during ablation. Left atrium is viewed from a posterior (panel A) and superior (panel B) orientation, with left atrium appendage on left. Dots represent sites of delivery of radiofrequency energy. Radiofrequency lesions encircle both left and right pulmonary veins, avoiding posterior wall of left atrium, and a line of radiofrequency ablation is seen along the mitral isthmus (region extending from left inferior pulmonary vein to mitral annulus)

populations studied, ablative techniques and end points utilised, and number of repeat ablations.

Moreover, substantially different methods for surveillance of rhythm were used, such as 12 lead electrocardiography, Holter monitoring, or event monitoring as prompted by symptoms. These methods have varying diagnostic accuracy for detecting occult arrhythmias. As few studies reported the incidence of recurrent asymptomatic atrial fibrillation after ablation, the benefits may have been overestimated. Available data show that asymptomatic recurrences occur in 2% to 16% of patients within the first year of the procedure (table 1),[15 16 18] although recurrences were prevalent in only 2% of patients with paroxysmal atrial fibrillation two years after ablation in one single centre analysis.[19]

A consensus statement by the Heart Rhythm Society, European Heart Rhythm Association, and European Cardiac Arrhythmia Society states that patients should be evaluated with electrocardiography within three months of ablation, every six months for the next two years, and assessed with event monitors if they have recurrent palpitations (box 2).[20] These are similar to recommendations made by the Venice Chart international consensus group.[22] The benefits of more extensive surveillance after ablation are unclear.

Which ablation technique is most efficacious?

Heterogeneity in the methods of published trials limits the ability to compare different techniques (table 1). A recent meta-analysis concluded that substrate ablation without pulmonary vein isolation was associated with no atrial fibrillation in 75% of patients at six months, whereas circumferential pulmonary vein isolation was successful in 67%.[23] Substrate ablation seems more

Table 1 Randomised controlled trials comparing efficacy of pulmonary vein isolation techniques (segmental ostial ablation versus circumferential pulmonary vein ablation) for prevention of recurrent atrial fibrillation

Study	No	Type of atrial fibrillation(%)	Additional substrate ablation	Rhythm monitoring*	Follow-up (months)	Freedom from recurrent atrial tachyarrhythmia (%)		Patients requiring repeat ablations for quoted success rate (%)		Overall frequency of asymptomatic atrial tachyarrhythmia after ablation	Overall frequency of major complications†
						CPVA	SOA	CPVA	SOA		
Oral et al 2003[14]	80	Paroxysmal (100)	CPVA group	Event monitoring if symptomatic	6	88	67	0	0	NR	0
Karch et al 2005[15]	100	Paroxysmal (89), persistent (11)	CPVA group	7 day Holter monitoring at 6 months	6	42	66	24	16	16	13
Nilsson et al 2006[16]	100	Paroxysmal (51), persistent (49)	None	14 day Holter monitoring at 3 months, event monitoring if symptomatic	12	57	31	74	74	2	4
Liu et al 2006[17]	110	Paroxysmal (100)	SOA group if inducible or residual atrial fibrillation	Periodic Holter monitoring	9	84	78	9	13	NR	7
Arentz et al 2007[18]	110	Paroxysmal (61), persistent (39)	None	Periodic Holter monitoring; further monitoring guided by symptoms	15	67	49	0	0	5	2

CPVA=circumferential pulmonary vein ablation; SOA=segmental ostial ablation; NR=not reported.

**Includes assessment at routine clinic appointments.*

†Includes death, cardiac tamponade, transient ischaemic attack or stroke, symptomatic or >50% pulmonary vein stenosis, atrio-oesophageal perforation, vascular complications, or phrenic nerve injury.

important with persistent or permanent atrial fibrillation than with paroxysmal disease, where isolation of triggers may suffice. None the less, a consensus statement by electrophysiological societies in the United States and Europe recognises that electrical pulmonary vein isolation forms the basis of most successful catheter ablations (box 2).[20] The ideal approach depends on individual patient characteristics and the chronicity of atrial fibrillation, and may require a combination of strategies (fig 5).

Is catheter ablation superior to medical therapy?

Although a strategy for rhythm control with antiarrhythmic drugs or electrical cardioversion offers no survival advantage over a rate control strategy, retrospective analyses of major trials show that maintenance of sinus rhythm may be associated with improved survival[24] and quality of life.[25] In the atrial fibrillation follow-up investigation of rhythm management (AFFIRM) trial, non-cardiovascular deaths in the rhythm control arm exceeded those in the rate control arm,[26] fuelling speculation that adverse effects of antiarrhythmic drugs may obscure the benefits of maintaining sinus rhythm and justifying the comparison of catheter ablation with medical therapy for achievement of sinus rhythm.

In a pilot trial of 70 patients with predominantly paroxysmal atrial fibrillation, pulmonary vein isolation was compared with antiarrhythmic drugs as first line therapy (table 2).[27] Freedom from symptomatic atrial fibrillation at one year after a single procedure was 87% compared with 37% for patients treated with antiarrhythmic drugs, most of whom received flecainide. In another study, pulmonary vein isolation in conjunction with antiarrhythmic drugs was compared with antiarrhythmic drugs alone in a group of 137 patients with mostly paroxysmal atrial fibrillation.[28] Freedom from atrial arrhythmias at one year was 56% in the ablation and antiarrhythmic drugs group and only 9% in the antiarrhythmic drugs alone group. More recently, pulmonary vein isolation was superior to a pharmacological strategy consisting of flecainide, sotalol, or amiodarone in a group of 198 patients with paroxysmal atrial fibrillation.[29] Daily transtelephonic monitoring and periodic Holter monitoring showed that freedom from atrial tachyarrhythmias at one year was 86% in the ablation group and 22% in the antiarrhythmic drug group.

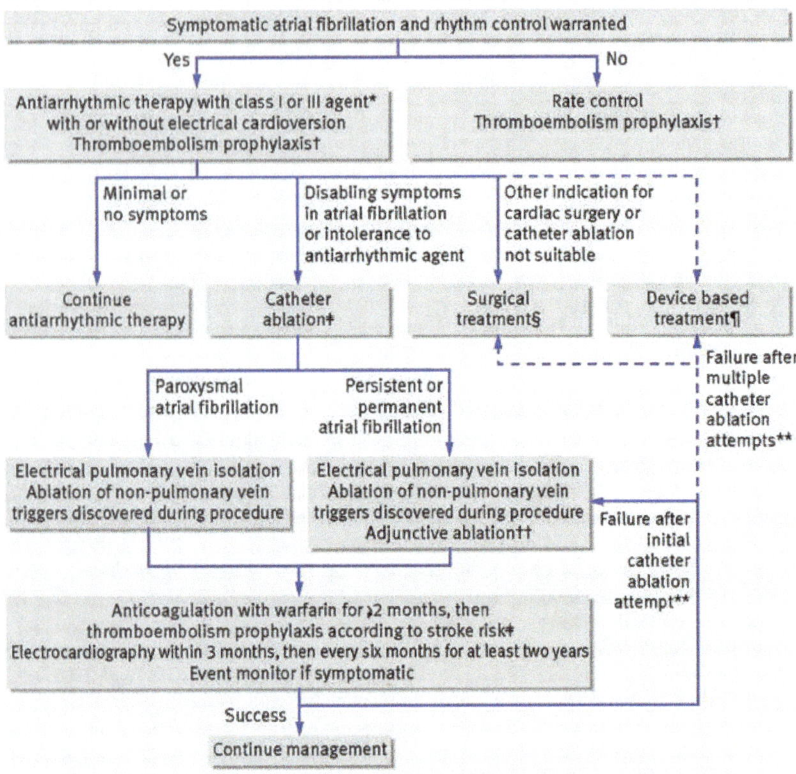

Fig 5 Proposed algorithm for management of symptomatic patients with atrial fibrillation referred for rhythm control. Solid lines represent established pathways supported by clinical evidence, guidelines, or expert consensus documents. Dashed lines represent less established pathways. *Appropriate antiarrhythmic drug therapy is outlined in practice guidelines.[1] †Underlying stroke risk can be assessed using the CHADS2 score[21]; one point each is assigned for a history of heart failure, hypertension, age >75, diabetes mellitus, and two points for previous cerebral ischaemia. Aspirin is generally recommended if the score is 0, aspirin or warfarin if the score is 1, and warfarin if the score is ≥2.[1] ‡First line therapy with catheter ablation may be appropriate for patients in whom long term antiarrhythmic drug therapy may be harmful or for those who want to avoid antiarrhythmic drugs. Presence of a left atrial thrombus is an absolute contraindication to catheter ablation. §Summary of surgical techniques for restoration of atrial fibrillation can be found in Heart Rhythm Society consensus document.[20] ¶Potential measures include permanent pacing or implantable atrial defibrillators for restoration of sinus rhythm.[1] **Repeat catheter ablations should generally be delayed until at least three months after the initial procedure. No consensus exists on what constitutes the maximum number for repeat attempts. ††Substrate ablation in form of linear ablation, or ablation of complex fractionated electrograms or sites of autonomic innervation. Adjunctive ablation may be appropriate in patients with paroxysmal atrial fibrillation in whom an initial attempt has been unsuccessful

BOX 2: SUMMARY OF A RECENT CONSENSUS STATEMENT ON CATHETER ABLATION OF ATRIAL FIBRILLATION*

Indications
- Symptomatic atrial fibrillation refractory or intolerant to at least one class I or III antiarrhythmic drug
- First line therapy for atrial fibrillation in rare clinical situations
- Selected symptomatic patients with heart failure or reduced ejection fraction

Contraindications
- Presence of a left atrial thrombus

Technique
- Electrical isolation of pulmonary veins is the cornerstone of most atrial fibrillation ablation procedures
- Non-pulmonary venous triggers should be ablated if discovered during the ablation procedure
- Ablation of the cavotricuspid isthmus is indicated in patients with typical or isthmus dependent atrial flutter

Thromboembolism prophylaxis after ablation
- Warfarin is recommended for at least two months after ablation
- Further thromboembolism prophylaxis should be based on a patient's underlying risk for stroke†

Minimal surveillance and monitoring after ablation
- Patients should be assessed with electrocardiography within three months of ablation, and then every six months for at least two years
- Patients with palpitations should be evaluated with an event monitor

Repeat procedures
- Owing to frequent and often transient early atrial tachyarrhythmias after ablation, repeat procedures should be delayed for at least three months, during which time antiarrhythmic drug therapy is appropriate for relief of symptoms
- *Adapted from an expert consensus statement by Heart Rhythm Society, European Heart Rhythm Association, and European Cardiac Arrhythmia Society[20]
- †Underlying risk can be assessed using the CHADS2 score[21]

The success of ablation improved to 93% when including second procedures. Two other randomised trials have reported results favouring ablation over medical therapy in patients with predominantly paroxysmal disease during one year of follow-up.[30 31] Catheter ablation specifically in persistent atrial fibrillation was addressed in a trial of 146 patients randomised to treatment with amiodarone and electrical cardioversion alone for up to three months, or in combination with pulmonary vein isolation.[32] Freedom from atrial fibrillation or atrial flutter one year after ablation was 74% in the absence of antiarrhythmic drugs, including repeat ablations in 32% of patients. In the intention to treat analysis, 58% of patients in the control arm were free of atrial fibrillation, although 77% crossed over to the ablation arm.

These trials also reported that ablation improves symptoms or quality of life,[27 30 31 32] enhances ejection fraction,[32] reduces left atrial size,[29 32] and decreases hospital admissions.[27 29] One non-randomised trial reported improved survival with ablation.[33]

Although traditional strategies for rhythm control do not seem to be cost effective when compared with rate control strategies for the management of atrial fibrillation,[34] a recent decision analysis comparing rate control, rhythm control with antiarrhythmic drugs, and catheter ablation in cohorts of patients aged 55 and 65 years, concluded that ablation is cost effective for patients at moderate risk of stroke but not at low risk.[35] A cost comparison of ablation and medical therapy using the Canadian Registry of Atrial Fibrillation showed that ablation was initially more expensive than medical therapy, although it was equivalent in cost about four years after ablation, justifying ablation as a "fiscally sensible alternative."[36] Ablation was associated with an initial cost ranging from $C16 278 (£8157; $10 661; €16 441) to $C21 294, with subsequent annual costs of $C1597 to $C2132, whereas costs for medical therapy ranged from $C4176 to $C5060 annually. Caution must be used in interpreting this analysis considering the lack of long-term follow up to support the durable effectiveness of ablation.

BOX 3: POTENTIAL MAJOR COMPLICATIONS OF CATHETER ABLATION OF ATRIAL FIBRILLATION

- Periprocedural death
- Cardiac tamponade
- Thromboembolism, including stroke or transient ischaemic attack
- Air embolism
- Atrio-oesophageal fistula
- Pulmonary vein stenosis
- Phrenic nerve injury
- Perioesophageal vagal nerve injury
- Vascular complications (haematoma, pseudoaneurysm, arteriovenous fistula, retroperitoneal bleeding)
- Acute coronary artery occlusion
- Mitral valve trauma

Table 2 Randomised controlled trials comparing efficacy of catheter ablation versus medical therapy for prevention of recurrent atrial fibrillation

Study	No	Single or multicentre trial	Pulmonary vein isolation technique	Primary control group therapy (%)	Type of atrial fibrillation (%)	Ablation as first line therapy?	Rhythm monitoring*	Follow-up (years)	Freedom from recurrent atrial tachyarrhythmia: Ablation	Freedom from recurrent atrial tachyarrhythmia: Medical	Overall frequency of major complications with ablation (%)†
Krittayaphong et al 2003[31]	30	Single	SOA	Amiodarone (100)	Paroxysmal (70), persistent (30)	No	Periodic Holter monitoring	1	79	40	7
Wazni et al 2005[27]sA	70	Multicentre	SOA	Flecainide (77), sotalol (23)	Paroxysmal (96), persistent (4)	Yes	Daily brief event monitoring during first and third months, and periodic Holter monitoring	1	87	37	3
Oral et al 2006[32]	146	Multicentre	CPVA	Amiodarone and up to two electrical cardioversions within three months of randomisation	Persistent or permanent (100)	No	Daily brief event monitoring	1	74	58	0
Stabile et al 2006[28]‡	137	Multicentre	CPVA	Amiodarone (62), flecainide (26), propafenone (10), disopyramide (2), sotalol (6)§	Paroxysmal (67), persistent (33)	No	Daily brief event monitoring during first three months, and periodic Holter monitoring	1	56	9	4
Pappone et al 2006[29]	198	Single	CPVA	Amiodarone (33), flecainide (33), sotalol (33)§	Paroxysmal (100)	No	Daily brief event monitoring, and periodic Holter monitoring	1	86	22	1
Jais et al 2006[30]	112	Multicentre	SOA	§¶	Paroxysmal (100)	No	Periodic Holter monitoring	1	75	6	4

CPVA=circumferential pulmonary vein ablation; SOA=segmental ostial ablation.

**Includes assessment at routine clinic appointments.*

†Includes death, cardiac tamponade, transient ischaemic attack or stroke, symptomatic or >50% pulmonary vein stenosis, atrio-oesophageal perforation, vascular complications, or phrenic nerve injury.

‡According to study protocol, patients treated with catheter ablation also received antiarrhythmic drug therapy.

§Various combinations of antiarrhythmic drugs were used.

¶Not specified but 88 class I, 39 class II, 59 class III, and 6 class IV agents were used.

ONGOING RESEARCH

- The catheter ablation versus antiarrhythmic drug therapy for atrial fibrillation (CABANA) trial will assess survival outcomes among patients treated with ablation compared with those treated with pharmacological rhythm or rate control
- The multicenter radiofrequency ablation versus antiarrhythmic drugs for atrial fibrillation treatment (RAAFT) trial will compare catheter ablation as first line therapy against antiarrhythmic drugs
- The catheter ablation for the cure of atrial fibrillation (CACAF-2) study will compare the efficacy of catheter ablation with combined right and left atrial lesions against antiarrhythmic drugs in patients with persistent atrial fibrillation refractory to at least one antiarrhythmic drug

ADDITIONAL EDUCATIONAL RESOURCES

- American College of Cardiology (www.acc.org)—2006 guidelines for the management of patients with atrial fibrillation from the American College of Cardiology, the American Heart Association, and the European Society of Cardiology
- Heart Rhythm Society (www.hrsonline.org)—Expert consensus statement on catheter and surgical ablation of atrial fibrillation from the Heart Rhythm Society, European Heart Rhythm Association, and European Cardiac Arrhythmia Society
- Natale A, Raviele A, Arentz T, Calkins H, Chen SA, Haissaguerre M, et al. Venice Chart international consensus document on atrial fibrillation ablation. *J Cardiovasc Electrophysiol* 2007;18:560-80.

Information for patients

- MedlinePlus (www.nlm.nih.gov/medlineplus/healthtopics.html)—Online patient information resource from the United States National Library of Medicine and National Institutes of Health
- American Heart Association (www.americanheart.org/) and Heart Rhythm Society (www.hrsonline.org)—Both contain resources for patients

TIPS FOR NON-SPECIALISTS

- Patients should be considered for referral for atrial fibrillation ablation when rhythm control therapy is indicated and attempts with at least one antiarrhythmic drug have failed
- A substantial proportion of patients may require repeat ablations owing to recurrences of atrial fibrillation or left atrial tachyarrhythmias resulting from the procedure itself
- Guidelines recommend anticoagulation with warfarin for at least two months after ablation, but the optimal strategy for thromboembolism prophylaxis has not been tested
- Guidelines advocate electrocardiography within three months after ablation, and every six months thereafter, although the merits of more rigorous surveillance remain untested

In summary, evidence from several small trials suggests that isolation of the pulmonary vein is more efficacious than medical rhythm control therapy in select patients with highly symptomatic, drug refractory atrial fibrillation, although long term outcomes remain unclear.

Is catheter ablation safe?

The most undesirable complications of ablation are atrio-oesophageal fistulae, pulmonary vein stenosis, cardiac tamponade, stroke, and phrenic nerve injury (box 3 and tables 1 and 2). In a randomised trial comparing pulmonary vein isolation techniques, the incidence of pulmonary vein stenosis was 9%, and cerebrovascular events occurred in up to 6% of patients.[15] In a worldwide survey of more than 7000 patients, major complications were reported in 6%.[2] These included periprocedural death (0.05%), cardiac tamponade (1.2%), stroke or transient ischaemic attack (0.9%), and pulmonary vein stenosis (1.6%). Although lower complication rates reported in many controlled trials are reassuring, procedures done outside of clinical trials and by less experienced operators might result in more adverse effects.

Is thromboembolism prophylaxis necessary after ablation?

In most trials of ablation, anticoagulation was stopped after three to six months in the absence of recurrent atrial fibrillation without any significant incidence of thromboembolism during follow-up. The baseline risk for stroke as measured by validated tools such as the CHADS2 index,[21] was not, however, reported. In a retrospective analysis of 755 patients, 65% of whom had paroxysmal atrial fibrillation, the incidence of thromboembolism was 0.9% within the two weeks after ablation, and 0.2% between six and 10 months afterwards.[37] None of the patients in whom anticoagulation was discontinued had a stroke, including about half of whom had at least one risk factor.

Recent guidelines call for mandatory warfarin therapy for at least two months after ablation (box 2),[20] although clinical trials have not specifically assessed the optimal antithrombotic strategy. Until further data confirm the reduced stroke risk and ensure the absence of recurrent atrial fibrillation in a large and heterogeneous population, patients should continue to receive thromboembolism prophylaxis on the basis of their initial stroke risk in accordance with published guidelines.[1, 20]

Who should be referred for catheter ablation?

The presence of a left atrial thrombus is an absolute contraindication to ablation,[20] whereas the inability to anticoagulate represents a relative contraindication. To date, participants enrolled in trials of atrial fibrillation ablation overwhelmingly had highly symptomatic, drug refractory, paroxysmal disease. Most were aged less than 65, had ejection fractions greater than 50%, and did not have markedly enlarged atria. The prevalence of structural heart disease was variable, occasionally constituting more than half of the participants. The duration of atrial fibrillation was generally between three and seven years. Only one randomised controlled trial has compared ablation as first line therapy with medical therapy, although the results were favourable.[27] Similarly, one non-randomised prospective controlled trial assessed ablation in patients with congestive heart failure.[38] The study showed achievement of sinus rhythm in 78% of patients after about one year, with repeat ablations required in half of the patients, and reported improvements in functional status, symptoms, and ejection fraction with ablation. Recommendations for ablation reflect trial characteristics (box 2).[20 22]

Conclusion

Rhythm control of atrial fibrillation is receiving a resurgence of attention with the recognition that catheter ablation may offer benefits not achieved with pharmacological therapy. At present, patients considering ablation must be willing to undergo a prolonged procedure with associated risks, and a significant likelihood of recurrent disease that may necessitate a repeat ablation. As the understanding of mechanisms of atrial fibrillation evolves, catheter ablation techniques will follow suit. Large scale controlled trials assessing ablation in diverse patient populations are necessary for more precise clinical guidelines for its application.

We thank Marc A Miller for his critical review of the manuscript. Figure 3 is courtesy of John Fallon.

Contributors: All authors planned and contributed to the writing of the manuscript. SAL is guarantor.

Competing interests: AF consults for and has received honorariums from Medtronic and receives research support from St Jude Medical.

Provenance and peer review: Not commissioned; externally peer reviewed.

1 Fuster V, Ryden LE, Cannom DS, Crijns HJ, Curtis AB, Ellenbogen KA, et al. ACC/AHA/ESC 2006 guidelines for the management of patients with atrial fibrillation: a report of the American College of Cardiology/American Heart Association Task Force on Practice Guidelines and the European Society of Cardiology Committee for Practice Guidelines

(Writing Committee to revise the 2001 Guidelines for the Management of Patients With Atrial Fibrillation): developed in collaboration with the European Heart Rhythm Association and the Heart Rhythm Society. *Circulation* 2006;114:e257-354.

2 Cappato R, Calkins H, Chen SA, Davies W, Iesaka Y, Kalman J, et al. Worldwide survey on the methods, efficacy, and safety of catheter ablation for human atrial fibrillation. *Circulation* 2005;111:1100-5.

3 Nathan H, Eliakim M. The junction between the left atrium and the pulmonary veins. An anatomic study of human hearts. *Circulation* 1966;34:412-22.

4 Haissaguerre M, Jais P, Shah DC, Takahashi A, Hocini M, Quiniou G, et al. Spontaneous initiation of atrial fibrillation by ectopic beats originating in the pulmonary veins. *N Engl J Med* 1998;339:659-66.

5 Haissaguerre M, Shah DC, Jais P, Hocini M, Yamane T, Deisenhofer I, et al. Electrophysiological breakthroughs from the left atrium to the pulmonary veins. *Circulation* 2000;102:2463-5.

6 Pappone C, Rosanio S, Oreto G, Tocchi M, Gugliotta F, Vicedomini G, et al. Circumferential radiofrequency ablation of pulmonary vein ostia: a new anatomic approach for curing atrial fibrillation. *Circulation* 2000;102:2619-28.

7 Chen YJ, Chen SA, Tai CT, Wen ZC, Feng AN, Ding YA, et al. Role of atrial electrophysiology and autonomic nervous system in patients with supraventricular tachycardia and paroxysmal atrial fibrillation. *J Am Coll Cardiol* 1998;32:732-8.

8 Pappone C, Santinelli V, Manguso F, Vicedomini G, Gugliotta F, Augello G, et al. Pulmonary vein denervation enhances long-term benefit after circumferential ablation for paroxysmal atrial fibrillation. *Circulation* 2004;109:327-34.

9 Nademanee K, McKenzie J, Kosar E, Schwab M, Sunsaneewitayakul B, Vasavakul T, et al. A new approach for catheter ablation of atrial fibrillation: mapping of the electrophysiologic substrate. *J Am Coll Cardiol* 2004;43:2044-53.

10 Oral H, Chugh A, Good E, Sankaran S, Reich SS, Igic P, et al. A tailored approach to catheter ablation of paroxysmal atrial fibrillation. *Circulation* 2006;113:1824-31.

11 Oral H, Knight BP, Ozaydin M, Tada H, Chugh A, Hassan S, et al. Clinical significance of early recurrences of atrial fibrillation after pulmonary vein isolation. *J Am Coll Cardiol* 2002;40:100-4.

12 Bertaglia E, Stabile G, Senatore G, Zoppo F, Turco P, Amellone C, et al. Predictive value of early atrial tachyarrhythmias recurrence after circumferential anatomical pulmonary vein ablation. *Pacing Clin Electrophysiol* 2005;28:366-71.

13 Ouyang F, Antz M, Ernst S, Hachiya H, Mavrakis H, Deger FT, et al. Recovered pulmonary vein conduction as a dominant factor for recurrent atrial tachyarrhythmias after complete circular isolation of the pulmonary veins: lessons from double Lasso technique. *Circulation* 2005;111:127-35.

14 Oral H, Scharf C, Chugh A, Hall B, Cheung P, Good E, et al. Catheter ablation for paroxysmal atrial fibrillation: segmental pulmonary vein ostial ablation versus left atrial ablation. *Circulation* 2003;108:2355-60.

15 Karch MR, Zrenner B, Deisenhofer I, Schreieck J, Ndrepepa G, Dong J, et al. Freedom from atrial tachyarrhythmias after catheter ablation of atrial fibrillation: a randomized comparison between 2 current ablation strategies. *Circulation* 2005;111:2875-80.

16 Nilsson B, Chen X, Pehrson S, Kober L, Hilden J, Svendsen JH. Recurrence of pulmonary vein conduction and atrial fibrillation after pulmonary vein isolation for atrial fibrillation: a randomized trial of the ostial versus the extraostial ablation strategy. *Am Heart J* 2006;152:537 e1-8.

17 Liu X, Long D, Dong J, Hu F, Yu R, Tang R, et al. Is circumferential pulmonary vein isolation preferable to stepwise segmental pulmonary vein isolation for patients with paroxysmal atrial fibrillation? *Circ J* 2006;70:1392-7.

18 Arentz T, Weber R, Burkle G, Herrera C, Blum T, Stockinger J, et al. Small or large isolation areas around the pulmonary veins for the treatment of atrial fibrillation? Results from a prospective randomized study. *Circulation* 2007;115:3057-63.

19 Oral H, Veerareddy S, Good E, Hall B, Cheung P, Tamirisa K, et al. Prevalence of asymptomatic recurrences of atrial fibrillation after successful radiofrequency catheter ablation. *J Cardiovasc Electrophysiol* 2004;15:920-4.

20 Calkins H, Brugada J, Packer DL, Cappato R, Chen S, Crijns HJ, et al. HRS/EHRA/ECAS Expert consensus statement on catheter and surgical ablation of atrial fibrillation: recommendations for personnel, policy, procedures and follow-up. A report of the Heart Rhythm Society (HRS) Task Force on catheter and surgical ablation of atrial fibrillation. *Heart Rhythm* 2007;4:816-61.

21 Gage BF, Waterman AD, Shannon W, Boechler M, Rich MW, Radford MJ. Validation of clinical classification schemes for predicting stroke: results from the National Registry of Atrial Fibrillation. *JAMA* 2001;285:2864-70.

22 Natale A, Raviele A, Arentz T, Calkins H, Chen SA, Haissaguerre M, et al. Venice Chart international consensus document on atrial fibrillation ablation. *J Cardiovasc Electrophysiol* 2007;18:560-80.

23 Fisher JD, Spinelli MA, Mookherjee D, Krumerman AK, Palma EC. Atrial fibrillation ablation: reaching the mainstream. *Pacing Clin Electrophysiol* 2006;29:523-37.

24 Corley SD, Epstein AE, DiMarco JP, Domanski MJ, Geller N, Greene HL, et al. Relationships between sinus rhythm, treatment, and survival in the atrial fibrillation follow-up investigation of rhythm management (AFFIRM) study. *Circulation* 2004;109:1509-13.

25 Hagens VE, Ranchor AV, Van Sonderen E, Bosker HA, Kamp O, Tijssen JG, et al. Effect of rate or rhythm control on quality of life in persistent atrial fibrillation. Results from the rate control versus electrical cardioversion (RACE) study. *J Am Coll Cardiol* 2004;43:241-7.

26 Steinberg JS, Sadaniantz A, Kron J, Krahn A, Denny DM, Daubert J, et al. Analysis of cause-specific mortality in the atrial fibrillation follow-up investigation of rhythm management (AFFIRM) study. *Circulation* 2004;109:1973-80.

27 Wazni OM, Marrouche NF, Martin DO, Verma A, Bhargava M, Saliba W, et al. Radiofrequency ablation vs antiarrhythmic drugs as first-line treatment of symptomatic atrial fibrillation: a randomized trial. *JAMA* 2005;293:2634-40.

28 Stabile G, Bertaglia E, Senatore G, De Simone A, Zoppo F, Donnici G, et al. Catheter ablation treatment in patients with drug-refractory atrial fibrillation: a prospective, multi-centre, randomized, controlled study (catheter ablation for the cure of atrial fibrillation study). *Eur Heart J* 2006;27:216-21.

29 Pappone C, Augello G, Sala S, Gugliotta F, Vicedomini G, Gulletta S, et al. A randomized trial of circumferential pulmonary vein ablation versus antiarrhythmic drug therapy in paroxysmal atrial fibrillation: the APAF study. *J Am Coll Cardiol* 2006;48:2340-7.

30 Jais P, Cauchemez B, Macle L, Daoud E, Waldo AL, Ruskin JN, et al. Atrial fibrillation ablation vs antiarrhythmic drugs: a multicenter randomized trial. *Heart Rhythm* 2006;3:1126.

31 Krittayaphong R, Raungrattanaamporn O, Bhuripanyo K, Sriratanasathavorn C, Pooranawattanakul S, Punlee K, et al. A randomized clinical trial of the efficacy of radiofrequency catheter ablation and amiodarone in the treatment of symptomatic atrial fibrillation. *J Med Assoc Thai* 2003;86(suppl 1):S8-16.

32 Oral H, Pappone C, Chugh A, Good E, Bogun F, Pelosi F Jr, et al. Circumferential pulmonary-vein ablation for chronic atrial fibrillation. *N Engl J Med* 2006;354:934-41.

33 Pappone C, Rosanio S, Augello G, Gallus G, Vicedomini G, Mazzone P, et al. Mortality, morbidity, and quality of life after circumferential pulmonary vein ablation for atrial fibrillation: outcomes from a controlled nonrandomized long-term study. *J Am Coll Cardiol* 2003;42:185-97.

34 Marshall DA, Levy AR, Vidaillet H, Fenwick E, Slee A, Blackhouse G, et al. Cost-effectiveness of rhythm versus rate control in atrial fibrillation. *Ann Intern Med* 2004;141:653-61.

35 Chan PS, Vijan S, Morady F, Oral H. Cost-effectiveness of radiofrequency catheter ablation for atrial fibrillation. *J Am Coll Cardiol* 2006;47:2513-20.

36 Khaykin Y, Morillo CA, Skanes AC, McCracken A, Humphries K, Kerr CR. Cost comparison of catheter ablation and medical therapy in atrial fibrillation. *J Cardiovasc Electrophysiol* 2007;18:907-13.

37 Oral H, Chugh A, Ozaydin M, Good E, Fortino J, Sankaran S, et al. Risk of thromboembolic events after percutaneous left atrial radiofrequency ablation of atrial fibrillation. *Circulation* 2006;114:759-65.

38 Hsu LF, Jais P, Sanders P, Garrigue S, Hocini M, Sacher F, et al. Catheter ablation for atrial fibrillation in congestive heart failure. *N Engl J Med* 2004;351:2373-83.

BMJ BPP UNIVERSITY SCHOOL OF HEALTH

Clopidogrel in acute coronary syndromes

Doson Chua, clinical pharmacotherapeutic specialist, Andrew Ignaszewski, head, division of cardiology

[1]St Paul's Hospital, Department of Pharmacy, Vancouver, BC V6Z 1Y6, Canada

Correspondence to: D Chua dchua@providencehealth.bc.ca

Cite this as: *BMJ* 2009;338:b1180

‹DOI› 10.1136/bmj.b1180
http://www.bmj.com/content/338/bmj.b1180

Clopidogrel is well established in the treatment of acute coronary syndromes and is ubiquitous in cardiology practice. Landmark studies have established the importance of clopidogrel in the treatment of non-ST and ST elevation myocardial infarction and in percutaneous coronary intervention by reducing death, reinfarction, and adverse cardiac events. Knowledge of the benefits, risks, and duration of clopidogrel treatment is important for clinicians caring for patients presenting with and recovering from acute coronary syndromes. This review examines the recent key trials of clopidogrel in the treatment of acute coronary syndromes, as well as current cardiac guidelines from several professional societies.

What is clopidogrel and how does it reduce cardiac ischaemia?

Clopidogrel is a thienopyridine platelet antagonist that requires hepatic activation to form the active molecule. It selectively and irreversibly inhibits the binding of adenosine diphosphate to platelet receptors. Platelet activation plays a crucial role in the pathophysiology of arterial thrombosis and subsequent cardiac ischaemia.[1 2] Inhibition of adenosine diphosphate receptor binding deactivates the platelet glycoprotein IIb-IIIa complex, thereby inhibiting platelet aggregation.[3] Clopidogrel is often given together with aspirin because they work synergistically as platelet antagonists by inhibiting different receptor mediated pathways that ultimately lead to platelet activation. Daily aspirin is indicated for patients who have already had or are at high risk for a cardiovascular event.

SOURCES AND SELECTION CRITERIA

We reviewed the most recent guidelines from the American College of Cardiology, National Institute for Health and Clinical Excellence, European Society of Cardiology, and American College of Chest Physicians on the use of clopidogrel in myocardial infarction. The landmark trials discussed in the above guidelines were retrieved for further review. We also searched for subsequent publications in this area by the key authors of the landmark trials. We searched Medline, Cochrane Library, and Embase using the terms "clopidogrel", "thienopyridine", "myocardial infarction", "acute coronary syndrome", "percutaneous coronary intervention", "coronary stent", and "coronary artery disease" for any additional landmark studies, reviews, or meta-analysis on the use of clopidogrel in myocardial infarction.

SUMMARY POINTS

- All patients presenting with acute coronary syndromes should be given a 300 mg loading dose of clopidogrel, then 75 mg daily
- Patients not undergoing percutaneous coronary intervention should receive clopidogrel for nine to 12 months for non-ST elevation myocardial infarction and 14 days for ST elevation myocardial infarction
- Patients given a bare metal stent should receive clopidogrel, in addition to aspirin, for at least one month and ideally for one year
- Patients given a drug eluting stent should receive clopidogrel, in addition to aspirin, for at least one year
- The duration of clopidogrel treatment must take into account the patient's risk of bleeding

Who should be treated with clopidogrel?

Patients with non-ST elevation myocardial infarction

The CURE randomised trial established the role of clopidogrel in the treatment of patients with non-ST elevation myocardial infarction.[4] In the trial, 12 562 patients with unstable angina or non-ST elevation myocardial infarction, who were largely medically managed, received aspirin and were randomly assigned to clopidogrel (300 mg loading dose, followed by 75 mg daily) or placebo. The absolute risk reduction in the composite end point of cardiovascular death, non-fatal myocardial infarction, and stroke for those who took both aspirin and clopidogrel was 2.1% ($P<0.001$; relative risk 0.8, 95% confidence interval 0.72 to 0.9). This benefit of clopidogrel was also seen in patients who received subsequent coronary artery bypass surgery or percutaneous coronary intervention. Despite a 1% absolute increase in major bleeding with dual aspirin and clopidogrel treatment, such treatment has become standard clinical practice in the management of non-ST elevation myocardial infarction. The latest guidance from the American College of Cardiology, American College of Chest Physicians, and European Society of Cardiology on non-ST elevation myocardial infarction strongly recommends the use of clopidogrel (level I A recommendation; see box).[5 6 7]

Patients with ST elevation myocardial infarction

Two landmark trials established the role of clopidogrel in the treatment of patients with ST elevation myocardial infarction. CLARITY randomised 3491 patients who presented with ST elevation myocardial infarction within 12 hours of the onset of chest pain to receive a 300 mg clopidogrel loading dose, followed by 75 mg daily, or matching placebo for 30 days.[8] All patients received aspirin, heparin, and fibrinolytics and then proceeded to coronary angiography. The primary composite end point (death, myocardial infarction, and infarct related occluded artery flow) was lower in the clopidogrel arm than in the placebo arm, with no difference in bleeding between the two groups.

Subsequently, the COMMIT randomised trial enrolled 45 852 patients who presented with ST elevation myocardial

CLASSIFICATION OF RECOMMENDATIONS AND LEVELS OF EVIDENCE

Recommendations

- Level I: Evidence and agreement that treatment is beneficial
- Level II: Conflicting evidence and divergence of opinion regarding benefits of treatment
- Level III: Evidence and agreement that treatment is not beneficial, and may cause harm

Evidence

- Level A evidence: Data derived from multiple randomised clinical trials or meta-analyses
- Level B evidence: Data derived from a single randomised trial or non-randomised studies
- Level C evidence: Consensus opinion or experts, case studies, or standard of care

infarction within 24 hours of onset of ischaemic pain but did not undergo percutaneous coronary intervention.[9] Patients were randomised to clopidogrel 75 mg daily or matching placebo for four weeks or until hospital discharge. All patients received aspirin, and fibrinolytic agents were used if clinically appropriate. The clopidogrel group had a 0.9% absolute risk reduction in the composite end point of death, reinfarction, and stroke (P=0.002; odds ratio 0.91, 0.86 to 0.97) and a 0.6% reduction in absolute risk of death (P=0.03; 0.93, 0.87 to 0.99) compared with the placebo group at 28 days. Subgroup analysis of COMMIT showed that the effects of clopidogrel were consistent across a wide range of patients and independent of other drugs used. No excess major bleeding or cerebral haemorrhage was seen in the clopidogrel group.

The findings of the CLARITY and COMMIT trials have led to clopidogrel becoming standard treatment for ST elevation myocardial infarction. Guidelines from the American College of Cardiology strongly recommend the use of clopidogrel in addition to aspirin for the management of ST elevation myocardial infarction (level I A recommendation).[10] A loading dose of clopidogrel 300 mg is encouraged in patients under 75 years, although this recommendation is based on expert opinion alone.

Patients undergoing percutaneous coronary intervention with coronary stenting

The CLASSICS trial established the role of clopidogrel after percutaneous coronary intervention by showing that clopidogrel was equivalent to ticlodipine in reducing adverse cardiac events after coronary stenting but had a better safety and tolerability profile.[11 12]

The PCI-CURE study, a subgroup analysis of the CURE trial, further established the role of clopidogrel after coronary stenting.[13] In this trial, 2658 patients with non-ST elevation myocardial infarction who subsequently underwent percutaneous coronary intervention with stenting were randomised to a 300 mg loading dose of clopidogrel, followed by 75 mg daily clopidogrel or matching placebo. All patients received aspirin. The use of clopidogrel reduced the composite end point (death from cardiac disease, myocardial infarction, and target vessel revascularisation at 30 days) compared with the placebo group. The role of clopidogrel in reducing adverse cardiac events after coronary stenting is established, and treatment with clopidogrel has become standard clinical practice.

For how long should treatment with clopidogrel continue?

After acute coronary syndromes

The ideal duration of clopidogrel treatment for non-ST elevation myocardial infarction is unclear, although the average length of treatment in the CURE trial was nine months. The latest American College of Cardiology and American College of Chest Physicians guidelines for ST elevation myocardial infarction recommend a 14 day course of clopidogrel treatment (level I B recommendation) on the basis of the average duration of treatment in the COMMIT trial.[10 14] These guidelines also suggest that up to one year of clopidogrel may be beneficial in ST elevation myocardial infarction, although this is based on extrapolation from other clopidogrel studies in coronary artery disease and expert opinion (level II C recommendation).

CHARISMA, a trial that randomised 15603 patients with multiple cardiac risk factors and clinically evident cardiovascular disease to either clopidogrel 75 mg daily or placebo plus background aspirin for two years, showed that prolonged treatment with clopidogrel did not reduce cardiac adverse events.[15] This trial enrolled a heterogeneous group of patients with cardiac disease, so it is difficult to know whether patients with documented coronary artery disease would benefit from long term dual antiplatelet therapy with aspirin and clopidogrel. Routine prolonged treatment with clopidogrel beyond current recommendations is not warranted at this time.

After coronary stenting

The optimal duration of clopidogrel after coronary stenting was still unclear at the end of the PCI-CURE study, which looked at the use of clopidogrel only up to 30 days after stenting. The CREDO trial randomised 2116 patients who underwent percutaneous coronary intervention with stenting to a 300 mg loading dose of clopidogrel, followed by 75 mg daily for 12 months or a placebo loading dose, followed by clopidogrel 75 mg daily for 28 days.[16] The composite end point of death, myocardial infarction, and stroke at 12 months was lower in the 12 month clopidogrel arm than in the 28 day clopidogrel arm. This showed that a longer rather than shorter course of treatment with clopidogrel is best after coronary stenting. Major bleeding at 12 months was not significantly different between the 12 month and 28 day clopidogrel groups. On the basis of PCI-CURE and CREDO, the most recent guidance from the American College of Cardiology, European Society of Cardiology, and American College of Chest Physicians on percutaneous coronary intervention strongly recommends clopidogrel for at least one month after bare metal stent insertion (level I A recommendation), with an ideal duration of one year (level I B recommendation).[17 18 19]

After drug eluting coronary stent placement

A longer duration of dual antiplatelet treatment with aspirin and clopidogrel is needed after placement of a drug eluting stent than a bare metal stent. Previous percutaneous coronary intervention guidelines recommended six to 12 months of such treatment, largely on the basis of randomised clinical trials of drug eluting stent studies and registry data.[20] Concerns have recently emerged about late stent thrombosis and subsequent adverse cardiac events with drug eluting stents. Several small observational studies and registry data suggest that mortality and the incidence of myocardial infarction may be higher with drug eluting stents than with bare metal stents, probably because of the greater chance of late stent thrombosis with drug eluting stents.[21 22] Observational studies and analysis of registry data show that premature discontinuation of clopidogrel is the biggest risk factor for late stent thrombosis.[22 23] The possibility of higher cardiac event rates associated with drug eluting stents has sparked much concern and debate.[24]

Because of these concerns, the American College of Cardiology has recommended that patients receive at least one year of dual antiplatelet treatment with aspirin and clopidogrel after implantation of any drug eluting stent. These recommendations are based largely on observational data and expert opinion (level I B recommendation).[22] The use of dual antiplatelet treatment is crucial and patients should be told about the importance of adhering to treatment with clopidogrel before implantation of a drug eluting stent.

The optimal treatment beyond one year is unknown, but studies to determine the optimal duration of clopidogrel after placement of a drug eluting stent are under way. Patients who are allergic to aspirin should take clopidogrel indefinitely.

What about bleeding?

Concerns about the risk of bleeding when using clopidogrel in addition to a fibrinolytic and aspirin still remain. Clopidogrel monotherapy has a similar risk of bleeding to that of aspirin monotherapy. Prolonged dual antiplatelet treatment carries a risk of increased bleeding. The CURE and CHARISMA trials showed around a 1% absolute increase in moderate to major bleeding with combined aspirin and clopidogrel versus aspirin alone. No increase in intracranial haemorrhage was seen with combined aspirin and clopidogrel treatment compared with aspirin alone in all the landmark trials. Dual antiplatelet treatment caused bleeding mostly in the gut. The risk is higher with increasing age, concurrent use of anticoagulant and anti-inflammatory drugs, a history of gastrointestinal bleeding, and other risk factors for bleeding.

An ongoing dilemma is the use of aspirin and clopidogrel in patients who also need warfarin. The addition of warfarin puts patients at further risk of significant bleeding. Little literature is available to guide clinicians, although expert consensus opinion recommends reducing the dose of aspirin (to 75-80 mg daily), targeting a lower international normalised ratio, and minimising the duration of dual antiplatelet treatment in these patients.[17] Temporary discontinuation of warfarin or use of one antiplatelet agent only may be considered if the risk of bleeding is deemed to exceed the benefits of treatment. Gastrointestinal prophylactic treatment should be initiated in all patients at high risk for gastrointestinal bleeding who are on dual antiplatelet treatment. These risks should be considered before placement of drug eluting stents and when determining the duration of treatment for individual patients.

RESEARCH QUESTIONS

Ongoing research

- The OASIS 7 trial is investigating the benefits of a 600 mg loading dose of clopidogrel, followed by 150 mg daily for one week, then 75 mg daily compared with the current standard of a 300 mg loading dose and 75 mg daily
- The DAPT trial is investigating the optimal duration of clopidogrel after placement of a drug eluting stent
- Other thienopyridine agents are in development

Questions for future research

- What advantages do newer thienopyridine platelet antagonists, such as prasugrel, have compared with clopidogrel?
- What is the optimal dose of clopidogrel for patients with diabetes?

TIPS FOR NON-SPECIALISTS

- Patients who are allergic to aspirin should take clopidogrel indefinitely
- If the patient had a recent acute coronary syndrome, find out whether percutaneous coronary intervention was performed and what type of stent was used because this determines the optimal duration of clopidogrel treatment
- Minimise the risk of bleeding in high risk patients (those on dual antiplatelet treatment or also taking anticoagulants or non-steroidal anti-inflammatory drugs) by reducing the dose of aspirin, targeting the lower range of the therapeutic international normalised ratio, minimising the duration of dual antiplatelet treatment, and prophylactically treating the patient with a proton pump inhibitor
- Clopidogrel should be stopped five days before scheduled surgery or dental extraction. A cardiologist should be consulted first if a drug eluting stent has recently been inserted
- Herbal remedies such as ginko should be avoided because they have antiplatelet activity and may increase the risk of bleeding in patients on dual antiplatelet treatment and warfarin
- Tell the patient about the importance of adhering to dual antiplatelet therapy with aspirin and clopidogrel after stent implantation

ADDITIONAL EDUCATIONAL RESOURCES

Resources for healthcare professionals

- American College of Chest Physicians (www.chestjournal.org/content/vol133/6_suppl/)– Latest guidelines from the ACCP on antithrombotic treatment
- American College of Cardiology (http://www.acc.org/qualityandscience/clinical/statements.htm)–ACC guidelines on non-ST elevation myocardial infarction, ST elevation myocardial infarction, and percutaneous coronary interventions
- European Society of Cardiology (www.escardio.org/guidelines-surveys/esc-guidelines/Pages/GuidelinesList.aspx)–ESC guidelines on acute coronary syndromes
- Emmons KL, Taylor NT. Contemporary issues in clopidogrel therapy: new evidence shaping clinical practice. *Pharmacotherapy* 2007;27:553-63
- Galla JM, Lincoff AM. The role of clopidogrel in the management of ischemic heart disease. *Curr Opin Cardiol* 2007;22:273-9

Resources for patients

- NHS Direct (http://cks.library.nhs.uk/patient_information_leaflet/anti_platelets_clopidogrel#)–Clopidogrel drug monograph
- NHS Direct (http://cks.library.nhs.uk/patient_information_leaflet/heart_attack)–Information about heart attacks
- NHS Choices (www.nhsdirect.nhs.uk/articles/article.aspx?articleId=112&sectionId=145)–Information about percutaneous coronary intervention

What is the optimal loading dose of clopidogrel?

The optimal loading dose of clopidogrel is still unclear. Although the landmark studies in myocardial infarction and percutaneous coronary intervention used a 300 mg loading dose, higher doses have recently been shown to produce faster and greater platelet inhibition, thereby reducing the risk of further cardiac events. The ARMYDA-2 randomised study showed that, in patients undergoing percutaneous coronary intervention, a 600 mg loading dose of clopidogrel was superior to 300 mg in reducing periprocedural myocardial infarction.[25] On the basis of emerging clinical trial data, the current American and European guidelines recommend 600 mg in patients undergoing percutaneous coronary intervention (level I C recommendation) and 300 mg in patients presenting with acute coronary syndromes.[17 18]

Contributors: DC conceived the idea for the article, wrote the article, and revised the manuscript. He is the primary author and guarantor. AI reviewed the manuscript for accuracy and content.

Funding: No funding was received to write this article.

Competing interests: None declared.

Provenance and peer review: Encouraged but not commissioned; externally peer reviewed.

1 Grech ED, Ramsdale DR. Acute coronary syndrome: unstable angina and non-ST segment elevation myocardial infarction. *BMJ* 2003;326:1259-61.

2 White HD, Chew P. Acute myocardial infarction. *Lancet* 2008;372:570-84.

3 Patrono C, Baigent C, Hirsh J, Roth G. Antiplatelet drugs: American College of Chest Physicians evidence-based clinical practice guidelines (8th edition). *Chest* 2008;133(6 suppl):199S-233S.

4 Yusuf S, Zhao F, Mehta SR, Chrolavicius S, Tognoni G, Fox KK. Effects of clopidogrel in addition to aspirin in patients with acute coronary syndromes without ST-segment elevation. *N Engl J Med* 2001;345:494-502.

5 Anderson JL, Adams CD, Antman EM, Bridges CR, Califf RM, Casey DE Jr, et al. ACC/AHA 2007 guidelines for the management of patients with unstable angina/non ST-elevation myocardial infarction: a report of the American College of Cardiology/American Heart Association task force on practice guidelines (writing committee to revise the 2002 guidelines for the management of patients with unstable angina/non ST-elevation myocardial infarction). *Circulation* 2007;116:e148-304.

6 Harrington RA, Becker RC, Cannon CP, Gutterman D, Lincoff AM, Popma JJ, et al. Antithrombotic therapy for non-ST-segment elevation acute coronary syndromes: American College of Chest Physicians evidence-based clinical practice guidelines (8th edition). *Chest* 2008;133:670S-707.

7 Task Force for Diagnosis and Treatment of Non-ST-Segment Elevation Acute Coronary Syndromes of European Society of Cardiology; Bassand JP, Hamm CW, Ardissino D, Boersma E, Budaj A, Fernández-Avilés F, et al. Guidelines for the diagnosis and treatment of non-ST-segment elevation acute coronary syndromes. *Eur Heart J* 2007;28:1598-660.

8 Sabatine MS, Cannon CP, Gibson CM, López-Sendón JL, Montalescot G, Theroux P, et al. Addition of clopidogrel to aspirin and fibrinolytic therapy for myocardial infarction with ST-segment elevation. *N Engl J Med* 2005;352:1179-89.

9 Chen ZM, Jiang LX, Chen YP, Xie JX, Pan HC, Peto R, et al. Addition of clopidogrel to aspirin in 45 852 patients with acute myocardial infarction: randomised placebo-controlled trial. *Lancet* 2005;366:1607-21.

10 2007 focused update of the ACC/AHA 2004 guidelines for the management of patients with ST-elevation myocardial infarction: a report of the American College of Cardiology/American Heart Association task force on practice guidelines: 2007 writing group to review new evidence and update the ACC/AHA 2004 guidelines for the management of patients with ST-elevation myocardial infarction, writing on behalf of the 2004 writing committee. *Circulation* 2008;117:296-329.

11 Bertrand ME, Rupprecht HJ, Urban P, Gershlick AH. Double-blind study of the safety of clopidogrel with and without a loading dose in combination with aspirin compared with ticlopidine in combination with aspirin after coronary stenting: the clopidogrel aspirin stent international cooperative study (CLASSICS). *Circulation* 2000;102:624-9.

12 Muller C, Buttner HJ, Petersen J, Roskamm H. A randomized comparison of clopidogrel and aspirin versus ticlodipine and aspirin after the placement of coronary-artery stents. *Circulation* 2000;101:590-3.

13 Mehta SR, Yusuf S, Peters RJ, Bertrand ME, Lewis BS, Natarajan MK, et al. Effects of pretreatment with clopidogrel and aspirin followed by long-term therapy in patients undergoing percutaneous coronary intervention: the PCI-CURE study. *Lancet* 2001;358:527-33.

14 Goodman SG, Menon V, Cannon CP, Steg G, Ohman EM, Harrington RA. Acute ST-segment elevation myocardial infarction: American College of Chest Physicians evidence-based clinical practice guidelines (8th edition). *Chest* 2008;133(6 suppl):708S-75S.

15 Bhatt DL, Fox KA, Hacke W, Berger PB, Black HR, Boden WE, et al. Clopidogrel and aspirin versus aspirin alone for the prevention of atherothrombotic events. *N Engl J Med* 2006;354:1706-17.

16 Steinhubl SR, Berger PB, Mann JT 3rd, Fry ET, DeLago A, Wilmer C, et al. Early and sustained dual oral antiplatelet therapy following percutaneous coronary intervention: a randomized controlled trial. *JAMA* 2002;288:2411-20.

17 King SB 3rd, Smith SC Jr, Hirshfeld JW Jr, Jacobs AK, Morrison DA, Williams DO, et al. 2007 focused update of the ACC/AHA/SCAI 2005 guideline update for percutaneous coronary intervention: a report of the American College of Cardiology/American Heart Association Task Force on Practice guidelines. *J Am Coll Cardiol* 2008;51:172-209.

18 Silber S, Albertsson P, Avilés FF, Camici PG, Colombo A, Hamm C, et al. Guidelines for percutaneous coronary interventions. The task force for percutaneous coronary interventions of the European Society of Cardiology. *Eur Heart J* 2005;26:804-47.

19 Harrington RA, Becker RC, Ezekowitz M, Meade TW, O'Connor CM, Vorchheimer DA, et al. Antithrombotic therapy for coronary artery disease: the seventh ACCP conference on antithrombotic and thrombolytic therapy. *Chest* 2004;126(3 suppl):513S-48S.

20 Smith SC Jr, Feldman TE, Hirshfeld JW Jr, Jacobs AK, Kern MJ, King SB 3rd, et al. ACC/AHA/SCAI 2005 guideline update for percutaneous coronary intervention: a report of the American College of Cardiology/American Heart Association task force on practice guidelines (ACC/AHA/SCAI writing committee to update 2001 guidelines for percutaneous coronary intervention). *Circulation* 2006;113:e166-286.

21 Pfisterer M, Brunner-La Rocca HP, Buser PT, Rickenbacher P, Hunziker P, Mueller C, et al. Late clinical events after clopidogrel discontinuation may limit the benefit of drug-eluting stents: an observational study of drug-eluting versus bare-metal stents. *J Am Coll Cardiol* 2006;48:2584-91.

22 Grines CL, Bonow RO, Casey DE Jr, Gardner TJ, Lockhart PB, Moliterno DJ, et al. Prevention of premature discontinuation of dual antiplatelet therapy in patients with coronary artery stents: a science advisory from the American Heart Association, American College of Cardiology, Society for Cardiovascular Angiography and Interventions, American College of Surgeons, and American Dental Association, with representation from the American College of Physicians. *Circulation* 2007;115:813-8.

23 Iakovou I, Schmidt T, Bonizzoni E, Ge L, Sangiorgi GM, Stankovic G, et al. Incidence, predictors, and outcome of thrombosis after successful implantation of drug-eluting stents. *JAMA* 2005;293:2126-30.

24 Maisel WH. Unanswered questions–drug-eluting stents and the risk of late thrombosis. *N Engl J Med* 2007;356:981-4.

25 Patti G, Colonna G, Pasceri V, Pepe LL, Montinaro A, Di Sciascio G. Randomized trial of high loading dose of clopidogrel for reduction of periprocedural myocardial infarction in patients undergoing coronary intervention: results from the ARMYDA-2 (Antiplatelet Therapy for Reduction of Myocardial Damage during Angioplasty) study. *Circulation* 2005;111:2099-106.

Anticipating and managing bleeding complications in patients with coronary stents who are receiving dual antiplatelet treatment

Neeraj Bhala, Medical Research Council health of the public research fellow and specialist registrar in gastroenterology[1], Jaspal S Taggar, specialist registrar and research fellow in general practice[2], Praveen Rajasekhar, Northern Regional Endoscopy Group research fellow and specialist registrar in gastroenterology[3], Amitava Banerjee, clinical lecturer in cardiovascular medicine[4]

[1]Clinical Trial Service Unit and Epidemiological Studies Unit, University of Oxford, Oxford OX3 7LF, UK and Translational Gastroenterology Unit, John Radcliffe Hospital, Oxford, OX3 9DU, UK

[2]Division of Primary Care, University of Nottingham, Queens Medical Centre, Nottingham, UK

[3]South Tyneside District Hospital, South Shields, UK

[4]University of Birmingham Centre for Cardiovascular Sciences, City Hospital, Birmingham, UK

Correspondence to: N Bhala nijbhala@doctors.org.uk

Cite this as: *BMJ* 2011;343:d4264

‹DOI› 10.1136/bmj.d4264
http://www.bmj.com/content/343/bmj.d4264

Coronary artery stents are used to treat the full spectrum of coronary heart diseases, from stable angina through to ST elevation myocardial infarctions, and stent insertions are common medical procedures, with more than 80 000 and 1.3 million performed in the United Kingdom and United States each year, respectively.[1 2] Both bare metal stents and drug eluting stents, which release anti-proliferative drugs and reduce restenosis, are commonly used. Although drug eluting stents have been associated with lower rates of medium term vascular complications, such as revascularisation, there have been concerns about other rarer later vascular outcomes. Of particular concern is the apparent small absolute risk of in-stent thrombosis with drug eluting stents.

To prevent these vascular complications, treatment with multiple antithrombotic drugs, including dual antiplatelet treatment (such as aspirin and clopidogrel), is an important part of acute stent management. To reduce the risk of in-stent thrombosis, longer periods of dual antiplatelet treatment are needed for drug eluting stents than for bare metal stents. However, antithrombotic treatments are associated with an increased risk of bleeding, which can vary from mild to potentially life threatening. This is partly because of the prolonged exposure to these drugs, but also because bleeding and atherosclerosis share many risk factors. As well as bleeding at the vascular access sites after stent insertion, bleeding mediated by platelet inhibition can affect other organs, such as intracranial vessels or, most commonly, the upper gastrointestinal tract. Management of bleeding complications in patients with coronary artery stents is especially challenging because of the need to consider vascular and bleeding risks.

Our narrative review of the risks and benefits of coronary stents and concomitant antiplatelet treatment is based on randomised controlled trials, meta-analyses, systematic reviews, and international guidelines. We focus on how to assess the risk of bleeding complications in patients with coronary artery stents and how to manage them, with particular emphasis on upper gastrointestinal bleeding—the most common bleeding medical emergency that presents to acute physicians.

SOURCES AND SELECTION CRITERIA

We searched PubMed for "coronary stents" and "managing bleeding complications" and used reference lists to identify key studies. We also consulted the Cochrane Library, the Cochrane Collaboration, consensus statements, and national guidelines. The evidence base informing bleeding complications is relatively strong and we gave priority to large well designed randomised controlled trials, systematic reviews, and meta-analyses. Evidence for the management of upper gastrointestinal bleeding after coronary stenting is relatively sparse, however, so other methodological designs were also cited where appropriate.

SUMMARY POINTS

- Cardiac catheterisation and insertion of coronary artery stents are common interventions in patients with coronary heart disease
- Compared with bare metal stents, drug eluting stents are associated with lower rates of restenosis but may be associated with later vascular complications, such as in-stent thrombosis
- Patients with coronary artery stents need multiple antithrombotic drugs at the time of insertion, including long term dual antiplatelets (such as aspirin and clopidogrel)
- Antithrombotic drugs are associated with bleeding at vascular access sites, intracranially, and the upper gastrointestinal tract
- Acute upper gastrointestinal bleeding is managed by patient resuscitation, endoscopy for diagnosis and treatment, and medical gastroprotectant treatments
- The management of emergency bleeding complications in patients with stents requires a multidisciplinary approach to balance bleeding versus long term vascular risks

What are coronary stents?

Coronary artery disease can be treated medically using smoking cessation, blood pressure lowering, cholesterol lowering, and antiplatelet drugs, but in many cases it also requires interventional procedures for reperfusion. Interventions for coronary artery disease include percutaneous coronary intervention and coronary artery bypass grafting. Percutaneous coronary intervention is less invasive than surgery and includes percutaneous transluminal coronary angioplasty, with or without insertion of coronary artery stents. Stents are expandable devices that are inserted within narrowed segments of coronary arteries after angioplasty and consist of a tubular wire mesh that forms a "scaffold."

Coronary stents fall into two broad categories—first generation bare metal stents and later drug eluting stents.[1] The main complication after stent insertion is restenosis of the stented artery, which may require revascularisation procedures. Restenosis is caused by proliferation of cells in the intima, a smooth muscle wall in the coronary vessel (neointimal hyperplasia), which together with clots (thromboses) can occlude the stented artery. To help reduce restenosis, drug eluting stents that release anti-proliferative agents—such as sirolimus, tacrolimus, paclitaxel, and zotarolimus—were developed and introduced at the beginning of the 21st century. Rates of revascularisation at one year for drug eluting stents within individual trials were less than 5% compared with 10-25% for bare metal stents.[2 3]

What is the evidence of benefit for coronary stents?

According to UK national audit data, by 2008, 92% of percutaneous coronary intervention procedures involved stents, with more than 60% of these using drug eluting stents.[4] Guidelines vary by country, but in the UK, drug eluting stents are recommended for the treatment of coronary artery disease if the artery to be treated is less than 3 mm wide or the lesion is longer than 15 mm, and if the drug eluting stent is no more than £300 (€335; $480) more expensive than the bare metal stent.[2] Although stents are sometime used to treat symptoms, a meta-analysis of randomised trials suggested no difference between percutaneous coronary intervention and conservative medical treatment in terms of death, myocardial infarction, or subsequent revascularisation rates in patients with angina symptoms only.[5] In coronary artery disease traditionally treated with bypass surgery (multi-vessel disease or left main stem disease), meta-analyses have confirmed that percutaneous coronary intervention seems to be equivalent in terms of mortality or major adverse vascular events, although the risk of later target vessel revascularisation is higher.[6 7]

Although restenosis is lower with drug eluting stents than with bare metal stents, they have been associated with late in-stent thrombosis.[8] In a meta-analysis of randomised controlled trials, the incidence of definite or probable in-stent thrombosis one to four years after implantation was 0.9% in the sirolimus and paclitaxel eluting stent groups versus 0.4-0.6% in the bare metal stent group, highlighting the relatively low absolute rates of this complication.[9] Although in-stent thrombosis has a slightly higher absolute rate (~1.5% per annum) in prospective observational studies,[10] meta-analyses of randomised controlled trials have shown that drug eluting stents are not associated with excess mortality after four to five years of follow-up.[8] It is still unclear which types of stents (and which specific antiproliferative drugs) offer the best long term management in different populations, so both types of stent are still widely used. Clinicians should use the appropriate national and international guidelines when considering the use of coronary stents.

What are the recommendations for concomitant antiplatelet drugs?

A wide range of antithrombotic drugs are used during the acute management of coronary intervention, such as heparin, glycoprotein IIb/IIIa inhibitors, and direct thrombin inhibitors. In the acute and longer term management of myocardial infarction and unstable angina, aspirin taken with other antiplatelet agents, such as clopidogrel, reduces the rate of major vascular events in patients with overt occlusive vascular disease.[11 12] Moreover, in patients with coronary artery stents, aspirin and clopidogrel dual antiplatelet treatment is prescribed to reduce the risks of in-stent thrombosis and restenosis. These dual antiplatelet regimens are prescribed for varying lengths of time depending on the type and sometimes the site of the coronary lesion. Because the risk of late in-stent thrombosis with the use of drug eluting stents is of particular concern,[1] dual antiplatelet treatments are generally recommended for longer with these stents. Although it is unclear how long dual antiplatelet treatment should last,[13] some guidelines recommend that patients with drug eluting stents should receive at least 12 months of dual treatment with aspirin and clopidogrel.[2] Recommendations may be revised if newer antiplatelet agents, such as prasugrel and ticagrelor, replace clopidogrel as a second antiplatelet agent.[14 15] Table 1 lists some of the antithrombotic drugs available.[16]

What are the main bleeding risks and how is bleeding managed?

The risks of bleeding associated with stent implantation are mainly related to antithrombotic drugs, including antiplatelet agents, anticoagulants, and fibrinolytics (although other factors, such as comorbidity, are also relevant). Hence, short term bleeding risks depend on the combination of antithrombotic drugs at the point of stent insertion, with longer term risks related to oral dual antiplatelets, usually aspirin and clopidogrel. Different scores have been used to define "bleeding," so it can be difficult to compare studies, although attempts are now being made to standardise recording of bleeding.[17] However, bleeding is commonly recorded at the vascular access site, intracranially, or within the gastrointestinal tract.

Data from three recent large randomised trials showed a 5% risk of major bleeding within 30 days of stent placement, with an associated threefold relative increase of overall mortality at one year.[18] Models have been developed to help stratify the risk of bleeding complications in patients with

Table 1 Commonly used antithrombotic agents

Drug class	Target	Examples
Antiplatelet agents		
Acetylsalicylic acid	Cyclo-oxygenase	Aspirin
Thienopyridines	ADP	Clopidogrel, prasugrel
P2Y12 receptor antagonists	ADP	Ticagrelor, cangrelor
Pyrimido-pyrimidine derivatives	cAMP	Dipyridamole
Glycoprotein IIb/IIIa receptor antagonists	Fibrinogen and von Willebrand factor	Eptifibatide, tirofiban, abciximab
Thromboxane inhibitors	Thromboxane	Terutroban
Anticoagulants		
Vitamin K antagonists	Clotting factors II, VII, IX, X	Warfarin
Heparins	Clotting factor Xa, others	Unfractionated heparin, low molecular weight heparin
Factor Xa inhibitors	Clotting factor Xa	Fondaparinux, indraparinux, apixaban
Direct thrombin inhibitors	Clotting factor II	Bivalirudin, argatroban, dabigatran
Fibrinolytics		
Plasminogen activators	Plasminogen	Alteplase, reteplase, tenecteplase
Other thrombolytics	Plasminogen	Streptokinase

Table 2 Commonly used agents for reversal of bleeding and their mechanism of action

Agent	Mechanism of action
Blood products	
Packed red cells	Replacement of red blood cells
Platelets	Supplies platelets
Fresh frozen plasma	Supplies clotting factors
Prothrombin complex concentrate	Supplies factors II, VII, IX, X
Cryoprecipitate	Supplies factor VII, von Willebrand factor, and fibrinogen
Drugs	
Desamino-D-arginine vasopressin	Releases von Willebrand factor
Vitamin K	Rejuvenates factors II, VII, IX, X
Protamine	Reverses heparin
Recombinant factor VIIa	Activates coagulation cascade
Tranexamic acid	Antifibrinolytic

intracoronary stents but have all used a composite outcome that includes all types of bleeding. Examples include registry models that predict major bleeding events in inpatients presenting with non-ST segment elevation myocardial infarction.[19] More recently, meta-analyses of large scale randomised trials have developed a scoring system that predicts the 30 day risk of bleeding in patients presenting with acute coronary syndromes.[20] In these studies, factors that confer greater risk of bleeding include increasing age, renal impairment, anaemia, and certain antithrombotic agents.

Because data on cause specific bleeding complications in patients with coronary stents are sparse, some of the evidence needs to be extrapolated from the wider population—for example, from large scale randomised trials of antithrombotic drugs.[11] Although treatments to reverse the effects of thrombosis (table 2) are available, they can be used only in specific settings, and the emergency focus is on resuscitation and treatment of the underlying cause.[16]

Bleeding from vascular access sites

Vascular access for percutaneous coronary interventions can be via the transfemoral, transradial, or transbrachial sites, although the last site is rarely used now because of the risk of upper limb ischaemia.[21 22] A recent large randomised trial assessing radial and femoral approaches found both to be safe and effective for percutaneous coronary intervention. However, at 30 days, 42 of 3507 patients in the radial group had large haematomas compared with 106 of 3514 in the femoral group (hazard ratio 0.40, 95% confidence interval 0.28 to 0.57; $P<0.0001$), so the radial approach, the default route in most European countries, may be preferable.[23]

The incidence of vascular access complications after percutaneous coronary intervention is reported to be 2-6%, with the highest risk in the first month; risk factors include increasing age, female sex, renal impairment, and certain antithrombotic agents.[18 19] Access site complications include haematoma, pseudoaneurysm, arteriovenous fistula formation, lower limb ischaemia, femoral artery infection, and retroperitoneal bleeding.[21 24] Mild bruises and small haematomas are common; these usually resolve with time without the need for specific investigation or treatment. However, a large or enlarging lump at the site of arterial access suggests an enlarging haematoma or the formation of a pseudoaneurysm, which requires investigation with vascular ultrasound imaging. If a large haematoma or pseudoaneurysm is found, it should be managed by the interventionist and may require surgical repair.

Retroperitoneal bleeding may occur after puncture of the femoral artery above the inguinal ligament, although this is rare (<1% of all percutaneous coronary interventions). Blood in the retroperitoneum may cause severe abdominal pain or back pain, with no obvious haematoma formation in the groin, and if not immediately recognised the patient may develop persistent hypotension. Treatment of a large retroperitoneal bleed is often conservative, with fluid replacement and careful monitoring of vital parameters, although it may need surgical evacuation and repair.[25]

Intracranial bleeding

Intracranial haemorrhage is one of the most severe complications associated with antiplatelet treatment and is associated with high mortality and morbidity. The risk of spontaneous intracranial haemorrhage is less well defined for patients with coronary artery stents, although it seems to be more likely with use of antithrombotic drugs. Evidence from meta-analyses of randomised trials suggests those taking aspirin alone or dual antiplatelet treatment have an increased relative risk of intracranial haemorrhage,[26 27] with a large randomised trial suggesting a low absolute rate (~0.3% a year) in patients receiving dual antiplatelet treatment.[28]

Because of the small subgroups available, evidence for the risk factors of intracranial haemorrhage specific to patients receiving multiple antithrombotics or coronary artery stents is limited. However, factors associated with spontaneous intracranial bleeds in the general population include hypertension, excess alcohol consumption, male sex, advanced age, and smoking.[29]

Although intracranial haemorrhage is uncommon, doctors should maintain a high index of suspicion in patients with coronary stents and promptly refer any patient with sudden onset of focal neurological signs for prompt radiological and physician review. The management of patients with intracranial haemorrhage is beyond the scope of this article but it broadly involves patient resuscitation, correction of coagulopathy, and specialist neurosurgical intervention. Antithrombotic agents are often withdrawn in the acute setting, although liaison with cardiology colleagues is required in later management. A previous *BMJ* article provides a comprehensive review on the management of spontaneous intracerebral haemorrhage.[30]

Upper gastrointestinal bleeding

The risk of gastrointestinal bleeding is increased in people taking dual antiplatelet drugs, although other comorbidities probably play a role. Bleeding can occur at any site in the gastrointestinal tract, but it is most common in the upper gastrointestinal tract. Acute upper gastrointestinal bleeding is the most common gastroenterological emergency or bleeding complication requiring hospital admission in the UK, with an estimated annual incidence of 50-100 per 100 000.[w1 w2] Patients usually present after vomiting fresh or altered blood (haematemesis) or passing dark tarry stools (melaena or digested blood), classically with epigastric pain. However, patients with coronary artery stents can present atypically as a result of severe volume loss, with anginal chest pain or postural dizziness.

Factors associated with a greater risk of such bleeding in patients taking antiplatelet drugs have been investigated as part of observational studies and post hoc analyses of randomised trials. Risk factors include a history of peptic ulcer disease; increasing age; male sex; concomitant use of anticoagulants, steroids, or non-steroidal anti-inflammatory drugs; *Helicobacter pylori* infection; baseline anaemia;

diabetes; and smoking.[w3 w4] Although the strongest and most consistent predictor is a history of upper gastrointestinal bleeding,[w5] the risk of complications is greater with an increasing number of risk factors.[20] A large case-control study to evaluate upper gastrointestinal bleeding in patients using single and dual antiplatelet drugs in the Danish population found an odds ratio for bleeding of 1.8 in people taking low dose aspirin alone, 1.1 in those taking clopidogrel alone, and 7.4 in those taking both.[w6] Increased dose and duration of dual antiplatelet treatment are also likely to affect the risk of upper gastrointestinal bleeding.[w7 w8] Although estimates from randomised trials in patients with coronary stents are rare, estimates of risk can be extrapolated from other studies. For example, in a randomised trial of clopidogrel plus aspirin in patients with acute coronary syndromes without ST segment elevation, gastrointestinal bleeding occurred in 1.3% of those on dual antiplatelet treatment at one month,[w9] with a reported 3% annual risk in patients taking low (≤100 mg) long term doses of aspirin.[w10] Subsequent observational analyses of patients having percutaneous coronary intervention in this trial suggest that this aspirin dose offers the best long term risk-benefit balance.[w11]

Can clopidogrel and proton pump inhibitors be used together to reduce the risk of bleeding?

The recent joint North American cardiology and gastroenterology consensus guidelines recommend that patients taking dual antiplatelet drugs who are at high risk of upper gastrointestinal bleeding (as outlined above) should be co-prescribed proton pump inhibitors, because of their considerable gastroprotective effect.[w3] Although retrospective studies had raised concerns that such treatment might reduce the cardiovascular efficacy of clopidogrel, this observation could be prone to biases.[w12 w13] A randomised controlled trial of 3627 patients taking aspirin and clopidogrel randomised to omeprazole or placebo found no difference in the rate of adverse vascular outcomes between groups.[w14] Pharmacodynamic studies in other randomised trials support these findings,[w15 w16] suggesting that proton pump inhibitors have little, if any, effect on the cardiovascular efficacy of clopidogrel. Hence, gastroprotectant therapy should not be withheld for prevention of bleeding in high risk groups or for treatment of acute bleeding.[w3]

How is acute upper gastrointestinal bleeding managed?

Guidelines, such as those published by the British Society of Gastroenterology,[w2] highlight the need for a team approach, with an experienced endoscopy team and a surgical team in close proximity. Circulatory resuscitation is vital, initially with crystalloid or colloid fluids, and consideration of blood products according to haemodynamic status.[w17] Baseline blood tests should include a full blood count, coagulation studies, biochemistry, and blood group for crossmatch. After resuscitation, haemodynamic status must be monitored carefully and may require involvement of specialist intensivists before moving to endoscopy (for diagnosis and potential treatment). Evidence from randomised trials supports the acute administration of gastroprotectants, such as intravenous proton pump inhibitors, in patients with confirmed peptic ulcer bleeds.[w18]

Risk stratification scores can be used to assess the patient's risk of a re-bleed or death.[w5 w19] Figure 1 shows an algorithm for the suggested management of a patient with coronary artery stents presenting with a large upper gastrointestinal bleed. This should also include prompt discussion with an interventional cardiologist after initial assessment.

What is the role of blood transfusion?

The purpose of blood transfusion is to correct global or regional oxygenation and to improve haemostasis. The role of blood transfusion in patients with exsanguinating haemorrhage is self evident, but its role in patients with less severe haemorrhage is unclear.[w20] The most recent British Society of Gastroenterology audit of blood use in upper gastrointestinal bleeding, which defined the appropriate threshold for transfusion as a serum haemoglobin of less than 100 g/L, found that 5-15% (depending on clinical setting) of transfusions were unnecessary.[w21] The current Scottish Intercollegiate Guidelines Network guideline for management of upper gastrointestinal bleeding recommends transfusion after the loss of 30% of the circulating volume, and provides guidance on how this can be estimated.[w17]

Systematic reviews of studies of blood transfusion in upper gastrointestinal bleeding have reported variable outcomes, including a higher re-bleeding rate and increased incidence of coagulopathy in patients receiving blood transfusions.[w22] Observational studies in populations with coronary stents suggest that blood transfusion carries a risk for ischaemic outcomes that is independent of bleeding itself.[w23] The reasons for this are unclear, but the effect of blood transfusion on coagulation could play a role. Although transfusion and blood products will continue to be used in this setting, especially for patients with haemodynamic compromise, their optimal role is uncertain.[w24]

How soon should upper gastrointestinal endoscopy take place?

The British Society of Gastroenterology recommends that all patients with suspected upper gastrointestinal bleeding should undergo upper gastrointestinal endoscopy within 24 hours of presentation, but that those at risk of haemodynamic compromise warrant prompt endoscopy out of hours.[w25] Small retrospective studies have shown endoscopy to be safe after acute coronary syndromes, although its timing should be considered on a case-by-case basis.[w26 w27]

Should antiplatelet agents be withheld in a major bleed?

After the acute episode of upper gastrointestinal bleeding has resolved, consider measures to reduce the risk of recurrent events, such as stopping concomitant non-steroidal anti-inflammatory drugs and eradicating *H pylori.* Although it may be intuitive to withhold dual antiplatelet treatment in this context, the patients' vascular risk must be evaluated and reduced appropriately. For example, although aspirin is stopped acutely in an upper gastrointestinal bleed, a small randomised trial found that continuation of aspirin with a proton pump inhibitor five days after endoscopic haemostasis reduced death at eight weeks, mainly through a reduction in vascular thrombotic events.[w28] Withholding antiplatelet drugs in patients with coronary stents affects the risk of stent thrombosis, so discussion with interventional cardiologists is vital in these patients. A systematic review suggested that continuation of one antiplatelet drug (potentially with gastroprotectant cover) may be beneficial after adequate haemostasis in patients with coronary artery stents, especially if bleeding

Upper gastrointestinal bleeding in a patient with coronary stents
Clinically shocked (such as systolic blood pressure <100 mm Hg or heart rate >100 beats/min)
Or other evidence of massive haemorrhage
Or other evidence of vascular complications (such as myocardial ischaemia)

↓

Admit for clinical assessment and resuscitation:
Consider supportive treatment on high dependency or coronary care unit
Perform baseline blood tests; consider liberal or restrictive blood transfusion

↓

If presumed upper gastrointestinal source: urgent endoscopy for diagnosis and therapeutic intervention
If upper gastrointestinal non-variceal bleed (eg, peptic ulcer) treat with a gastroprotectant drug (such as intravenous proton pump inhibitor)
Withhold other drugs relevant to bleeding (such as NSAIDs); consider correcting other abnormalities (such as deranged clotting); consider temporary cessation of antiplatelet treatment, after discussion with a cardiologist

↓

Consider risks associated with antiplatelet treatment or cessation (gastrointestinal bleeding versus stent thromboses)

↓

Stent thromboses: Risks include diabetes, left ventricular systolic function, renal failure, stent length, site, inserted <30 days

Gastrointestinal bleeding: Use Rockall score (see below: such as age, shock, comorbidity, endoscopic findings, etc)

↓

Lower risk of recurrent bleeding (eg, Rockall score ≤3)
Continue both antiplatelets but investigate and treat for other causes, such as *Helicobacter pylori*

Higher risk of recurrent bleeding (eg, Rockall score ≥4)
Withhold aspirin alone (aim to restart within 5-7 days) and investigate and treat for other causes

Continued gastrointestinal bleeding
Withhold aspirin and clopidogrel (aim to restart within 5 days) and investigate and treat for other causes; reassess daily

Rockall scoring system for risk of rebleeding and death after admission to hospital with acute gastrointestinal bleeding

Score	0	1	2	3
Clinical findings on presentation				
Age (years)	<60	60-79	>80	
Shock	No shock: systolic blood pressure >100 mm Hg, heart rate <100 beats/min	Tachycardic: heart rate >100 beats/min, systolic blood pressure >100 mm Hg	Shocked: systolic blood pressure <100 mm Hg, heart rate >100 beats/min	
Comorbidity	Nil major		Cardiac failure, coronary heart disease	Renal failure, liver failure, disseminated malignancy
Endoscopic findings				
Diagnosis	No lesion, Mallory Weiss tear with no stigmata of recent haemorrhage	All other diagnoses	Malignancy of upper gastrointestinal tract	
Major stigmata of recent haemorrhage	None or dark spot		Blood in upper gastrointestinal tract, adherent clot, visible or spurting vessel	

Suggested algorithm for assessing and treating patients with coronary artery stents on dual antiplatelet treatments presenting with upper gastrointestinal bleeding. *Assessment may be influenced by the effect of drugs (such as β blockers) on blood pressure or pulse. NSAIDs=non-steroidal anti-inflammatory drugs

occurs more than a month after coronary intervention.[w29] Careful consideration must be given to balancing the risk of stent thrombosis (after antiplatelet withdrawal) and that of bleeding (with antiplatelet continuation). Although the evidence on which to base a decision in a high risk patient with continued bleeding is limited, we would suggest withholding aspirin and using clopidogrel in some settings, because of clopidogrel's relatively safer gastrointestinal profile (fig 1).

Many of the risk factors for upper gastrointestinal bleeding are shared with those for vascular thrombotic events—for example, analyses of a large randomised trial (using multiple antithrombotics) found that in-stent thrombosis at one year after stent insertion was more likely in patients with a history of gastrointestinal bleeding (5.8%) than in those without (2.4%).[w4] The reasons for this association include the presence of shared risk factors, reduced coronary perfusion as a result of haemodynamic compromise, and cessation of antiplatelets at the time of bleeding and at discharge. Other independent predictors for in-stent thrombosis include inadequate stent expansion at insertion, bifurcation lesions, renal failure, diabetes, and impaired left ventricular ejection fraction.[w30] However, the most important risk factor for in-stent thrombosis is the

QUESTIONS FOR FUTURE RESEARCH

- Which coronary artery stents are the safest and most efficacious in the long term management of stenotic occlusive heart disease—bare metal stents or drug eluting stents (and if the second type, which type of drug)?
- What are the optimal antithrombotic treatments and longer term antiplatelet treatments?
- As well as reliable estimates of associated complications, including restenosis, in-stent thrombosis, and bleeding complications, what is the safest duration of antiplatelet treatment in these patients?
- What are the safest roles for blood products, given uncertainties about increased mortality in patients with bleeding complications?
- Do gastroprotectants (such as proton pump inhibitors) have any clinically relevant vascular interactions with antithrombotics?
- What interventions could help prevent or treat post-procedural or intracranial haemorrhage?

TIPS FOR NON-SPECIALISTS

- In a patient with bleeding after insertion of a coronary stent first deal with the basics of cardiorespiratory support, adequate intravenous access, and appropriate fluid management
- Then institute appropriate diagnostic and therapeutic strategies to locate and treat the cause of bleeding (for example, upper gastrointestinal endoscopy for an upper gastrointestinal bleed, interventional cardiology for a post-procedural bleed)
- Although patients with exsanguinating bleeding complications may need blood products, they should be used with caution in those who are clinically stable. Other medical treatments can be used depending on the aetiology of bleeding (such as gastroprotectants for upper gastrointestinal ulcers)
- Deal with the patient's immediate bleeding problem. This may include reappraising drug treatment, but bear in mind that these patients are usually at high risk for vascular events. Discussion with specialists (such as an interventional cardiologist) may help prevent later vascular complications (such as stent thrombosis)
- Close liaison between the admitting physician, cardiologists, gastroenterologists, radiologists, intensivists, and others as appropriate is essential to ensure optimal management

ADDITIONAL EDUCATIONAL RESOURCES

Resources for healthcare professionals

- British Cardiovascular Society (www.bcs.com)—UK organisation that supports and represents all those working in cardiovascular care and research; includes a portal to relevant guidelines
- British Society of Gastroenterology (www.bsg.org.uk)—UK society focused on the promotion of gastroenterology, including guidelines
- National Institute for Health and Clinical Excellence. Coronary artery disease—drug-eluting stents: guidance. 2008. http://guidance.nice.org.uk/TA152/Guidance/pdf/English
- American College of Cardiology/American Heart Association. ACC/AHA guidelines for the management of patients with ST-elevation myocardial infarction (updating the 2004 guideline and 2007 focused update) and ACC/AHA/SCAI guidelines on percutaneous coronary intervention (updating the 2005 guideline and 2007 focused update). 2009. http://content.onlinejacc.org/cgi/content/full/j.jacc.2009.10.015

Resources for patients

- British Heart Foundation (www.bhf.org.uk)—UK charity that funds research, education, care, and awareness campaigns aimed at preventing heart disease
- CORE (www.corecharity.org.uk/Peptic-ulcers.html)—UK charity that funds research into diseases of the gut, liver, and pancreas; provides patient information leaflets

cessation of dual antiplatelet treatment: the risk increases with greater time off treatment, particularly more than five days, and if treatment is stopped within the first month of the procedure.[w25 w29 w31]

Current and future scenarios

This review has focused on the emergency management of bleeding, but multidisciplinary discussions would also be relevant in other scenarios, such as emergency surgery. Bleeding complications can also be anticipated and managed for elective procedures, such as non-cardiac surgery after placement of a coronary stent. Anaesthetic and surgical liaison with a cardiologist, ideally well in advance of the procedure, could help ensure appropriate management.

In the future, the management of bleeding complications in patients with coronary stents will be even more complex. For example, the effects of commonly used long term treatments that can exacerbate bleeding, such as non-steroidal anti-inflammatory drugs, must be carefully considered.[w32] Another increasingly common clinical scenario is that of the patient with a coronary artery stent who needs long term oral anticoagulation for indications such as atrial fibrillation. Current consensus guidelines advocate the use of triple therapy (dual antiplatelet drugs and oral anticoagulants), which, although potentially beneficial for the prevention of vascular outcomes,[w33] is even more likely to increase the risk of bleeding.[w34 w35] The risk-benefit balance of concomitant warfarin in patients with atrial fibrillation, venous thromboembolism, and metallic heart valves (mitral and aortic) must be considered on a case by case basis. Although further randomised evidence is needed, consideration needs to be given to stratification and treatment to reduce the risk of bleeding complications when assessing these patients.

The complexity of deciding the appropriate treatment in patients with coronary stents is already challenging. More potent antiplatelets (such as prasugrel and ticagrelor), newer anticoagulants (such as bivalirudin, dabigatran, fondaparinux, and idraparinux), and newer types of coronary stents are being developed for widespread use, and they will require even more careful evaluation of their associated benefits and hazards. Ongoing research is needed to provide further reliable evidence for the appropriate use of stents, associated medical treatments, and complications. Patients admitted with bleeding complications will continue to need multidisciplinary management for the prevention and treatment of haemorrhagic and vascular sequelae.

We would like to acknowledge comments made by Vipul Jairath and suggestions for the figure made by Simon Travis and Andy Veitch.

Contributors: All authors helped draft and critically revise the article and all approved the final version. Each author contributed on the basis of their clinical expertise. NB is guarantor.

Competing interests: All authors have completed the Unified Competing Interest form at http://www.icmje.org/coi_disclosure.pdf (available on request from the corresponding author) and declare: no support from any organisation for the submitted work; no financial relationships with any organisations that might have an interest in the submitted work in the previous three years, no other relationships or activities that could appear to have influenced the submitted work.

Provenance and peer review: Commissioned; externally peer reviewed.

The views expressed in this clinical review reflect those of the authors and not their institutions or funding bodies; the CTSU has a staff policy of not accepting honorariums.

1 Greenhalgh J, Hockenhull J, Rao N, Dundar Y, Dickson RC, Bagust A. Drug-eluting stents versus bare metal stents for angina or acute coronary syndromes. *Cochrane Database Syst Rev* 2010;5:CD004587.
2 National Institute for Health and Clinical Excellence. Drug-eluting stents for the treatment of coronary artery disease. Technology Appraisal Guidance 152. 2008. www.nice.org.uk/nicemedia/pdf/TA152Guidance.pdf.
3 Meads C, Cummins C, Jolly K, Stevens A, Burls A, Hyde C. Coronary artery stents in the treatment of ischaemic heart disease: a rapid and systematic review. *Health Technol Assess* 2000;4:1-153.
4 Ludman P. BCIS—British Cardiovascular Intervention Society. BCIS audit returns. Adult interventional procedures. Jan 2008 to Dec 2008. 2009. www.bcis.org.uk/resources/documents/BCIS%20Audit%202008%20for%20web%2016-10-09%20version%201.pdf.
5 Katritsis DG, Ioannidis JP. Percutaneous coronary intervention versus conservative therapy in nonacute coronary artery disease: a meta-analysis. *Circulation* 2005;111:2906-12.
6 Naik H, White AJ, Chakravarty T, Forrester J, Fontana G, Kar S, et al. A meta-analysis of 3,773 patients treated with percutaneous coronary intervention or surgery for unprotected left main coronary artery stenosis. *JACC Cardiovasc Interv* 2009;2:739-47.
7 From AM, Al Badarin FJ, Cha SS, Rihal CS. Percutaneous coronary intervention with drug-eluting stents versus coronary artery bypass

surgery for multivessel coronary artery disease: a meta-analysis of data from the ARTS II, CARDia, ERACI III, and SYNTAX studies and systematic review of observational data. *EuroIntervention* 2010;6:269-76.
8 Bavry AA, Bhatt DL. Appropriate use of drug-eluting stents: balancing the reduction in restenosis with the concern of late thrombosis. *Lancet* 2008;371:2134-43.
9 Mauri L, Hsieh WH, Massaro JM, Ho KK, D'Agostino R, Cutlip DE. Stent thrombosis in randomized clinical trials of drug-eluting stents. *N Engl J Med* 2007;356:1020-9.
10 Iakovou I, Schmidt T, Bonizzoni E, Ge L, Sangiorgi GM, Stankovic G, et al. Incidence, predictors, and outcome of thrombosis after successful implantation of drug-eluting stents. *JAMA* 2005;293:2126-30.
11 Antithrombotic Trialists' (ATT) Collaboration. Collaborative meta-analysis of randomised trials of antiplatelet therapy for prevention of death, myocardial infarction, and stroke in high risk patients. *BMJ* 2002;324:71-86.
12 Mehta SR, Yusuf S, Peters RJ, Bertrand ME, Lewis BS, Natarajan MK, et al. Effects of pretreatment with clopidogrel and aspirin followed by long-term therapy in patients undergoing percutaneous coronary intervention: the PCI-CURE study. *Lancet* 2001;358:527-33.
13 Sorensen R, Abildstrom SZ, Weeke P, Fosbol EL, Folke F, Hansen ML, et al. Duration of clopidogrel treatment and risk of mortality and recurrent myocardial infarction among 11 680 patients with myocardial infarction treated with percutaneous coronary intervention: a cohort study. *BMC Cardiovasc Disord* 2010;10:6.
14 Wallentin L, Becker RC, Budaj A, Cannon CP, Emanuelsson H, Held C, et al. Ticagrelor versus clopidogrel in patients with acute coronary syndromes. *N Engl J Med* 2009;361:1045-57.
15 Montalescot G, Wiviott SD, Braunwald E, Murphy SA, Gibson CM, McCabe CH, et al. Prasugrel compared with clopidogrel in patients undergoing percutaneous coronary intervention for ST-elevation myocardial infarction (TRITON-TIMI 38): double-blind, randomised controlled trial 38. *Lancet* 2009;373:723-31.
16 Neuner M, Davis J. How to reverse an antithrombotic agent. *Emergency Medicine* 2011. www.emedmag.com/html/pre/fea/features/041060008.asp.
17 Mehran R, Rao SV, Bhatt DL, Gibson CM, Caixeta A, Eikelboom J, et al. Standardized bleeding definitions for cardiovascular clinical trials: a consensus report from the bleeding academic research consortium 1. *Circulation* 2011;123:2736-47.
18 Verheugt FW, Steinhubl SR, Hamon M, Darius H, Steg PG, Valgimigli M, et al. Incidence, prognostic impact, and influence of antithrombotic therapy on access and nonaccess site bleeding in percutaneous coronary intervention. *JACC Cardiovasc Interv* 2011;4:191-7.
19 Subherwal S, Bach RG, Chen AY, Gage BF, Rao SV, Newby LK, et al. Baseline risk of major bleeding in non-ST-segment-elevation myocardial infarction: the CRUSADE (Can Rapid risk stratification of Unstable angina patients Suppress ADverse outcomes with Early implementation of the ACC/AHA Guidelines) Bleeding Score 1. *Circulation* 2009;119:1873-82.
20 Mehran R, Pocock SJ, Nikolsky E, Clayton T, Dangas GD, Kirtane AJ, et al. A risk score to predict bleeding in patients with acute coronary syndromes. *J Am Coll Cardiol* 2010;55:2556-66.
21 Agostoni P, Biondi-Zoccai GG, De Benedictis ML, Rigattieri S, Turri M, Anselmi M, et al. Radial versus femoral approach for percutaneous coronary diagnostic and interventional procedures; systematic overview and meta-analysis of randomized trials. *J Am Coll Cardiol* 2004;44:349-56.
22 Archbold RA, Robinson NM, Schilling RJ. Radial artery access for coronary angiography and percutaneous coronary intervention. *BMJ* 2004;329:443-6.
23 Jolly SS, Yusuf S, Cairns J, Niemela K, Xavier D, Widimsky P, et al. Radial versus femoral access for coronary angiography and intervention in patients with acute coronary syndromes (RIVAL): a randomised, parallel group, multicentre trial 1. *Lancet* 2011;377:1409-20.
24 Muller DW, Shamir KJ, Ellis SG, Topol EJ. Peripheral vascular complications after conventional and complex percutaneous coronary interventional procedures. *Am J Cardiol* 1992;69:63-8.
25 Wong EM, Wu EB, Chan WW, Yu CM. A review of the management of patients after percutaneous coronary intervention. *Int J Clin Pract* 2006;60:582-9.
26 Baigent C, Blackwell L, Collins R, Emberson J, Godwin J, Peto R, et al. Aspirin in the primary and secondary prevention of vascular disease: collaborative meta-analysis of individual participant data from randomised trials. *Lancet* 2009;373:1849-60.
27 Serebruany VL, Malinin AI, Ferguson JJ, Vahabi J, Atar D, Hennekens CH. Bleeding risks of combination vs. single antiplatelet therapy: a meta-analysis of 18 randomized trials comprising 129,314 patients. *Fundam Clin Pharmacol* 2008;22:315-21.
28 Bhatt DL, Fox KA, Hacke W, Berger PB, Black HR, Boden WE, et al. Clopidogrel and aspirin versus aspirin alone for the prevention of atherothrombotic events. *N Engl J Med* 2006;354:1706-17.
29 Ariesen MJ, Claus SP, Rinkel GJ, Algra A. Risk factors for intracerebral hemorrhage in the general population: a systematic review. *Stroke* 2003;34:2060-5.
30 Al-Shahi SR, Labovitz DL, Stapf C. Spontaneous intracerebral haemorrhage 1. *BMJ* 2009;339:b2586.

Related links

bmj.com/archive

Previous articles in this series

- Anticipating and managing postoperative delirium and cognitive decline in adults (2011;343:d4331)
- Contemporary management and recent advances in paediatric hydrocephalus (2011;343:d4191)
- Endometrial cancer (2011;343:d3954)
- Clinical management of stuttering in children and adults (2011;342:d3742)
- Management of nausea and vomiting in pregnancy (2011;342:d3606)

doc2doc.bmj.com

- Discuss coronary stents on doc2doc's cardiology forum

BMJ BPP UNIVERSITY SCHOOL OF HEALTH

Cardiac resynchronisation therapy for chronic heart failure and conduction delay

Richard M Cubbon, lecturer in cardiology[1], Klaus K A Witte, senior lecturer in cardiology and honorary consultant cardiologist[1]

[1]Division of Cardiovascular and Diabetes Research, University of Leeds, Leeds LS2 9JT

Correspondence to: K K A Witte klauswitte@hotmail.com

Cite this as: BMJ 2009;338:b1265

‹DOI› 10.1136/bmj.b1265
http://www.bmj.com/content/338/bmj.b1265

Chronic heart failure is common, affecting about 900 000 people in the United Kingdom and with a prevalence of about 6-10% in people aged over 65 years[1]; despite modern drug treatment, it carries a high morbidity and a 10% annual mortality. About a third of patients with chronic heart failure have a left ventricular ejection fraction ≤35%,[2] up to 40% of whom are at risk of worse outcomes and more severe heart failure identified by conduction delay (QRS duration on a surface electrocardiogram of >120 ms).[3]

A recent addition to therapeutic algorithms for chronic heart failure is cardiac resynchronisation therapy (also known as biventricular pacing). Cardiac resynchronisation therapy is a well proved treatment for patients with heart failure who have left ventricular systolic dysfunction and conduction delay, and it can reduce symptoms and admission to hospital and improve quality of life and prognosis. Clear mortality benefits have moved it from a treatment for intractable symptoms to one that, alongside β blockers, angiotensin converting enzyme inhibitors, and aldosterone antagonists, is now a routine therapy for patients with current or previous severe chronic heart failure.

Identifying suitable patients is straightforward; there is no upper age limit of benefit; the implant technique is of low risk; and the treatment is highly cost effective. This article reviews the evidence and indications for cardiac resynchronisation therapy, discusses the clinical features that should alert general physicians and general practitioners to patients who may benefit from this therapy, and considers future directions for such therapy for heart failure ("device therapy") in the UK.

SOURCES AND SELECTION CRITERIA

We searched Medline and the Cochrane database for evidence from systematic reviews and clinical trials. We also used our personal experience of clinical trials, cardiac imaging, and device implantation and searched for relevant reports from the Healthcare Commission.

SUMMARY POINTS

- Consider cardiac resynchronisation therapy for any patient with chronic heart failure if they have, or have recently had, moderate or severe symptoms of heart failure; if their left ventricular ejection fraction is ≤35%; and if their QRS duration is ≥150 ms or 120-149 ms with dyssynchrony measured on echocardiography
- Cardiac resynchronisation therapy can improve symptoms and prognosis
- Advanced age does not reduce the effectiveness of the therapy
- All healthcare professionals involved in the management of heart failure need to be aware of the potential benefits of cardiac resynchronisation therapy and who to refer
- Evaluation of the QRS duration and heart rhythm on the electrocardiogram should be part of the standard management of any patient with heart failure and repeated at least yearly

What is cardiac resynchronisation therapy?

Cardiac resynchronisation therapy is a form of cardiac pacing that aims to improve the coordination of the atria and both ventricles. Pacing leads are placed into the right atrial appendage, at the right ventricular apex, which is also the anterior wall of the left ventricle, and, via a lateral tributary of the coronary sinus, into the left ventricular posterolateral wall (fig 1). Venous access is through the subclavian vein as for normal pacing, and the procedure is usually done under local anaesthetic through an infraclavicular incision. The target vein on the lateral wall is identified by retrograde balloon venography of the coronary sinus (fig 2; see videoclip 1 on bmj.com).

The leads are connected to a subcutaneous generator, which can then be programmed to deliver simultaneous left ventricular and right ventricular pacing. To over-ride intrinsic conduction, the atrioventricular delay is set shorter than the intrinsic PR interval. In selected patients cardiac resynchronisation therapy can be combined with additional protection from sudden cardiac death by implantation of an automatic implantable cardioverter defibrillator.[4]

How does cardiac resynchronisation therapy work?

Conduction system disease is common in patients with chronic heart failure and can be identified by a broad QRS complex on a surface electrocardiogram (fig 3). This is commonly accompanied by dyssynchronous, inefficient cardiac contraction, increased mitral regurgitation, and regional ischaemia, all of which contribute to further adverse remodelling and a downward spiral of cardiac function (see videoclip 2 on bmj.com).

By pacing both sides of the left ventricle, thereby improving the coordination of left (and right) ventricular contraction, cardiac resynchronisation thpy can improve cardiac output, reduce mitral regurgitation during rest and exercise,[5] and improve regional perfusion defects (see videoclip 3 on bmj.com).

What is the evidence for cardiac resynchronisation therapy?

Early double blind randomised controlled clinical trials of cardiac resynchronisation therapy (achieved by implanting a full system but randomly allocating patients to having the left ventricular lead switched off) found that during biventricular pacing there were improvements in cardiac function, left ventricular dimensions, mitral regurgitation,[5] [6] [7] and exercise capacity.[8] [9] The largest study (CARE-HF), published in 2005, randomised 813 patients either to optimal drug treatment or to optimal drug treatment plus cardiac resynchronisation therapy. Over the 29 month follow-up period, 30% of those receiving only the drug treatment died, compared with 20% of those also receiving biventricular pacemakers (absolute risk reduction of 10 percentage points). Biventricular pacing was associated

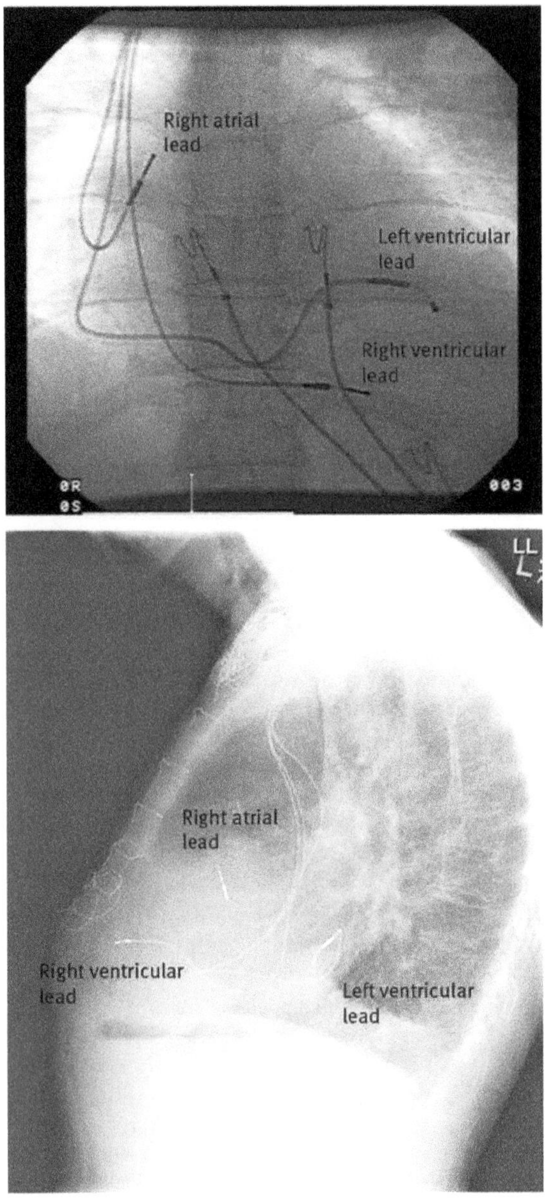

Fig 1 Top: Anteroposterior chest fluoroscopy image showing right ventricular, right atrial, and left ventricular leads (the left ventricular lead is advanced through the coronary sinus and placed in a lateral vein). Bottom: Lateral chest radiograph showing right ventricular, right atrial, and left ventricular leads in position

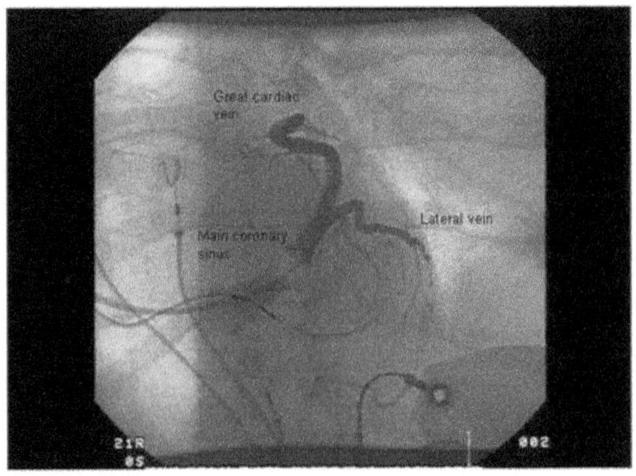

Fig 2 Contrast venogram of coronary sinus showing lateral vein suitable for left ventricular lead placement

with lower mortality resulting from both heart failure and sudden death. Every nine devices implanted (for cardiac resynchronisation) prevented one death and three admissions to hospital over the follow-up period (fig 4).[4 10 11] Morbidity related to the implanted device was uncommon (about 10%), and there was only one death related to the device (this was caused by deteriorating heart failure owing to lead displacement). An economic analysis using a model populated by data from the CARE-HF study showed that cardiac resynchronisation therapy is cost effective, with an estimated cost per quality of life year gained of about £7000 (€7500; $10 000).[12]

Who is suitable for cardiac resynchronisation therapy?

Before the publication of the CARE-HF study, cardiologists tried to select patients most likely to have a symptomatic response. Since the publication of data showing mortality benefits, selection has become much easier.

American and European guidelines recommend cardiac resynchronisation therapy for patients with New York Heart Association (NYHA) classes III and IV heart failure (table), an ejection fraction ≤35%, and a QRS duration of ≥120 ms.[13] Guidelines published by the National Institute for Health and Clinical Excellence (NICE; www.nice.org.uk/TA120), differ slightly and include patients with "recent or persistent" moderate or severe (classes III and IV) heart failure despite optimal drug treatment, and a QRS duration of >150 ms. In the UK, patients with a shorter QRS duration (120-149 ms) should have confirmation of mechanical dyssynchrony by echocardiography. Current UK guidelines also require the presence of sinus rhythm, but patients with atrial fibrillation probably fare no worse than those in sinus rhythm provided that intrinsic conduction can be suppressed pharmacologically or by atrioventricular node ablation.[14] Although randomised controlled trials have focused on patients with left bundle branch block, guidelines do not distinguish between patients with right and left bundle branch block, and patients with right bundle branch block and important symptoms may be considered for biventricular pacing.

Age is unrelated to improvements in mortality and morbidity from heart failure treatments, including cardiac resynchronisation therapy (but not implantable cardioverter defibrillators),[15] so advanced age alone should not affect a decision on whether to refer for possible cardiac resynchronisation therapy.

Electrocardiography, a simple non-invasive test that can be performed and interpreted by non-specialists and

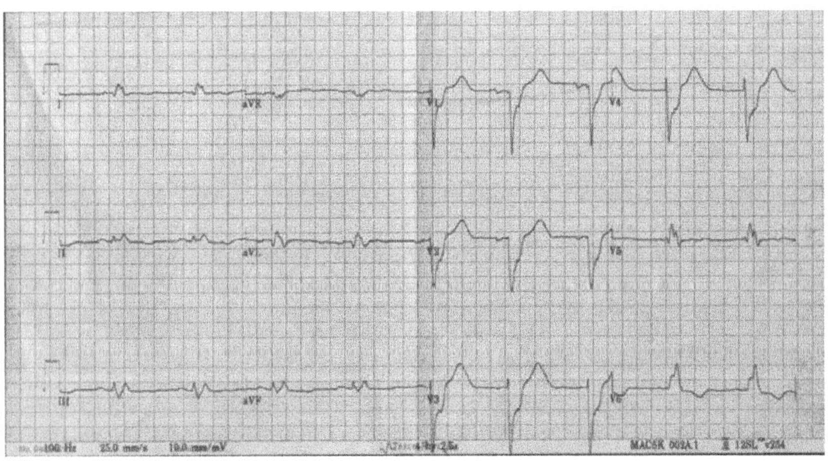

Fig 3 Electrocardiogram showing the characteristic R-R pattern in V5 and V6 of left bundle branch block and a QRS duration of 200 ms in a patient with heart failure

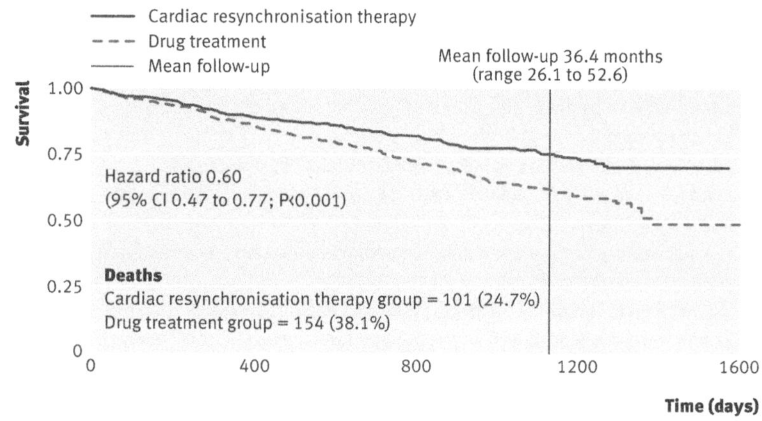

No at risk							
Cardiac resynchronisation therapy	409	383	358	338	209	85	9
Drug treatment	404	372	331	298	178	63	6

Fig 4 Kaplan-Meier curves from the CARE-HF study showing reductions in mortality with cardiac resynchronisation therapy compared with optimal drug treatment. Adapted from Cleland et al[10]

repeated easily, means that non-specialists can screen their patients with chronic heart failure for the potential to benefit from cardiac resynchronisation therapy.

Do all patients with conduction delay benefit from cardiac resynchronisation therapy?

Between 60% and 70% of patients with chronic heart failure who have left bundle branch block show an improvement in symptoms after biventricular pacing. The degree of improvement in any individual is unpredictable, although an improvement by one class of the NYHA classification of heart failure is common.

The consequence of a perceived "failure to respond" of 30-40% before the publication of the CARE-HF study was the development of many echocardiographic measures of mechanical dyssynchrony, which in observational studies seemed to identify patients with a greater likelihood of an improvement in symptoms and cardiac function. None of these measures has proved useful when applied in a larger multicentre trial,[16] probably because the presence of dyssynchrony at baseline identifies patients with a better overall prognosis,[17] because dyssynchrony is not fixed,[18] and because dyssynchrony measures have poor inter-observer reproducibility and cannot be assessed in all subjects.[16] The best predictor of symptomatic response remains a surface electrocardiogram showing a QRS duration of ≥120 ms.

Now that we know that biventricular pacing brings mortality benefits, cardiac resynchronisation therapy also now focuses on mortality and morbidity outcomes (and is no longer just a treatment primarily for symptoms). This shift in indication implies that in any individual it is impossible to say whether they have had no response at all to biventricular pacing, as this might manifest merely as a stabilisation or slowing of the condition (fig 5). Even "non-responders" deteriorate when the device is temporarily switched off, implying an underlying progression of the disease. Hence a failure to improve after cardiac resynchronisation therapy in an individual is not equivalent to a failure to respond. Whether patients with a short QRS duration (<120 ms) experience a mortality benefit from biventricular pacing remains unknown.

The New York Heart Association's classification of symptoms in chronic heart failure

Class	Symptoms
I	No limitation: ordinary physical exercise does not cause undue fatigue, dyspnoea, or palpitations
II	Slight limitation of physical activity: comfortable at rest, but ordinary exercise results in fatigue, palpitations, or dyspnoea
III	Marked limitation of physical activity: comfortable at rest, but less than ordinary activity results in symptoms
IV	Unable to carry out any physical activity without discomfort: symptoms of heart failure are present even at rest, with increased discomfort with any physical activity

What are the complications of cardiac resynchronisation therapy?

Major morbidity and death as a consequence of biventricular pacing are rare. Failure to implant the left ventricular lead is <5% in large series, and lead displacement after successful implantation is about 1%. The course of the left phrenic nerve over the posterolateral wall of the heart occasionally leads to uncomfortable diaphragmatic stimulation. If this is identified during implantation the lead can be repositioned; if it occurs after implantation, the discomfort can often be limited by reprogramming. The serious though uncommon (around 1%) major complication of the procedure—infection and the attendant risks of extraction—is closely related to procedure time and hence to the experience of the cardiologist doing the procedure. Patients with a biventricular pacemaker should not drive for one week after the implantation (one month if combined with an implantable cardioverter defibrillator).

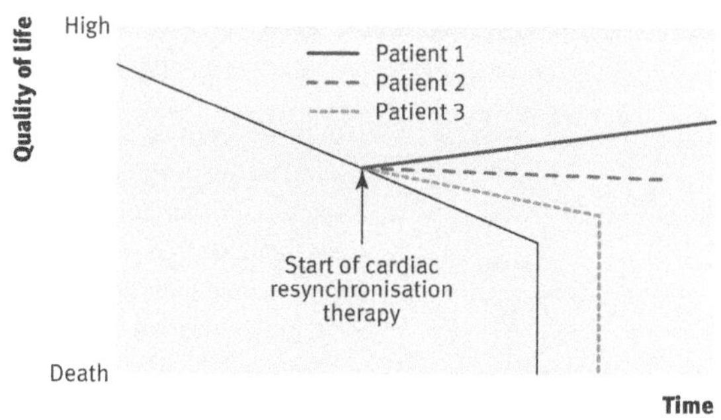

Fig 5 Representation of quality of life in patients with heart failure, showing potential outcomes after cardiac resynchronisation therapy. Patient 1 is a traditional responder, with an improvement in quality of life and prognosis; patients 2 and 3 are patients with no symptomatic improvement, traditionally labelled "failure to respond," but both have prognostic benefits, and symptomatic deterioration is slowed

ADDITIONAL EDUCATIONAL RESOURCES

For patients

- Arrhythmia Alliance (www.heartrhythmcharity.org.uk/)—UK charity with patient orientated information on arrhythmias and their treatment
- Leeds Institute of Genetics, Health and Therapeutics (www.leeds.ac.uk/light/research/cdr/Clinical%20Research%20Section.html)—Information about the Leeds heart failure clinic and research currently under way
- St Jude Medical (www.sjm.com/procedures/procedure.aspx?name=Cardiac+Resynchronization+Therapy+(CRT))—Information about cardiac resynchronisation therapy
- Boston Scientific (www.bostonscientific-international.com/procedure/ProcedureLanding.bsci/,,/navRelId/1000.1002/method/Procedure/id/10084822/seo.serve)—Cardiac pacemaker company with patient information about pacemakers and the implantation procedure

For healthcare professionals

- *Cardiac resynchronisation therapy for the treatment of heart failure* (www.nice.org.uk/Guidance/TA120)—Guidelines from the National Institute for Health and Clinical Excellence
- Medtronic (www.medtronic.com/physician/hf/)—Website by a manufacturer of devices with images and explanations
- Cardiac Network Device Survey Group (www.devicesurvey.com/)—Website providing yearly updated survey of UK implant rates for pacemakers, implantable cardioverter defibrillators, and cardiac resynchronisation therapy

QUESTIONS FOR FURTHER RESEARCH

- Does cardiac resynchronisation therapy improve prognosis in patients with mild chronic heart failure and is the New York Heart Association's classification of heart failure sufficient to identify those who should and should not be offered such therapy?
- Does cardiac resynchronisation therapy improve outcomes in patients with QRS of short duration?
- Should all patients with a standard pacemaker and requiring a high percentage of pacing receive an upgrade at the time they get their pacemaker generator replaced?

TIPS FOR NON-SPECIALISTS

- High risk features in chronic heart failure include more severe (or worsening) symptoms; recent decompensation; left bundle branch block; renal impairment; hypotension (systolic pressure <90 mm Hg)
- Need for increasing amounts of diuretic is a sign of impending or current instability
- Early referral to a heart failure clinic can prevent admission
- Older patients benefit from intensive heart failure therapy as much as younger patients
- Patients intolerant of optimal drug treatment such as β blockers and angiotensin converting enzyme inhibitors will often tolerate higher doses of these after biventricular pacing with additional prognostic and symptomatic benefit

PATIENT'S STORY

In 2002, aged 27, I began to experience shortness of breath and fatigue. I was repeatedly reassured (that I was "out of shape") but I knew something was wrong. I tried to overcome the fatigue by going to the gym more frequently. I was putting on weight rapidly and I felt lazy. I became increasingly depressed. Eventually, I was admitted to hospital, and heart failure was diagnosed.

My care was transferred to the heart failure unit in Toronto, where I was told that I might need a heart transplant. This had a terrible impact on me. I became withdrawn and increasingly frustrated and angry. I lost motivation in my executive career path and I quit my job.

In 2004, I was told I was suitable for a new type of pacemaker (a biventricular pacemaker defibrillator). The implant procedure took place under local anaesthetic. I could feel the doctor's movements and hear him talk. The procedure left a scar about two inches long below my collar bone and a bulge the size of a small cigarette lighter under my skin. Three leads had been placed in my heart, and the device was programmed to improve the heart's function and also give a shock in the event of fast, life threatening irregular heart rhythms.

The improvement was immediate. Within 24 hours, I was able to get up and walk around. For the first time in years, I could sleep without four pillows to keep me upright. It was as though a light switch had been thrown. I actually felt alive again. I enrolled in a cardiac rehabilitation programme and soon I was walking three miles a day and cycling. I finally felt well enough to resume my life and I went back to my job.

During 2007 I received inappropriate shocks from the defibrillator. The cause was a failing pacemaker lead, and this was replaced. However, the fear of further shocks became disabling, and I requested that the defibrillator portion was turned off. I am told my heart function has returned almost to normal.

I'm back at work, doing a fulfilling job I enjoy, and the overall trajectory of my life finally feels right again.Matt Nelson, Canada

Should every patient also receive an implantable cardioverter defibrillator?

The use of implantable cardioverter defibrillators in patients with ischaemic heart disease and severe heart failure without a previous arrhythmic event (primary prevention) remains controversial. Subgroup analysis of large trials suggests mortality benefits from these devices only in patients with mild chronic heart failure (NYHA class I or II). The current NICE guidelines recommend that patients with symptoms "no worse than class III," left ventricular dysfunction (left ventricular ejection fraction <30%), and conduction delay with a QRS duration of >120 ms should receive a cardioverter defibrillator (www.nice.org.uk/Guidance/TA95). The NICE guidelines for cardiac resynchronisation therapy and for implantable cardioverter defibrillators overlap therefore only in patients with class III heart failure. Despite this, many cardiologists think that a single procedure is prudent in patients with class II symptoms as many will deteriorate over the lifetime of the device. Such patients often therefore receive a device capable of both defibrillation and biventricular pacing. In contrast, the decision to implant a cardioverter defibrillator in a patient with class III symptoms must be considered carefully. Although such devices reduce sudden death in these patients, there is an increased frequency of deaths from heart failure, such that overall mortality is unchanged. In addition, implantable cardioverter defibrillators are associated with a higher complication rate than cardiac resynchronisation therapy alone, including inappropriate discharges (with an associated increased mortality[19]) and a higher chance of lead failure. Therefore, frank discussions are needed with patients with NYHA class III symptoms, those aged over 75 years,[20] and those with very poor ventricular function (<10%)[21] about how and where they might like to die.

The findings of three primary prevention trials and a subsequent meta-analysis of use of implantable cardioverter defibrillators in patients with non-ischaemic cardiomyopathy were neutral,[22] and although there was a trend towards improved outcomes in the device arm of non-ischaemic subgroups of larger trials,[4 23] no consensus yet exists on whether these patients should receive implantable cardioverter defibrillators. In patients tolerating high dose β blockade, particularly young patients in whom lead complications and inappropriate discharges are more frequent, biventricular pacing alone might be sufficient.

What about patients with existing pacemakers?

Left ventricular dysfunction and heart failure are common in patients with standard right ventricular pacemakers.[24] Right ventricular pacing induces dyssynchrony that is the same as that seen with intrinsic left bundle branch block[25] and can induce new or worsen existing left ventricular dysfunction. The risk of hospital admission for heart failure is directly related to the percentage of paced beats required.[26] No randomised controlled trial of upgrading right ventricular pacemakers to biventricular pacemakers has been performed, but the frequency and magnitude of increases in left ventricular ejection fraction and improvements in symptoms are the same in patients with previous right ventricular pacemakers as in those with intrinsic left bundle branch block.[25]

Are the indications for cardiac resynchronisation therapy expanding?

The UK indications for cardiac resynchronisation therapy are likely to broaden in the future to include patients with a QRS duration of ≥120 ms whether or not there is echocardiographic dyssynchrony.[27] Patients with less severe heart failure symptoms (NYHA classes I and II) have improvements in left ventricular function and exercise capacity of a similar magnitude to those in patients with NYHA classes III and IV symptoms,[28] and the relative risk reduction from cardiac resynchronisation therapy in the CARE-HF study was larger in patients with less severe heart failure.[29] Further, severity and nature of symptoms at baseline do not seem to be a good marker of prognostic benefit.[30 31] The MADIT-CRT study examining "early" cardiac resynchronisation therapy in patients with mild or no symptoms of heart failure and who are also having a cardioverter defibrillator implanted has completed recruitment and will report in 2009. Symptoms may soon be less frequently used to identify patients suitable for biventricular pacing. Randomised studies with hard end points are needed in patients with a QRS duration of <120 ms.

Who should refer patients for possible cardiac resynchronisation therapy and when?

All individuals involved in the care of patients with chronic heart failure must be aware of the indications, potential benefits, and cost effectiveness[12] of device therapy. A systematic approach to the long term follow-up of patients with chronic heart failure both in the community and by general physicians is required to identify patients needing treatment in a timely fashion. Mortality after hospital admission with heart failure is particularly high. Patients with a recent or persistent episode of moderate or severe heart failure should have 12 lead electrocardiography at follow-up and those with a QRS duration of ≥120 ms (three or more small squares on a standard recording at 25 mm/s) should be referred for consideration of cardiac resynchronisation therapy. Patients with chronic heart failure who are not initially considered suitable for biventricular pacing should be reassessed with electrocardiography after each exacerbation, or yearly if stable, as conduction delay develops as chronic heart failure progresses.[3]

Contributors: Both authors wrote the article; KKAW is the guarantor.

Competing interests: KKAW has received research funding and speaker's honorariums from Medtronic and Boston Scientific, which manufacture cardiac resynchronisation devices.

Provenance and peer review: Commissioned; externally peer reviewed

Patient consent obtained.

1 Cowie MR, Mosterd A, Wood DA. The epidemiology of heart failure. *Eur Heart J* 1997;18:208-25.
2 Khan NK, Goode KM, Cleland JG, Rigby AS, Freemantle N, Eastaugh J, et al. Prevalence of ECG abnormalities in an international survey of patients with suspected or confirmed heart failure at death or discharge. *Eur J Heart Fail* 2007;9:491-501.
3 Clark AL, Goode K, Cleland JG. The prevalence and incidence of left bundle branch block in ambulant patients with chronic heart failure. *Eur J Heart Fail* 2008;10:696-702.
4 Bristow MR, Saxon LA, Boehmer J, Krueger S, Kass DA, de Marco T, et al. Cardiac-resynchronization therapy with or without an implantable defibrillator in advanced chronic heart failure. *N Engl J Med* 2004;350:2140-50.
5 Witte KK, Sasson Z, Persaud JA, Jolliffe R, Wald RW, Parker JD. Biventricular pacing: impact on exercise-induced increases in mitral insufficiency in patients with chronic heart failure. *Can J Cardiol* 2008;24:379-84.
6 Abraham WT, Fisher WG, Smith AL, Delurgio DB, Leon AR, Loh E, et al. Cardiac resynchronization in chronic heart failure. *N Engl J Med* 2002;346:1845-53.
7 Young JB, Abraham WT, Smith AL, Leon AR, Lieberman R, Wilkoff B, et al. Combined cardiac resynchronization and implantable cardioversion defibrillation in advanced chronic heart failure: the MIRACLE-ICD Trial. *JAMA* 2003;289:2685-94.
8 Cazeau S, Leclercq C, Lavergne T, Walker S, Varma C, Linde C. Effects of multisite biventricular pacing in patients with heart failure and intraventricular conduction delay. *N Engl J Med* 2001;344:873-80.
9 Freemantle N, Tharmanathan P, Calvert MJ, Abraham WT, Ghosh J, Cleland JG. Cardiac resynchronisation for patients with heart failure due to left ventricular systolic dysfunction—a systematic review and meta-analysis. *Eur J Heart Fail* 2006;8:433-40.
10 Cleland JG, Daubert JC, Erdmann E, Freemantle N, Gras D, Kappenberger L, et al. The effect of cardiac resynchronization on morbidity and mortality in heart failure. *N Engl J Med* 2005;352:1539-49.
11 Cleland JG, Daubert JC, Erdmann E, Freemantle N, Gras D, Kappenberger L, et al. Longer-term effects of cardiac resynchronization therapy on mortality in heart failure [the CArdiac REsynchronization-Heart Failure (CARE-HF) trial extension phase]. *Eur Heart J* 2006;27:1928-32.
12 Yao G, Freemantle N, Calvert MJ, Bryan S, Daubert JC, Cleland JG. The long-term cost-effectiveness of cardiac resynchronization therapy with or without an implantable cardioverter-defibrillator. *Eur Heart J* 2007;28:42-51.
13 Task Force for Diagnosis and Treatment of Acute and Chronic Heart Failure 2008 of European Society of Cardiology, Dickstein K, Cohen-Solal A, Filippatos G, McMurray JJ, Ponikowski P, et al. ESC guidelines for the diagnosis and treatment of acute and chronic heart failure 2008: the Task Force for the Diagnosis and Treatment of Acute and Chronic Heart Failure 2008 of the European Society of Cardiology. Developed in collaboration with the Heart Failure Association of the ESC (HFA) and endorsed by the European Society of Intensive Care Medicine (ESICM). *Eur Heart J* 2008;29:2388-442
14 Upadhyay GA, Choudhry NK, Auricchio A, Ruskin J, Singh JP. Cardiac resynchronization in patients with atrial fibrillation: a meta-analysis of prospective cohort studies. *J Am Coll Cardiol* 2008;52:1239-46.
15 Foley PW, Chalil S, Khadjooi K, Smith RE, Frenneaux MP, Leyva F. Long-term effects of cardiac resynchronization therapy in octogenarians: a comparative study with a younger population. *Europace* 2008;10:1302-7.
16 Chung ES, Leon AR, Tavazzi L, Sun JP, Nihoyannopoulos P, Merlino J, et al. Results of the Predictors of Response to CRT (PROSPECT) trial. *Circulation* 2008;117:2608-16.
17 Cleland J, Freemantle N, Ghio S, Fruhwald F, Shankar A, Marijanowski M, et al. Predicting the long-term effects of cardiac resynchronization therapy on mortality from baseline variables and the early response. A report from the CARE-HF (Cardiac Resynchronization in Heart Failure) Trial. *J Am Coll Cardiol* 2008;52:438-45.
18 Chattopadhyay S, Alamgir MF, Nikitin NP, Fraser AG, Clark AL, Cleland JG. The effect of pharmacological stress on intraventricular dyssynchrony in left ventricular systolic dysfunction. *Eur J Heart Fail* 2008;10:412-20.
19 Daubert JP, Zareba W, Cannom DS, McNitt S, Rosero SZ, Wang P, et al. Inappropriate implantable cardioverter-defibrillator shocks in MADIT II: frequency, mechanisms, predictors, and survival impact. *J Am Coll Cardiol* 2008;51:1357-65.
20 Healey JS, Hallstrom AP, Kuck KH, Nair G, Schron EP, Roberts RS, et al. Role of the implantable defibrillator among elderly patients with a history of life-threatening ventricular arrhythmias. *Eur Heart J* 2007;28:1746-9.
21 Yap YG, Duong T, Bland JM, Malik M, Torp-Pedersen C, Køber L, et al. Optimising the dichotomy limit for left ventricular ejection fraction in selecting patients for defibrillator therapy after myocardial infarction. *Heart* 2007;93:832-6.
22 Desai AS, Fang JC, Maisel WH, Baughman KL. Implantable defibrillators for the prevention of mortality in patients with nonischemic cardiomyopathy: a meta-analysis of randomized controlled trials. *JAMA* 2004;292:2874-9.
23 Bardy GH, Lee KL, Mark DB, Poole JE, Packer DL, Boineau R, et al. Amiodarone or an implantable cardioverter-defibrillator for congestive heart failure. *N Engl J Med* 2005;352:225-37.
24 Thackray SD, Witte KK, Nikitin NP, Clark AL, Kaye GC, Cleland JG. The prevalence of heart failure and asymptomatic left ventricular systolic dysfunction in a typical regional pacemaker population. *Eur Heart J* 2003;24:1143-52.
25 Witte KK, Pipes RR, Nanthakumar K, Parker JD. Biventricular pacemaker upgrade in previously paced heart failure patients—

improvements in ventricular dyssynchrony. *J Cardiol Fail* 2006;12:199-204.

26 Sweeney MO, Hellkamp AS, Ellenbogen KA, Greenspon AJ, Freedman RA, Lee KL, et al. Adverse effect of ventricular pacing on heart failure and atrial fibrillation among patients with normal baseline QRS duration in a clinical trial of pacemaker therapy for sinus node dysfunction. *Circulation* 2003;107:2932-7.

27 Beshai JF, Grimm RA, Nagueh SF, Baker JH 2nd, Beau SL, Greenberg SM, et al. Cardiac-resynchronization therapy in heart failure with narrow QRS complexes. *N Engl J Med* 2007;357:2461-71.

28 Linde C, Abraham WT, Gold MR, St John Sutton M, Ghio S, Daubert C, et al. Randomized trial of cardiac resynchronization in mildly symptomatic heart failure patients and in asymptomatic patients with left ventricular dysfunction and previous heart failure symptoms. *J Am Coll Cardiol* 2008;52:1834-43.

29 Uretsky BF, Thygesen K, Daubert JC, Erdmann E, Freemantle N, Gras D, et al. Predictors of mortality from pump failure and sudden cardiac death in patients with systolic heart failure and left ventricular dyssynchrony: results of the CARE-HF trial. *J Cardiol Fail* 2008;14:670-5.

30 Witte KK, Clark AL. Dyspnoea versus fatigue: Additional prognostic information from symptoms in chronic heart failure? *Eur J Heart Fail* 2008;10:1224-8.

31 Cleland JG, Freemantle N, Daubert JC, Toff WD, Leisch F, Tavazzi L. Long-term effect of cardiac resynchronisation in patients reporting mild symptoms of heart failure: a report from the CARE-HF study. *Heart* 2008;94:278-83.

Degenerative aortic stenosis

Radhakrishnan Ramaraj, resident physician[1], Vincent L Sorrell, professor of clinical medicine and radiology, and Allan C Hudson and Helen Lovaas chair of cardiac imaging[2]

[1]Department of Internal Medicine, Section of Cardiology, Sarver Heart Center, University of Arizona College of Medicine, 1501, N Campbell Avenue, Tucson, AZ 85724, USA

[2]Section of Cardiology, Sarver Heart Center, University of Arizona College of Medicine

Correspondence to: R Ramaraj drkutty2@gmail.com

Cite this as: *BMJ* 2008;336:550-5

‹DOI› 10.1136/bmj.39478.498819.AD
http://www.bmj.com/content/336/7643/550

Aortic stenosis is the most common valvular lesion in Europe and North America. It primarily presents as calcific aortic stenosis in 2-7% of the population aged ›65 years.[1] About 80% of adult patients with symptomatic aortic stenosis are male. As 1-2% of the population is born with a congenital bicuspid aortic valve and populations are ageing, aortic stenosis is becoming more common. By 2020, about 3.5 million people in England are expected to have aortic sclerosis and 150000 will have severe aortic stenosis.[2] Here we provide an overview to help diagnosis and a summary of the management of AS and its sequelae. Many of the points made in this review are based on randomised controlled trials. However, observational studies and the guideline recommendations of the American Heart Association and the American College of Cardiology and of the European Society of Cardiology are also included to provide comprehensive overviews that are beyond the scope of this article.

What are the factors leading to aortic stenosis?

The most common cause of aortic stenosis in adults is calcification of a normal trileaflet (fig 1). Calcific aortic stenosis is thought to be a degenerative process that shares many features with coronary artery disease, such as lipid accumulation, inflammation, and calcification. The abnormal architecture of the bicuspid or unicuspid aortic valve makes the leaflets susceptible to haemodynamic stress, leading to valvular thickening, calcification, and increased rigidity and narrowing of the aortic orifice.

Aortic stenosis may also be secondary to rheumatic inflammation of the valve leaflets. Investigators have found histological similarities between the lesion of aortic stenosis and atheromatous coronary artery disease and have documented an association between traditional atherosclerotic risk factors and the development of calcific aortic valve disease.[3] Mature lamellar bone formation and osteopontin bone expression are present in calcified aortic valves. Researchers have also shown that hypercholesterolaemia can induce both cellular proliferation and osteoblast phenotype expression that may lead to progression of aortic valvular disease.[4]

How is the haemodynamic severity of aortic stenosis classified?

In 2006 the American Heart Association and the American College of Cardiology jointly provided the guidelines in grading aortic stenosis (box 1) as mild, moderate, and severe (figs 2 and 3) (see www.americanheart.org.)[5]

Recently, the European Society of Cardiology (ESC) has also published guidelines (a summary is at www.escardio.org).[6] Aortic stenosis produces a systolic gradient between the left ventricular outflow tract and the aorta. Aortic sclerosis is distinguished from aortic stenosis by the valve thickening and calcification without obstruction (no significant gradient) (fig 1). However, 16% of patients with aortic sclerosis will progress to aortic stenosis in seven years time.[7]

How do we diagnose aortic stenosis?

Clinical diagnosis

The patient's history and physical examination are essential in diagnosing aortic stenosis. Identifying symptoms such as exertional shortness of breath, angina, dizziness, or syncope is important for proper management. The characteristic systolic murmur guides further diagnostic investigations. An early peaking murmur is usually associated with a less stenotic valve, whereas a late peaking murmur has a more severe degree of stenosis. This is because a more stenotic valve takes longer for the ventricle to generate the pressures needed to force the blood past the lesion. Occasionally, the murmur may be faint and primary presentation may be heart failure of unknown cause. The disappearance of the second aortic sound is specific to severe aortic stenosis, although not a sensitive sign.[7] The murmur of aortic

SOURCES AND SELECTION CRITERIA

The literature search included Medline and PubMed from 2003 to the present. The terms searched were "aortic stenosis", "diagnosis", "aortic valve replacement", and "grading" in various combinations. We scrutinised the articles identified by this search and selected high quality randomised controlled trials and retrospective studies. We examined citation lists from these for further relevant articles. To identify the factors contributing to aortic stenosis, we did a complete search of the Medline database. When appropriate, we also considered publications from before 2003. We included some review articles, websites, and book chapters because they provide comprehensive overviews that are beyond the scope of this article.

SUMMARY POINTS

- Although aortic stenosis is common, its diagnosis may be missed
- Calcific aortic stenosis shares many common features with atherosclerosis
- After the onset of symptoms, the average survival is two to three years, and patients with symptoms of syncope, angina, and dyspnoea need prompt aortic valve replacement
- Endocarditis prophylaxis is indicated in all patients with aortic stenosis
- Echocardiography should be performed once aortic stenosis is suspected.
- Coronary artery angiography is usually needed before aortic valve replacement, except in young patients
- Careful exercise testing should be considered in asymptomatic patients with severe aortic stenosis who are sedentary or unable to give a clear history

BOX 1 GRADING OF AORTIC STENOSIS[5]

Mild stenosis

- Area ›1.5 cm^2
- Mean gradient ‹25 mm Hg
- Aortic jet velocity ‹3 m/s

Moderate stenosis

- Area 1.0-1.5 cm^2
- Mean gradient 25-40 mm Hg
- Aortic jet velocity 3-4 m/s

Severe stenosis

- Area ‹1.0 cm^2
- Mean gradient ›40 mm Hg
- Aortic jet velocity ›4 m/s

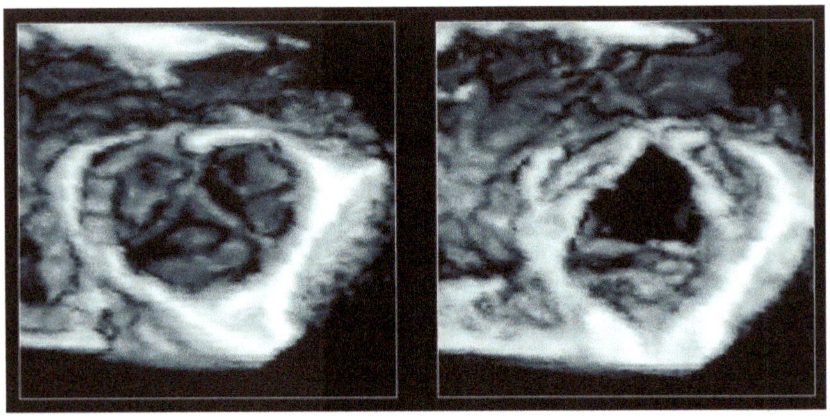

Fig 1 Three dimensional transoesophageal echocardiographic image at the level of the tricuspid aortic valve, displayed from the perspective of the aortic root (looking into the left ventricular cavity) in a patient with a widely patent trileaflet aortic valve (left panel shows diastole, right panel shows systole)

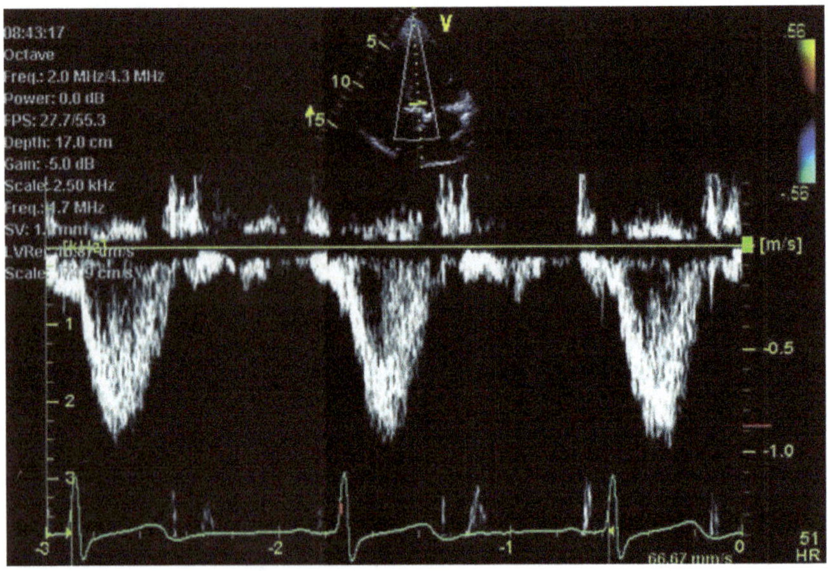

Fig 2 Pulsed wave Doppler echocardiogram in patient with severe aortic stenosis: transthoracic, two dimensional, apical, five chamber view (inset). A pulsed wave Doppler region of interest (sample volume) is placed proximal to the stenotic aortic valve in the left ventricular outflow tract, and the spectral display is shown. At 1.0 m/s, the blood flow velocity in the left ventricular outflow tract is equivalent to a gradient of 4 mm Hg

stenosis is often "missed" (or not understood for what it is) in many patients, especially in those who are obese or have underlying obstructive lung diseases (where the murmur is muffled) and in those with left ventricular dysfunction (where the murmur is blunted).

Radiological diagnosis

Echocardiography has become the key diagnostic tool to confirm the presence of aortic stenosis; assess the degree of valve calcification, left ventricular function, and wall thickness; detect the presence of other associated valve disease; and provide prognostic information. Doppler echocardiography is the preferred technique for assessing severity. Aortic stenosis with a valve area <1.0 cm² is considered severe; however, when patients have unusually small or large body surface area, a cut-off value of 0.6 cm²/m² is helpful.[8]

What is the natural course of aortic stenosis?

The process of maintaining cardiac output against the aortic stenosis gradient leads to left ventricular hypertrophy. Increased muscle mass of the left ventricle raises myocardial oxygen consumption. In severe aortic stenosis, even in the absence of narrowing of the coronary arteries, the increased stress on the left ventricular wall and workload demands, coupled with direct ventricular pressure compressing the coronary arteries during diastolic flow, may exceed adequate coronary perfusion pressure and cause myocardial ischaemia and angina. Left ventricular diastolic dysfunction is widespread, and left ventricular systolic dysfunction is not uncommon; both these conditions produce symptoms of congestive cardiac failure.

After the onset of symptoms, the average survival is only two to three years. On the basis of the data obtained at postmortem examination in patients not treated surgically, the average time to death after the onset of various symptoms was as follows: angina, three years; syncope, three years; dyspnoea, two years; and congestive cardiac failure, one and a half to two years. Conversely, asymptomatic patients even with severe aortic stenosis have an excellent prognosis without aortic valve replacement. However, the duration of the asymptomatic phase varies widely among individuals. Unfortunately, at least 1-2% of asymptomatic patients die suddenly or have very rapid rate of progression to symptomatic stage and then to sudden death.[9] Among patients with congenital or degenerative disease, progression to valve replacement occurs earliest if the patient has a unicuspid valve, later in the case of a bicuspid valve, and latest with a tricuspid valve.

What are the medical treatments for aortic stenosis?

When symptoms develop, mortality rises sharply, so standard therapeutic guidelines recommend surgery.[5] [6] No effective drug treatment exists for severe aortic stenosis, and only a few drugs are available to alleviate symptoms. Patients with evidence of pulmonary congestion can benefit from cautious treatment with digitalis or diuretics, or both. A recent observational, drug withdrawal, single blinded study, with randomisation of the order of tests supports the concept that angiotensin converting enzyme inhibitors are safe and may provide short term benefit to patients with aortic stenosis.[10] In patients with aortic stenosis, the afterload reduction caused by angiotensin converting enzyme inhibitors is partially blunted by a parallel increase in the transvalvular pressure gradient. However, angiotensin converting enzyme inhibitors favourably affect stress haemodynamic variables in most hypertensive patients with aortic stenosis. A prospective, single blinded study conducted at Cleveland clinic, Ohio, showed that in patients with acute pulmonary oedema, left ventricular systolic dysfunction, and aortic stenosis nitroprusside infusion may help to reduce congestion and improve symptoms.[11] Atrial fibrillation has an adverse effect on atrial pump function and ventricular rate, hence prompt cardioversion is beneficial. Endocarditis prophylaxis is indicated in all patients with aortic stenosis.[12]

No medical treatment has been proved to prevent or delay the disease process in the aortic valve leaflets. The association of aortic stenosis with clinical features similar to atherosclerosis has led to the hypothesis that aggressive modification of risk factors, as for coronary heart disease, may slow or prevent disease progression in the valve leaflets. Despite this hope, recent reports using statins have shown mixed results: one study failed to show a beneficial effect,[13] whereas another study showed that rosuvastatin can slow the haemodynamic progression of aortic stenosis.[14]

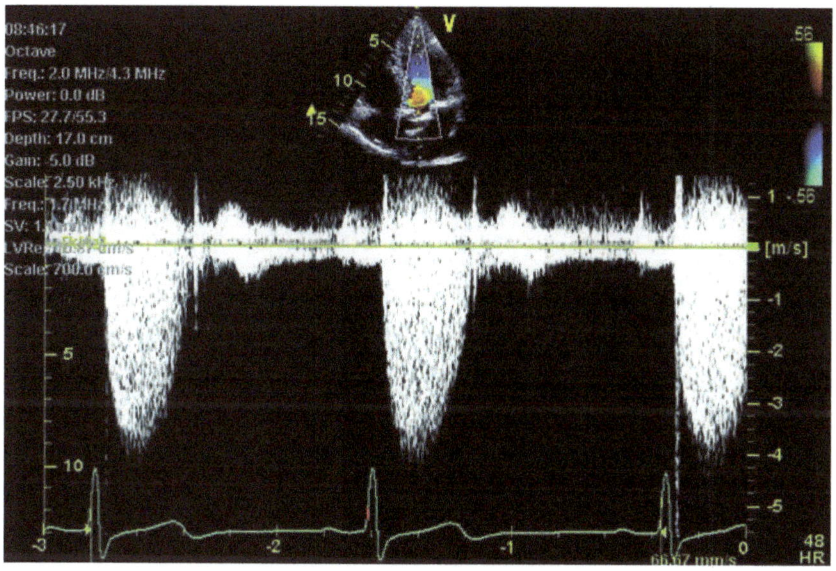

Fig 3 Continuous wave Doppler echocardiogram in patient with severe aortic stenosis (same patient as in figure 2). Transthoracic, two dimensional, apical, five chamber view (inset). A continuous wave Doppler records the maximal velocity across the narrowest point of the stenotic aortic valve and the spectral display is shown. The ratio of the velocity of the blood flow in the left ventricular outflow tract (1 m/s) to the aortic jet velocity (4.5 m/s) is <0.25, which is consistent with severe aortic stenosis

BOX 2 JOINT RECOMMENDATIONS OF AMERICAN HEART ASSOCIATION AND AMERICAN COLLEGE OF CARDIOLOGY FOR AORTIC VALVE REPLACEMENT IN PATIENTS WITH AORTIC STENOSIS[5]

Aortic valve replacement indicated

- In patients with severe aortic stenosis with its classic "SAD" symptoms (syncope, angina, and/or dyspnoea
- In patients with severe aortic stenosis who are having coronary artery bypass grafting
- In patients with severe aortic stenosis having surgery on the aorta or other heart valves
- In patients with severe aortic stenosis with left ventricular systolic dysfunction (ejection fraction <50%)

Aortic valve replacement possibly indicated

- In patients with moderate aortic stenosis having coronary artery bypass grafting or surgery on the aorta or other heart valves
- In patients with asymptomatic severe aortic stenosis with abnormal response to exercise (such as development of symptoms or asymptomatic hypotension)
- In patients with asymptomatic severe aortic stenosis if there is likelihood of rapid progression (age, calcification, and coronary artery disease) or if surgery might be delayed at the time of symptom onset
- In patients with mild aortic stenosis having coronary artery bypass grafting when there is evidence of moderate to severe calcification, suggesting that progression is likely and may be rapid
- In patients with asymptomatic extreme severe aortic stenosis (aortic valve area <0.6 cm², mean gradient >60 mm Hg, or a jet velocity >5 m/s) when the patient's expected operative mortality is ≤1%

What is the definitive treatment for aortic stenosis?

Aortic stenosis is a mechanical obstruction, hence requires mechanical correction. Studies have shown that once symptoms develop, a patient's life span is severely shortened unless the valve is replaced (fig 4). In contrast, age corrected 10 year survival rates among patients who had surgery for aortic valve replacement approach the survival rate in the normal population.[16] Therefore, in the absence of any serious comorbid conditions, aortic valve replacement is indicated in virtually all symptomatic patients with severe aortic stenosis, even in very elderly people.[5] Balloon valvuloplasty is not recommended in adults but can be used as a bridge to surgery in haemodynamically unstable patients who are at high risk of surgery or in patients with

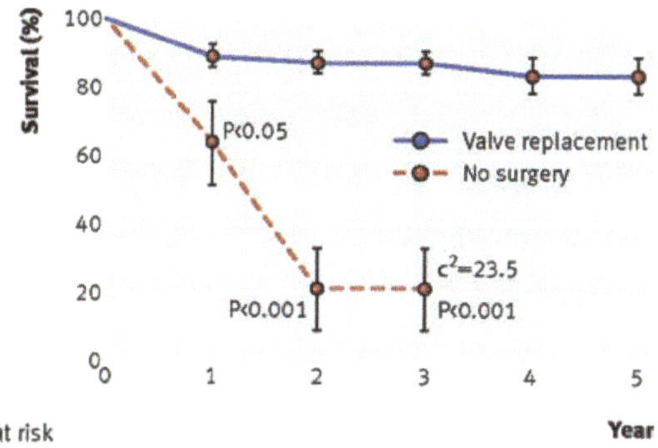

No at risk						
Valve replacement	125	87	51	35	9	0
No surgery	19	8	2	1	0	0

Fig 4 Kaplan-Meier survival curve for patients with severe symptomatic aortic stenosis who had valve replacement and similar patients who declined surgery. Adapted from Schwarz F et al[15]

BOX 3 RECOMMENDATIONS OF EUROPEAN SOCIETY OF CARDIOLOGY FOR FOLLOW-UP IN PATIENTS WITH AORTIC STENOSIS[6]

- Follow-up visits should include echocardiographic assessment
- Patients with moderate to severe calcification of the valve and peak aortic jet velocity >4 m/s should be re-evaluated every six months
- If peak aortic jet velocity increases by >0.3 m/s per year or if other evidence of haemodynamic progression is present, surgery should be considered
- If the patient remains asymptomatic, clinical re-evaluations every six months and echocardiographic re-evaluations every six to 12 months are recommended

symptomatic severe aortic stenosis who require urgent, major non-cardiac surgery.[6]

Most patients aged >40-45 years require coronary angiography before aortic valve replacement to exclude coexistent coronary artery disease. Grading or reconfirmation of aortic stenosis is also possible during this procedure if the diagnosis remains uncertain after echocardiography. About 40% of patients having aortic valve replacement have severe coronary artery disease and require concurrent coronary bypass grafting. Preliminary reports show that percutaneous aortic valve replacement is feasible, but this procedure is not often done yet and further studies are needed to evaluate its potential role.[17] Asymptomatic patients with severe aortic stenosis generally have an excellent prognosis without aortic valve replacement. In patients with left ventricular dysfunction and severe aortic stenosis, the outcome after replacement surgery is excellent despite the presence of a reduced ejection fraction preoperatively.[18] Excessive afterload may contribute to the left ventricular dysfunction, which often returns to normal once obstruction is relieved.

Is age a contraindication for aortic valve replacement?

A prospective Swedish study and an observational study show that aortic valve replacement improves symptoms and survival in patients with severe aortic stenosis.[16 18] Age is not a contraindication to surgery, with studies showing similar outcomes to those in age matched normal subjects in very elderly people. The operative risks can be estimated with readily available and a well validated online risk calculator from the European System for Cardiac Operative Risk Evaluation (www.euroscore.org).[19] Indications for aortic

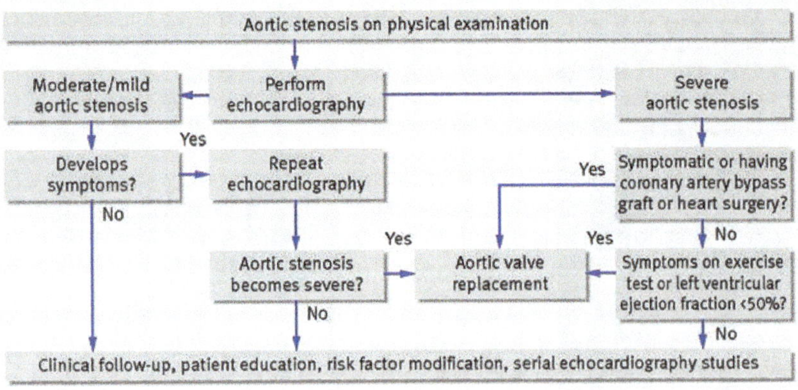

Fig 5 Proposed algorithm of treatment of aortic stenosis based on 2006 guidelines of American Heart Association and American College of Cardiology for management of patients with valvular heart disease

TIPS FOR NON-SPECIALISTS

- Careful physical examination of elderly patients can help to identify aortic stenosis
- Use SAD criteria (syncope, angina, and dyspnoea) to evaluate symptoms
- Aortic valve replacement is indicated for symptomatic aortic stenosis, regardless of age, and can save lives
- Aortic valve replacement is not indicated in the absence of symptoms
- An early peaking murmur is usually associated with a less stenotic valve, whereas a late peaking murmur has a more severe degree of stenosis
- The murmur of critical aortic stenosis is soft when the patient has left ventricular dysfunction
- Perform echocardiography whenever aortic stenosis is considered, and repeat according to onset or progression of symptoms
- Coronary angiography is usually needed before aortic valve replacement, except in young patients
- Endocarditis prophylaxis is indicated in all patients with aortic stenosis

ADDITIONAL EDUCATIONAL RESOURCES

- Joint guidelines from the American Heart Association and the American College of Cardiology and guidelines from the European Society of Cardiology for the treatment of valvular heart diseases are available at www.americanheart.org and www.escardio.org respectively
- Article on aortic stenosis from cardiology department in Cleveland clinic, Ohio, at www.clevelandclinicmeded.com

UNANSWERED RESEARCH QUESTIONS

- Does calcific aortic valve stenosis have an active process of progression, similar to atherosclerosis, that medical treatment may be proved to modify?
- Can lifestyle modifications or the use of hydroxymethylglutaryl coenzyme A reductase inhibitors (statins) retard the progression of aortic stenosis?
- Do patients with asymptomatic mild or moderate aortic stenosis who are having cardiac surgery need valve replacement?
- Given the low operative mortality, will elective aortic valve replacement ever be recommended for asymptomatic severe aortic stenosis to reduce subsequent morbidity and mortality?

ONGOING RESEARCH

Some of the many trials currently testing the effects of statins in aortic valve disease are listed below.

- *STOP-AS*—Stop aortic stenosis (Cleveland Clinic, Cleveland, Ohio, USA)
- *SEAS*—Simvastatin and the ezetimibe in aortic stenosis (Europe)
- *ASTRONOMER*—Aortic stenosis progression observation measuring effects of rosuvastatin (Canada)

BOX 4 PREDICTORS OF PROGRESSION OF AORTIC STENOSIS[6]

Clinical

- Older age
- Atherosclerotic risk factors

Echocardiography

- Valve calcification
- Peak aortic jet velocity (increase of 0.3 m/s per year)
- Decrease in left ventricular ejection fraction
- Haemodynamic progression
- Increase in gradient with exercise

Exercise testing

- Development of symptoms on exercise testing
- Abnormal blood pressure response
- ST segment depression

valve replacement (fig 5) are given in the guidelines of the American Heart Association and the American College of Cardiology (box 2)[5] and of the European Society of Cardiology.[6] Doppler echocardiography should be done for the initial evaluation of patients suspected of having aortic stenosis, as well as in patients with established disease if symptoms develop or physical signs change. Box 3 outlines the European Society of Cardiology's recommendations for follow-up in patients with aortic stenosis.

How can the progression of aortic stenosis be predicted?

The rate of progression of aortic stenosis in an individual patient cannot be predicted but is reportedly more rapid in patients with degenerative calcific disease than in those with congenital or rheumatic disease. Some studies suggest that the rate of haemodynamic progression is faster when the patient is aged over 50 years and has severe calcification or concurrent coronary heart disease.[20] Preliminary studies have shown that natriuretic peptides predict symptom-free survival in aortic stenosis.[21] Box 4 summarises the predictors of the progression of aortic stenosis and therefore of poor outcome in asymptomatic patients.[6]

The presence of low cardiac output may lead clinicians to an incorrect assessment of the severity of the aortic stenosis. Patients with low cardiac output usually have small aortic valve areas (suggesting severe aortic stenosis) but also low aortic valve gradients (suggesting a mild or moderate condition). This discrepancy can be distinguished by recalculating the valve area after increasing cardiac contractility with inotropic stimulation (usually dobutamine). Truly severe aortic stenosis shows only small changes in valve area (increase $<0.2\ cm^2$) with increasing flow rate but a substantialincrease in gradients (mean gradient >50 mm Hg). "Pseudosevere" aortic stenosis, however, shows a marked increase in valve area but only minor changes in gradients.[22] Patients with true severe aortic stenosis benefit from aortic valve replacement, but those with pseudosevere aortic stenosis would not benefit and could be harmed. Decreased contractile response (<20% of stroke volume) to inotropic infusion indicates a very poor clinical outcome and high mortality.

Conclusion

Clinicians should aim to diagnose aortic stenosis early in the physical examination, to document the severity with echocardiography while the patient is apparently asymptomatic, and try to predict whether the patient has the highest likelihood of developing symptoms. Elective surgery should be planned at the earliest onset of symptoms and requires careful clinical observation. When the history is unclear or the patient is sedentary, carefully supervised exercise tests should be done to identify the early onset of cardinal symptoms. As explained earlier, age is not a contraindication to aortic valve replacement.

Differences between the European and the US guidelines*

- Mild, moderate, and severe aortic stenosis are defined in the US guidelines, but only severe and moderate aortic stenosis are defined in the European guidelines
- The US guidelines recommend follow-up of patients with aortic stenosis as below, but the European guidelines are different (see box 3):
  - In patients with severe aortic stenosis, echocardiography every year may be appropriate
  - In patients with moderate aortic stenosis, serial studies every one to two years are satisfactory
  - Inpatients with mild AS, serial studies can be performed every 3 to 5 years.
- The US guidelines do not recommend using balloon valvuloplasty in adults because of high rate of complications (>10%) and restenosis. But the European guidelines recommend balloon valvuloplasty in certain circumstances, such as in haemodynamically unstable patients who are at high risk surgically or in patients with symptomatic severe aortic stenosis who require urgent, major non-cardiac surgery

*The guidelines of the European Society of Cardiology, and the joint guidelines of the American Heart Association and American College of Cardiology.Contributors: Both authors conceived and designed the article. RR did the literature search and wrote the article. VLS revised the article critically for important intellectual content and also added important figures. Parkavi Chellappa helped to revise the article and suggested modifications for the article. Both authors approved the final version of the manuscript. RR is the guarantor.

Funding: No specific funding.

Competing interests: None declared.

Provenance and peer review: Not commissioned; externally peer reviewed.

1 Lung B, Baron G, Butchart EG, Delahaye F, GohLke-Barwolf C, Levang OW, et al. A prospective survey of patients with valvular heart disease in Europe: the Euro heart survey on valvular heart disease. *Eur Heart J* 2003;24:1231-43.
2 Chambers J. Aortic stenosis. *BMJ* 2005;330:801-2.
3 Glader CA, Birgander LS, Söderberg S, Ildgruben HP, Saikku P, Waldenström A, et al. Lipoprotein(a), Chlamydia pneumoniae, leptin and tissue plasminogen activator as risk marker for valvular aortic stenosis. *Eur Heart J* 2003;24:198-208.
4 Chan KL. Is aortic stenosis a preventable disease? *J Am Coll Cardiol* 2003;42:593-9.
5 American College of Cardiology/American Heart Association Task Force on Practice Guidelines, Society of Cardiovascular Anesthesiologists, Society for Cardiovascular Angiography and Interventions, Society of Thoracic Surgeons, et al. ACC/AHA 2006 guidelines for the management of patients with valvular heart disease: a report of the American College of Cardiology/American Heart Association Task Force on Practice Guidelines (writing committee to revise the 1998 Guidelines for the Management of Patients With Valvular Heart Disease): developed in collaboration with the Society of Cardiovascular Anesthesiologists: endorsed by the Society for Cardiovascular Angiography and Interventions and the Society of Thoracic Surgeons. *Circulation* 2006;114:e84-231
6 Vahanian A, Baumgartner H, Bax J, Butchart E, Dion R, Filippatos G, et al. Guidelines on the management of valvular heart disease: the Task Force on the Management of Valvular Heart Disease of the European Society of Cardiology. *Eur Heart J* 2007;28:230-68.
7 Cosmi JE, Kort S, Tunick PA, Rosenzweig BP, Freedberg RS, Katz ES, et al. The risk of the development of aortic stenosis in patients with "benign" aortic valve thickening. *Arch Intern Med* 2002;162:2345-7.
8 Quinones MA, Otto CM, Stoddard M, Waggoner A, Zoghbi WA, for the Doppler Quantification Task Force of the Nomenclature Standards Committee of the American Society of Echocardiography. Recommendations for quantification of Doppler echocardiography: a report from the Doppler Quantification Task Force of the Nomenclature and Standards Committee of the American Society of Echocardiography. *J Am Soc Echocardiogr* 2002;15:167-84.
9 Pellikka PA, Sarano ME, Nishimura RA, Malouf JF, Bailey KR, Scott CG, et al. Outcome of 622 adults with asymptomatic, hemodynamically significant aortic stenosis during prolonged follow-up. *Circulation* 2005;111:3290-5.
10 Jiménez-Candil J, Bermejo J, Yotti R, Cortina C, Moreno M, Cantalapiedra JL, et al. Effects of angiotensin converting enzyme inhibitors in hypertensive patients with aortic valve stenosis: a drug withdrawal study. *Heart* 2005;91:1311-8.
11 Khot UN, Novaro GM, Popovic ZB, Mills RM, Thomas JD, Tuzcu EM, et al. Nitroprusside in critically ill patients with left ventricular dysfunction and aortic stenosis. *N Engl J Med* 2003;348:1756-63.
12 Horstkotte D, Follath F, Gutschik E, Lengyel M, Oto A, Pavie A, et al. Guidelines on prevention, diagnosis and treatment of infective endocarditis executive summary: the Task Force on Infective Endocarditis of the European Society of Cardiology. *Eur Heart J* 2004;25:267-76.
13 Cowell SJ, Newby DE, Prescott RJ, Bloomfield P, Reid J, Northridge DB, et al. A randomized trial of intensive lipid-lowering therapy in calcific aortic stenosis. *N Engl J Med* 2005;352:2389-97.
14 Moura LM, Ramos SF, Zamorano JL, Barros IM, Azevedo LF, Rocha-Gonçalves F, et al. Rosuvastatin affecting aortic valve endothelium to slow the progression of aortic stenosis. *J Am Coll Cardiol* 2007;49:554-61.
15 Schwarz F, Baumann P, Manthey J, Hoffmann M, Schuler G, Mehmel HC, et al. The effect of aortic valve replacement on survival. *Circulation* 1982;66:1105-10.
16 Kvidal P, Bergstrom R, Horte LG, Stahle E. Observed and relative survival after aortic valve replacement. *J Am Coll Cardiol* 2000;35:747-56.
17 Cribier A, Eltchaninoff H, Tron C, Bauer F, Agatiello C, Nercolini D, et al. Treatment of calcific aortic stenosis with the percutaneous heart valve: mid-term follow-up from the initial feasibility studies: the French experience. *J Am Coll Cardiol* 2006;47:1214-23.
18 Pereira JJ, Lauer MS, Bashir M, Afridi I, Blackstone EH, Stewart WJ, et al. Survival after aortic valve replacement for severe aortic stenosis with low transvalvular gradients and severe left ventricular dysfunction. *J Am Coll Cardiol* 2002;39:1356-63.
19 Nashef SA, Roques F, Hammill BG, Peterson ED, Michel P, Grover FL, et al. Validation of European system for cardiac operative risk evaluation (EuroSCORE) in North American cardiac surgery. *Eur J Cardiothorac Surg* 2002;22:101-5.
20 Rosenhek R, Klaar U, Schemper M, Scholten C, Heger M, Gabriel H, et al. Mild and moderate aortic stenosis. Natural history and risk stratification by echocardiography. *Eur Heart J* 2004;25:199-205.
21 Bergler-Klein J, Klaar U, Heger M, Rosenhek R, Mundigler G, Gabriel H, et al. Natriuretic peptides predict symptom-free survival and postoperative outcome in severe aortic stenosis. *Circulation* 2004;109:2302-8.
22 Monin JL, Quere JP, Monchi M, Petit H, Baleynaud S, Chauvel C, et al. Low-gradient aortic stenosis, operative risk stratification and predictors for long-term outcome: a multicenter study using dobutamine stress hemodynamics. *Circulation* 2003;108:319-24.

BMJ BPP UNIVERSITY SCHOOL OF HEALTH

Evaluating cardiovascular risk assessment for asymptomatic people

Ian A Scott, associate professor of medicine

[1]Department of Internal Medicine and Clinical Epidemiology, Princess Alexandra Hospital, Brisbane, QLD 4102, Australia

Correspondence to: I A Scott ian_scott@health.qld.gov.au

Cite this as: BMJ 2009;338:a2844

‹DOI› 10.1136/bmj.a2844
http://www.bmj.com/content/338/bmj.a2844

Clinician assessment of future risk of cardiovascular events in asymptomatic individuals is often inaccurate without formal risk prediction tools.[1] Prediction tools that are easy to use and that integrate Framingham criteria of age, sex, serum cholesterol, blood pressure, smoking status, diabetes, and left ventricular hypertrophy into one global risk score have evolved to aid risk assessment.[2] In recent decades, new putative risk factors have been described, including clinical risk factors such as chronic kidney disease and metabolic syndrome, as well as numerous laboratory markers of disease (box 1).[3 4 5] Each new risk factor attracts studies evaluating whether a certain ancillary test shows an incrementally higher cardiovascular risk after adjusting for traditional risk factors.[6] This review asks whether ancillary testing in asymptomatic adults improves the accuracy of predicting cardiovascular risk in individuals, and what effects it might have on patients' care, behaviour, and clinical outcomes.

What are the drawbacks of large scale testing?

Indiscriminate testing could waste resources on tests that will not affect intended management (and that may cause anxiety) and on treatment, started as a result of positive tests, in populations for whom efficacy has not been proved. In the 35% of adults deemed to be at low risk of cardiovascular events (10 year risk <5%), further tests, even with abnormal results, may not justify further investigation or treatment.[7] Conversely, in the 25% of patients at high risk (10 year risk ≥20%), even normal test results should not necessarily prompt discontinuation of aggressive preventive strategies. The 40% of patients at intermediate risk (5% to 20%) are the most likely to benefit from testing. This review does not consider investigations used to screen for or diagnose existing disease (rather than risk) in asymptomatic people.

How do we assess the value of tests that predict cardiovascular risk?

A positive or abnormal value for a new risk factor test will be more useful in estimating disease risk if:

- The more abnormal the test value, the greater the risk of an event (as expressed by the relative risk, odds ratio, or hazard ratio)
- This strong association persists as a further contribution to risk after the contribution of traditional risk factors has been taken into account or adjusted for
- The test discriminates well between individuals who will have an event in the future and those who will not (expressed as a C statistic or C index, with values of 0.5 being no better than chance and 1.0 representing perfect discrimination)
- For tests integrated into risk scoring tools or algorithms, the tools are well calibrated, with predicted and observed risk estimates being similar for each stratum of risk such that ratios of predicted to observed risk are close to 1.0
- The testing method is reliable and standardised across different laboratories
- The test value (or related scoring tool) leads to a change in risk estimates large enough to justify altering the intended management
- Results of clinical trials predict that the altered management plan will improve outcomes.

In general, tests are clinically useful if they correctly predict an event or non-event in 70% or more of cases (C-index ≥0.70), which requires a strong association between test value and disease risk (unadjusted relative risk or odds ratio ≥10.0).[8]

How accurate is risk assessment based on clinical risk factors?

Conventional risk factors and Framingham models

The Framingham risk score underpins most contemporary models of cardiovascular risk prediction that use conventional risk factors (box 2).[9] Models based on the Framingham risk score discriminate best in white Western females (C-statistic 0.79) and worst in non-white African males (0.63).[10]

New clinical risk models and clinical risk factors

New prediction models such as QRISK[11] and ASSIGN[12] aim to supersede Framingham based models by using data from more contemporary cohorts of individuals, many of whom are receiving treatment for known risk factors, and by including additional risk variables (box 2). The C-indices

SOURCES AND SELECTION CRITERIA

I searched Medline, Cochrane Library, BMJ Updates, and BMJ Clinical Evidence over the past 10 years using keywords "cardiovascular risk", "primary prevention", "screening", "risk prediction", "asymptomatic" and "prospective cohort studies", "controlled trials", and "systematic reviews". The content dealing with risk prediction is mainly based on prospective cohort studies; that dealing with effect of risk assessment and feedback on health outcomes and risk profiles is based on controlled trials

SUMMARY POINTS

- Risk prediction tools based on the Framingham score are the most widely used for determining individuals' absolute risk based on clinical risk factors, although newer tools are better calibrated
- The clinical label metabolic syndrome and abnormalities on the resting electrocardiograph do not add prognostic information beyond that obtained by traditional risk factors
- Exercise stress electrocardiography that generates a positive or negative result based on ST deviation alone is not predictive, although scores that integrate several electrocardiographic and clinical variables may be predictive in patients at intermediate risk
- Laboratory biomarkers, even in the form of multimarker panels, are not helpful in refining clinical risk estimates
- Imaging of subclinical atherosclerosis with computed coronary angiography can identify patients at significantly increased risk, but only a small proportion of patients screened fall into this group
- No randomised evidence to date has shown that informing clinicians and patients of absolute risk of cardiovascular events leads to changes in care or improvement in outcomes

BOX 1 NEW DISEASE MARKERS FOR ASSESSING CARDIOVASCULAR RISK

Markers of inflammation, endothelial dysfunction, oxidative stress

- Highly sensitive C reactive protein
- Homocysteine
- Folate
- Serum vitamin B-6
- Interleukin 6
- Intracellular adhesion molecule 1
- Tissue inhibitor of metalloproteinase
- Matrix metalloproteinase 1
- E-selectin
- Leptin
- Antibodies to infectious agents (cytomegalovirus, herpes simplex virus, chlamydia)

Cardiac injury markers

- Troponin

Markers of neurohormonal activation

- Brain natriuretic peptide
- Aldosterone

Renal injury markers

- Cystatin C
- Ratio of urinary albumen to creatinine

Procoagulant markers

- Fibrinogen
- Activated factor VIII
- Prostacyclin
- Thromboxane A2
- D-dimer
- Plasminogen activator inhibitor type 1
- Tissue plasminogen activator
- Thrombomodulin

Dyslipidaemic markers

- Lipoprotein (a)
- Ratio of apolipoprotein B to apolipoprotein A 1
- Lipoprotein associated phospholipase

Glycaemic markers

- Glycated haemoglobin

BOX 2 COMPARISON OF MODELS OF CLINICAL RISK

Framingham risk score[9]
Assigns points to each of several risk factors identified by a Cox proportional hazards regression analysis of the previously untreated Framingham cohort (5209 white, middle class individuals who were studied in the US over two decades, starting in 1948. Number of points (positive or negative) assigned to each variable accords with its β-coefficient in the original Framingham regression equations. Variables include age (with points varying by sex), high density lipoprotein cholesterol, total cholesterol, systolic blood pressure, cigarette smoking, diabetes, and left ventricular hypertrophy on electrocardiography. Points are summed to give an estimate of the 5 year and 10 year probability of a coronary event. More recent modifications include existing treatment for hypertension and family history of premature coronary disease as risk factors.

QRISK[11]
Derived from Cox regression modelling of data from two million patients attending primary care clinics in the United Kingdom between 1995 and 2007. Variables included in the first version were age, sex, smoking status, systolic blood pressure, ratio of total serum cholesterol to high density lipoprotein, body mass index, family history of coronary heart disease in first degree relatives younger than 60, area measure of deprivation (Townsend score), and existing treatment with antihypertensive agent. A more recent version (QRISK2) has additional variables of self assigned ethnicity, type 2 diabetes, rheumatoid arthritis, renal disease, and atrial fibrillation. Event risk at 10 years is calculated with interactive web based software. Recently endorsed by the National Institute for Health and Clinical Excellence (NICE) as the preferred risk prediction tool for UK citizens.

ASSIGN[12]
Derived from Cox regression modelling of data from 13‹thin ›297 individuals aged 30-74 who were initially free of cardiovascular disease and randomly chosen from 25 districts of Scotland between 1984 and 1987. Includes all Framingham variables along with family history of premature cardiovascular disease, cigarette dosage in smokers, and a measure of social deprivation (Scottish index of multiple deprivation).

do not differ much between the models, but QRISK is better calibrated than the Framingham risk score and ASSIGN, producing more accurate estimates in patients at low (<5%) and high (≥20%) 10 year risk (table).[11]

The clinical label of metabolic syndrome (defined as varying combinations of fasting plasma glucose, triglycerides, lipoprotein ratios, blood pressure, and measures of visceral adiposity) increases cardiovascular risk by 50% (relative risk 1.5) after adjustment for traditional risk factors.[13] However, most studies note little or no added improvement in predicting risk in individuals,[14] and its value in this context remains unclear.

What is the added value of resting and exercise electrocardiography?

Major abnormalities on the resting electrocardiogram—such as Q waves, left bundle branch block, and atrial fibrillation—are associated with up to a 3.5-fold increased risk of cardiovascular death at 10 years, but outcomes are incorrectly classified in a third of cases (C-statistics ≤0.67).[15] Similarly, exercise stress tests that report a positive or negative result based simply on ST segment deviation are little better than Framingham based models in predicting event risk. Among 25 927 asymptomatic men at low risk (mean age 43 years; 8 year coronary mortality rate 0.6%), an abnormal stress electrocardiogram, which occurred in only 4.3% of cases, incorrectly predicted death in almost 40% of cases, although accuracy improved with increasing number of risk factors (relative risk 21 for no risk factors, 80 for three or more factors).[16] More sophisticated stress electrocardiogram scores based on multiple variables (exercise time, extent of ST deviation, provocation of chest pain) and clinical risk factors (age, sex, diabetes, smoking status) show more promise, with C-statistics for 5 year survival up to 0.83.[17]

In patients who cannot undergo exercise stress electrocardiography (uninterpretable baseline electrocardiogram; inability to exercise; characteristics such as anaemia or left ventricular hypertrophy that predispose to false-positive ST segment changes), the prognostic value of pharmacologically induced stress imaging (echocardiography, myocardial perfusion scanning) has not been well studied but, to date, seems to be low even in populations at high risk.[18]

Summary statistics comparing Framingham, QRISK, and ASSIGN equation for 10 year risk of cardiovascular events (applied to QRISK validation cohort)

	Framingham	QRISK	ASSIGN
C-index			
Women	0.774	0.788	0.784
Men	0.760	0.767	0.764
Ratio of predicted to observed risk			
Women	1.18	1.02	1.38
Men	1.47	1.00	1.35

What is the added value of laboratory testing?

Biomarkers

Attention has shifted to readily assayable biomarkers, either singly or in combinations known as multimarker panels (box 1). Several studies have assessed the association of such markers with risk in populations, but the few that have assessed the predictive use of single biomarkers in individual patients have all shown no incremental value beyond traditional risk factors.[5] Multimarker panels have been claimed to have greater discriminatory power than single markers, but most studies,[19 20 21] although not all,[22] have reported disappointing results.

Non-invasive imaging tests

Can prediction be improved by directly imaging subclinical vascular atherosclerosis?

Coronary artery imaging

Using electron beam or multislice computed tomography, coronary artery calcium scanning visualises calcium accretions in atherosclerotic plaque lining the walls of coronary arteries, and computes a volumetric score (Agatston score) between 0 (no accretions) and over 1000 (heavy wall calcification).[23] Other studies using multidetector tomography identify substantial obstructive coronary disease (>50% luminal stenosis), which includes non-calcified plaque.[24]

The largest study to date of coronary artery calcium scanning measured scores and all cause mortality over seven years in 25<thin space>253 asymptomatic individuals, in whom scores above 10 were independently predictive of mortality after adjustment for traditional risk factors, with relative risk increasing from 3.6 for a score of 11-100 to 9.4 for a score of ≥1000.[23] These values corresponded to 12 year event rates of ≤5.5% for scores of 11-400, 7.0% for scores of 401-1000, and 23.1% for scores >1000. However, only 10% of all patients, in whom multiple risk factors were present, had scores greater than 400. After adjustment for conventional risk factors (dichotomised sex adjusted age, family history, hypertension, lipids, smoking, diabetes), scores retained greater accuracy in predicting risk than did risk factors alone (C-statistic 0.76 versus 0.61; P=0.03). However, when scores were compared with age alone as a continuous variable, the discrimination difference was attenuated (C-statistic 0.81 *v* 0.77), implying age is the single most important predictor of both death and extent of coronary artery calcification.

Current expert consensus recommends avoiding computed angiography in risk assessment for asymptomatic people at low risk, because of the carcinogenic risk associated with radiation (up to 2% for annual scanning over a lifespan),[25] and the possibility of iatrogenic morbidity incurred by invasive investigation—pulmonary lesions are incidentally detected in 20% of people who undergo scanning, but most are benign.[26]

Carotid and peripheral artery imaging

In asymptomatic populations, thickening of the intima media of the carotid artery or reduced arterial flow in the leg (low ankle brachial index), as assessed by ultrasound, is associated with as much as a threefold increase in cardiovascular risk after adjustment for traditional risk factors.[27] However, studies of incremental predictive value in individuals are few and no recommendations exist for the routine use of vascular ultrasound in risk prediction.

What is the evidence that risk prediction alters clinical management or outcomes?

A systematic review found eleven studies, including five randomised controlled trials with reasonable methodological quality, that had evaluated the clinical benefits and harms of applying Framingham based risk scores to the care of asymptomatic people.[28] None of the five showed a significant overall change in care or risk factors, although no harmful effects were seen. In one trial, an a priori subgroup analysis of patients at high risk showed significant improvements in prescribing of lipid lowering agents (absolute increase 11%) and antihypertensive drugs (absolute increase 13%).[29] Two other trials showed improvements in systolic blood pressure (4.6 mm Hg decrease)[30] and uptake of physical exercise (11% increase).[31] A more recent trial not included in the above review found a significant but small (0.08 mmol/l) decrease in low density lipoprotein cholesterol.[32] No effects on event rates have been reported; studies have been underpowered to detect such effects.

No trials have directly assessed the effects of stress testing or laboratory biomarkers on control of risk factors or on clinical outcomes compared with no investigation. As many as 3% of patients undergoing stress electrocardiography in cohort studies subsequently showed severe coronary disease prompting revascularisation,[12] but no trials have confirmed benefit from revascularisation in asymptomatic populations. Moreover, in populations at lower risk (<10% event risk at 5 years), at least 75% of positive test results are false positives, potentially resulting in unwarranted testing and anxiety.

One trial assessed the effect of coronary artery calcium scanning in 450 asymptomatic US army personnel (mean age 42 years, mean 10 year risk of coronary events 5.9%), of whom 15% had positive scores.[33] Using a factorial design that randomised participants to usual care or intensive case management with or without feedback to doctor or patient about the coronary artery calcium score, awareness of the score had no effect on risk profile or lifestyle. Another trial, which randomised 1005 people with raised coronary artery calcium scores (above 80th percentile) to a statin and vitamins C and E or matching placebo, found no treatment effect on scores or cardiovascular event rates at four year follow-up.[34]

Implications for clinical practice

According to the available evidence, ancillary testing in most asymptomatic people adds little to the prediction of individual cardiovascular risk, and does not affect care, lifestyle, adherence, or clinical outcomes. Randomised trials are needed to assess whether the improved accuracy of risk categorisation provided by some tests leads to therapeutic reductions of risk in patients not previously identified, or to reductions in the number of patients needing treatment by identifying low risk groups. Other areas in need of studies are the potential harms and cost effectiveness of

CASE SCENARIO

A 58 year old man who smokes and is being treated for hypertension with an angiotensin converting enzyme inhibitor comes in for review, driven by new concern about his cardiovascular risk since his 54 year old brother recently had a heart attack. You have been caring for him for some years and have been trying to get him to stop smoking. He is also overweight (body mass index 27) and has an unhealthy diet, with a ratio of total cholesterol to high density lipoprotein cholesterol of 4.0 while receiving statin therapy. He has read in the lay press about new blood tests that might give a better indication of his cardiovascular risk, and he is aware of new radiography techniques that can apparently show calcified plaque in coronary arteries. He asks whether these tests might be relevant to him. You hesitate, unsure about how useful these tests would be, and noting that no reference is made to them in recent NICE guidelines on risk assessment (see "Additional educational resources"). You are also worried that if such tests yield a negative result he might be even less motivated to alter his lifestyle than he is already. On the other hand, if the tests show a positive result, you are not sure what part of your current management plan you would change in response.

ADDITIONAL EDUCATIONAL RESOURCES

For healthcare professionals

- National Institute for Health and Clinical Excellence. Lipid modification: cardiovascular risk assessment and the modification of blood lipids for the primary and secondary prevention of cardiovascular disease. 2008. www.nice.org.uk/CG67 (risk assessment process recommended for primary care, although modifications of Framingham risk estimates based on premature family history of cardiovascular disease and ethnicity are controversial)
- QRISK risk calculator (www.qr2.dyndns.org)—Developed by QResearch and Hippisley-Cox et al[11]
- New Zealand Guideline Group. New Zealand cardiovascular risk assessment chart. http://www.nzgg.org.nz/guidelines/0035/CVD_Risk_Chart.pdf (Framingham based risk assessment matrix that combines 5 year absolute cardiovascular risk estimates with absolute risk reductions achievable with antihypertensive and lipid lowering therapy)
- British Cardiac Society, British Hyperlipidaemia Association, British Hypertension Society and Diabetes UK. Joint British societies coronary risk prediction chart. *Heart* 1998;80:S1-29
- The National Vascular Disease Prevention Alliance (Diabetes Australia, Kidney Health Australia, National Heart Foundation of Australia, and National Stroke Foundation of Australia). Consensus statement for the prevention of vascular disease. 2004. www.heartfoundation.org.au/document/NHF/nvdpa_04.pdf (comprehensive consensus statement on assessing and managing risk of CVD)
- US Preventive Services Task Force. Screening for coronary heart disease. 2004. www.ahrq.gov/clinic/uspstf/uspsacad.htm (evidence based recommendations for screening for heart disease, including avoidance of ancillary testing in low risk populations)
- American College of Cardiology Foundation/American Heart Association. 2007 clinical expert consensus document: coronary artery calcium scoring by computed tomography in global cardiovascular risk assessment. 2007. www.americanheart.org/downloadable/heart/1168626471943CECD%20on%20EBCT%20rev3.pdf (comprehensive review with recommendations that CAC scanning be avoided in low risk patients, although it may have a role in intermediate risk patients)

For patients

- QRESEARCH (www.qresearch.org/Public/qrisk.aspx)—website for QRISK2 risk calculator and answers to frequently asked questions by patients
- American Heart Association Heart Attack/Coronary Heart Disease Risk Assessment tool (www.americanheart.org/presenter.jhtml?identifier=3003499)—interactive web based tools that allow patients to calculate their own cardiovascular risk level

additional testing, generalisability of results to populations with different ethnicities and comorbidities, standardisation of test assays in maximising precision and validation of population norms to guide interpretation of results, and observer bias and reliability.

A case may be made for further testing in patients at intermediate or high risk who are younger (<35 years), older (>75 years), or come from population groups not included in cohorts used to derive and validate current clinical risk models. However, ancillary testing in most middle aged people is premature and potentially wasteful of resources. An alternative strategy, which needs to be studied in randomised trials, is to ensure that all adult patients (and their doctors) are aware of their cardiovascular risk by using simple, accessible clinical risk calculators (such as QRISK) and adopt a management plan appropriate to their level of risk. In the case scenario presented, the 10 year cardiovascular event risk using QRISK2 is 33%, which should provide sufficient motivation for this patient and his doctor to optimise lifestyle and preventive treatments, making further testing unnecessary.

I thank Chris del Mar, Jenny Doust, and Rod Jackson for their helpful comments on earlier drafts, and Peter Hawkins for giving me the idea for this review.

Contributors: JAS is the sole contributor.

Funding: None received.

Competing interests: None declared.

Provenance and peer review: Not commissioned; externally peer reviewed.

Patient consent not required (patient anonymised, dead, or hypothetical).

1 Friedmann PD, Brett AS, Mayo-Smith MF. Differences in generalists' and cardiologists' perceptions of cardiovascular risk and the outcomes of preventive therapy in cardiovascular disease. *Ann Intern Med* 1996;124:414-21.
2 Jackson R. Updated New Zealand cardiovascular disease risk-benefit prediction guide. *BMJ* 2000;320:709-10.
3 Astor BC, Coresh J, Heiss G, Pettitt D, Sarnak MJ. Kidney function and anemia as risk factors for coronary heart disease and mortality: the Atherosclerosis Risk in Communities (ARIC) Study. *Am Heart J* 2006;151:492-500.
4 Wilson PW, D'Agostino RB, Parise H, Sullivan L, Meigs JB. Metabolic syndrome as a precursor of cardiovascular disease and type 2 diabetes mellitus. *Circulation* 2005;112:3066-72.
5 Tsimikas S, Willerson JT, Ridker PM. C-reactive protein and other emerging blood biomarkers to optimize risk stratification of vulnerable patients. *J Am Coll Cardiol* 2006;47(suppl 8):C19-31.
6 Hackham DG, Anand SS. Emerging risk factors for atherosclerotic vascular disease. A critical review of the evidence. *JAMA* 2003;290:932-40.
7 Greenland P, Smith SC Jr, Grundy SM. Improving coronary heart disease risk assessment in asymptomatic people: role of traditional risk factors and noninvasive cardiovascular tests. *Circulation* 2001;104:1863-7.
8 Pepe MS, Janes H, Longton G, Leisenring W, Newcomb P. Limitations of the odds ratio in gauging the performance of a diagnostic, prognostic, or screening marker. *Am J Epidemiol* 2004;159:882-90.
9 Anderson KM, Odell PM, Wilson PW, Kannel WB. Cardiovascular disease risk profiles. *Am Heart J* 1991;121:293-8.
10 D'Agostino RB Sr, Vasan RS, Pencina MJ, Wolf PA, Cobain M, Massaro JM, et al. General cardiovascular risk profile for use in primary care: the Framingham Heart Study. *Circulation* 2008;117:743-53.
11 Hippisley-Cox J, Coupland C, Vinogradova Y, Robson J, May M, Brindle P. Derivation and validation of QRISK, a new cardiovascular disease risk score for the United Kingdom: prospective open cohort study. *BMJ* 2007;335:136.
12 Woodward M, Brindle P, Tunstall-Pedoe H, SIGN group on risk estimation. Adding social deprivation and family history to cardiovascular risk assessment: the ASSIGN score from the Scottish Heart Health Extended Cohort (SHHEC). *Heart* 2007;93:172-6.
13 Gami AS, Witt BJ, Howard DE, Erwin PJ, Gami LA, Somers VK, et al. Metabolic syndrome and risk of incident cardiovascular events and death: a systematic review and meta-analysis of longitudinal studies. *J Am Coll Cardiol* 2007;49:403-14.
14 Kahn R, Buse J, Ferrannini E, Stern M, American Diabetes Association; European Association for the Study of Diabetes. The metabolic syndrome: time for a critical appraisal: joint statement from the American Diabetes Association and the European Association for the Study of Diabetes. *Diabetes Care* 2005;28:2289-304.
15 Fowler-Brown A, Pignone M, Pletcher M, Tice JA, Sutton SF, Lohr KN, et al. Exercise tolerance testing to screen for coronary heart disease: a systematic review for the technical support for the U.S. Preventive Services Task Force. *Ann Intern Med* 2004;140:W9-24.
16 Gibbons LW, Mitchell TL, Wei M, Blair SN, Cooper KH. Maximal exercise test as a predictor of risk for mortality from coronary heart disease in asymptomatic men. *Am J Cardiol* 2000;86:53-8.
17 Lauer MS, Pothier CE, Magid DJ, Smith SS, Kattan MW. An externally validated model for predicting long-term survival after exercise treadmill testing in patients with suspected coronary artery disease and a normal electrocardiogram. *Ann Intern Med* 2007;147:821-8.
18 Blumenthal RS, Becker DM, Yanek LR, Aversano TR, Moy TF, Kral BG, Becker LC. Detecting occult coronary disease in a high-risk asymptomatic population. *Circulation* 2003;107:702-7.
19 Wang TJ, Gona P, Larson MG, Tofler GH, Levy D, Newton-Cheh C, et al. Multiple biomarkers for the prediction of first major cardiovascular events and death. *N Engl J Med* 2006;355:2631-9.
20 Folsom AR, Chambless LE, Ballantyne CM, Coresh J, Heiss G, Wu KK, et al. An assessment of incremental coronary risk prediction using C-reactive protein and other novel risk markers: the atherosclerosis risk in communities study. *Arch Intern Med* 2006;166:1368-73.

21 Shlipak MG, Fried LF, Cushman M, Manolio TA, Peterson D, Stehman-Breen C, et al. Cardiovascular mortality risk in chronic kidney disease: comparison of traditional and novel risk factors. *JAMA* 2005;293:1737-45.

22 Zethelius B, Berglund L, Sundström J, Ingelsson E, Basu S, Larsson A, et al. Use of multiple biomarkers to improve the prediction of death from cardiovascular causes. *N Engl J Med* 2008;358:2107-16.

23 Budoff MJ, Shaw LJ, Liu ST, Weinstein SR, Mosler TP, Tseng PH, et al. Long-term prognosis associated with coronary calcification: observations from a registry of 25,253 patients. *J Am Coll Cardiol* 2007;49:1860-70.

24 Bachar GN, Atar E, Fuchs S, Dror D, Kornowski R. Prevalence and clinical predictors of atherosclerotic coronary artery disease in asymptomatic patients undergoing coronary multidetector computed tomography. *Coron Art Dis* 2007;18:353-60.

25 Brenner DJ, Elliston CD. Estimated radiation risks potentially associated with full-body CT screening. *Radiology* 2004;232:735-8.

26 Burt JR, Iribarren C, Fair JM, Norton LC, Mahbouba M, Rubin GD, et al. Atherosclerotic Disease, Vascular Function, and Genetic Epidemiology (ADVANCE) Study. Incidental findings on cardiac multidetector row computed tomography among healthy older adults: prevalence and clinical correlates. *Arch Intern Med* 2008;168:756-61.

27 Van der Meer IM, Bots ML, Hofman A, del Sol AI, van der Kuip DAM, Witteman JCM. Predictive value of non-invasive measures of atherosclerosis for incident myocardial infarction. The Rotterdam Study. *Circulation* 2004;109:1089-94.

28 Sheridan SL, Crespo E. Does the routine use of global coronary heart disease risk scores translate into clinical benefits or harms? A systematic review of the literature. *BMC Health Services Research* 2008;8:60-73.

29 Hall LM, Jung RT, Leese GP. Controlled trial of effect of documented cardiovascular risk scores on prescribing. *BMJ* 2003;326:251-2.

30 Montgomery AA, Fahey T, Peters TJ, MacIntosh C, Sharp DJ. Evaluation of computer based clinical decision support system and risk chart for management of hypertension in primary care: randomised controlled trial. *BMJ* 2000;320:686-90.

31 Van Steenkiste B, van der Weijden T, Stoffers HE, Kester AD, Timmermans DR, Grol R. Improving cardiovascular risk management: a randomised, controlled trial on the effect of a decision support tool for patients and physicians. *Eur J Cardiovasc Prev Rehabil* 2007;14:44-50.

32 Grover SA, Lowensteyn I, Joseph L, Kaouache M, Marchand S, Coupal L, et al. Patient knowledge of coronary risk profile improves the effectiveness of dyslipidemia therapy: the CHECK-UP study: a randomized controlled trial. *Arch Intern Med* 2007;167:2296-303.

33 O'Malley PG, Feuerstein IM, Taylor AJ. Impact of electron beam tomography, with or without case management, on motivation, behavioral change, and cardiovascular risk profile: a randomized controlled trial. *JAMA* 2003;289:2215-23.

34 Arad Y, Spadaro LA, Roth M, Newstein D, Guerci AD. Treatment of asymptomatic adults with elevated coronary calcium scores with atorvastatin, vitamin C, and vitamin E: the St. Francis Heart Study randomized clinical trial. *J Am Coll Cardiol* 2005;46:166-72.

BMJ BPP UNIVERSITY SCHOOL OF HEALTH

Inherited cardiomyopathies

Hariharan Raju, cardiology fellow[1], Corinna Alberg, project manager[2], Gurdeep S Sagoo, epidemiologist[2], Hilary Burton, director[2], Elijah R Behr, senior lecturer and honorary consultant cardiologist[1]

[1]Cardiac and Vascular Division, St George's University of London, London SW17 0RE, UK

[2]PHG Foundation, Cambridge, UK

Correspondence to: E R Behr ebehr@sgul.ac.uk

Cite this as: *BMJ* 2011;343:d6966

<DOI> 10.1136/bmj.d6966
http://www.bmj.com/content/343/bmj.d6966

Inherited cardiac conditions include primary electrical, myocardial, and structural heart diseases, in addition to vascular conditions. The presentation, diagnosis, and management of the different categories of inherited cardiac disease vary greatly. In this review we focus on inherited heart muscle disorders, known as cardiomyopathies. Collectively, they affect about one in 390 people (table).[1] However, the true prevalence of each condition is difficult to determine because evidence of disease may be subtle in asymptomatic patients.[2 3 4]

Cardiomyopathies can lead to sudden death as a result of fatal ventricular arrhythmias.[5] Disease of the heart muscle may also progress with age and lead to heart failure.[2 6] Early diagnosis and modification of risk factors for premature death may prevent such outcomes and are important. The diagnostic process has improved in recent years, with advances in clinical cardiological evaluation,[2 6 7] and particularly genetic testing.[2 3 8] We review the diagnosis and management of patients with cardiomyopathy for non-specialist doctors and discuss the value of genetic testing in the management of affected families. This article is based mainly on the findings of medium and large cohort studies, which form the evidence base of the consensus statements of professional bodies.

Which inherited cardiomyopathies might general clinicians encounter?

On the basis of international estimates (table), an average primary care practice in the United Kingdom of 7380 patients would include about 15 patients with hypertrophic cardiomyopathy, the most common cardiomyopathy. Patients with less common conditions are likely to cluster in practices with affected families.[1]

Hypertrophic cardiomyopathy is defined as unexplained cardiac hypertrophy, and it often shows an asymmetric pattern—affecting mainly the interventricular septum.[6] Arrhythmogenic right ventricular cardiomyopathy causes replacement of myocardium with fibro-fatty tissue, particularly in the right ventricle, although the left ventricle may also be affected. Electrophysiological changes, including arrhythmias, can often pre-date overt structural and functional changes.[2] Dilated cardiomyopathy is characterised by dilation and impaired contraction of the left or both ventricles, and it is hereditary in about a quarter of cases.[9] End stage arrhythmogenic right ventricular cardiomyopathy and hypertrophic cardiomyopathy may be difficult to distinguish from dilated cardiomyopathy because left ventricular systolic dysfunction may complicate diagnosis. Different cardiomyopathic features can overlap in individual families, as seen in our patient case study.

SOURCES AND SELECTION CRITERIA

We reviewed the literature using OMIM (online mendelian inheritance in man, a database of human genes and genetic disorders); Gene Reviews; and National Institutes of Health PubMed searches using key words "hypertrophic cardiomyopathy", "dilated cardiomyopathy", "arrhythmogenic right ventricular cardiomyopathy", and "sudden cardiac death". This was supplemented with references from the authors' personal archives.

SUMMARY POINTS

- Primary care doctors play a key role in identifying those at risk of inherited cardiomyopathy
- People who present with symptoms of heart disease, relatives of an affected person, those with a family history of premature sudden death, and those with incidental electrocardiographic abnormalities are at risk of cardiomyopathy
- Most cardiomyopathies are inherited in an autosomal dominant manner
- Disease severity varies owing to variable penetrance
- Specialists should evaluate suspected cases, and pathways to specialist care should be tailored to local healthcare systems
- Mutation analysis allows accurate identification of carriers, but diagnosis and risk prediction still rely on clinical markers

What is the role of the family doctor?

Symptomatic patients

Patients may present to their primary care doctor with symptoms caused by myocardial ischaemia, arrhythmia, or heart failure, which can include chest pain, syncope, dyspnoea, palpitations, or stroke. However, a pilot study of the feasibility of heart screening for sudden cardiac arrest in healthy children found that history and physical examination alone are poor predictors of disease in young people, although it is still important to take a family history.[10] Initial investigation with electrocardiography, with a view to requesting cardiac imaging in the face of an abnormality, is warranted in any patient with worrying symptoms. "Red flag" symptoms (box) include palpitations and exertional dyspnoea accompanied by syncope or seizures in a young person.

After a definitive diagnosis, family doctors are often the first point of contact when patients deteriorate. Cardiomyopathies are progressive disorders and complications are a risk as patients age.[4 11 12] Any worsening in symptoms of heart failure, signs of ischaemia, or unheralded syncope warrants urgent specialist re-evaluation.

Asymptomatic case finding

Electrocardiographic abnormalities suggestive of cardiomyopathy may be identified incidentally, such as during preoperative risk evaluation or personal health assessment, or as a result of population based screening programmes that are available in some countries.[10]

Patients may seek medical advice directly after discovering a positive family history of cardiomyopathy or premature sudden death, or the family doctor may discover a family history of cardiomyopathy on careful history taking. It is always prudent to refer first degree blood relatives of an affected individual to a specialist for cardiological or genetic evaluation (or both), as recommended by the PHG Foundation UK working group and international consensus.[1 6] Because affected families may cluster in general practices, the family practitioner may be uniquely placed to discover "at risk" people. Referral of more distant relatives for evaluation depends on patterns of inheritance of the disease and is not routine practice in primary care. Because death certification may not always identify affected people who are asymptomatic and apparently undiagnosed before a sudden death, particularly those under 40 years,[13 14 15 16] it is important to consider cardiomyopathy as a potential cause of death if a patient reports the sudden and unexplained death of a relative. A recent population based study from Europe found that that relatives are often not referred for evaluation of inherited cardiac conditions after a premature death in the family.[7] Good communication between primary care doctors and cardiogenetic specialists, and clear patient pathways, are needed to facilitate appropriate evaluation of families and identification of family members at potential risk of inherited cardiomyopathy.

What is the role of the cardiogenetics specialist centre?

Evaluation and management of patients with cardiomyopathy should ideally be undertaken by specialists with appropriate expertise in cardiomyopathies, perhaps at a regional or national centre. We advocate a multidisciplinary approach, with liaison between a cardiovascular genetics service and adult and paediatric cardiologists to ensure that family groups are managed in a coordinated manner.[1] Although it is usual for genetics services to be planned around the investigation of family units, clinical cardiology services may need to be reorganised to fit this model. An integrated approach may improve diagnostic certainty in families where results are equivocal in multiple members. This model also allows family-wide education and counselling on inheritance patterns, diagnosis, and management, thereby promoting informed choices by affected and unaffected members of a family.

Reported prevalence of inherited cardiomyopathies[1]

Condition	Prevalence
Hypertrophic cardiomyopathy	1 in 500 (Europe)
Arrhythmogenic right ventricular cardiomyopathy	1 in 1000 to 1 in 10 000 (Europe)
Dilated cardiomyopathy	36.5 in 100 000 (United States)*

**This estimate of prevalence is based on sparse literature and is thought to be an underestimate; it is calculated on the assumption that about 25% of cases of dilated cardiomyopathy are familial.*

A PATIENT'S PERSPECTIVE

In November 2008, I collapsed while playing tennis at a sports club. I was resuscitated by a quick thinking attendant with a defibrillator. I spent a month at three local hospitals before eventually having a cardiac defibrillator implanted at St George's Hospital, just before my 50th birthday.

The members of my family were tested and my sons were found to have a similar heart condition. They are 20 and 16, and have both been fitted with a defibrillator as a precaution. I also have a younger brother who survived a similar collapse around 25 years ago. This was largely unexplained at the time, but he has now been fitted with a defibrillator.

The diagnosis has been uncertain for all concerned. I had a full range of tests while in hospital and my family has had the same. We feel protected by the cardiac defibrillators without knowing clearly what the underlying problem is.

My defibrillator went off in my first year when I was walking in the Lake District but it was found to be an inappropriate shock, the settings were altered, and I've had no incidents since. At the time it was reassuring to have immediate contact with the pacing clinic at St George's, to download the defibrillator data by telephone, and to pay a quick visit to hospital to sort the problem out.

Our ongoing treatment consists of a six monthly family visit to St George's, supplemented by remote downloads by telephone from home. It's a very "light touch" and doesn't disrupt our lives too much.

The defibrillators do not have that much impact on our daily lives. My sons have to steer clear of overly physical and competitive exercise. It is a minor inconvenience when passing through airports, and we check all travel destinations for "defibrillator friendly" hospitals.

But it is a worry. No doubt, as parents, we would worry anyway as our children negotiate their teenage years—late nights out, theme parks, different sports, terms away at college, foreign holidays, gap years, and so on. But the defibrillators add an extra dimension.

ADVICE FOR NON-SPECIALISTS: RED FLAG SYMPTOMS AND SIGNS

Consider priority referral for specialist evaluation in the following situations:

- Exertional syncope or seizures
- Exertional chest pain in a young person
- Palpitations associated with impaired consciousness
- Family history of cardiomyopathy
- Family history of premature sudden cardiac death
- Incidental finding of an unexpected electrocardiographic abnormality suggestive of cardiomyopathy

How is cardiomyopathy diagnosed?

Electrocardiography

In patients clinically affected by cardiomyopathy the resting electrocardiograph is rarely normal. In gene carriers who seem to be clinically unaffected (incomplete gene expression) the electrocardiograph is usually normal.[2 17] Classically, large voltage QRS complexes with ST depression and deep T wave inversion (figure; part A) are seen in patients with hypertrophic cardiomyopathy, although non-specific electrocardiographic changes may also be seen and may be the only initial indication of disease. In patients with arrhythmogenic right ventricular cardiomyopathy, subtle abnormalities may be evident on electrocardiography (figure; part B) in the right precordial leads (V1-V3). These abnormalities include T wave inversion and broadening of the QRS and the "epsilon wave" (notch in the ST segment), which reflect the predilection of the disease for right ventricular muscle. Changes can be more extensive in severe arrhythmogenic right ventricular cardiomyopathy. Patients with dilated cardiomyopathy may also show non-specific abnormalities on electrocardiography (figure; part C).

Specialist investigations

A cardiologist will request echocardiography or magnetic resonance imaging to make a definitive diagnosis in patients with hypertrophic cardiomyopathy and dilated cardiomyopathy; these investigations can identify characteristic ventricular hypertrophy or dilation and impaired systolic function, respectively.[6 9] Wide variability in gene expression in arrhythmogenic right ventricular cardiomyopathy has led experts to develop a complex diagnostic scoring system that is used to determine the likelihood of disease (http://qstatistic.com/pdg/public.php?rep=arvc_cri).[2]

Excluding other conditions

The cardiologist will need to exclude conditions that may mimic inherited cardiomyopathies because these will require different management strategies from the inherited conditions they resemble. Athlete's heart (as a result of chronic exercise training) and cardiac changes secondary to hypertension and amyloid may mimic hypertrophic cardiomyopathy, and coronary artery disease and chronic alcohol excess may lead to cardiac muscle changes that mimic dilated cardiomyopathy.[4 6 9]

Dilated cardiomyopathies pose a particular difficulty, given that only some are inherited; the familial nature of dilated cardiomyopathy can be established only by reviewing family history, which may require investigation of blood relatives.[4 9]

What is the approach to management of people with inherited cardiomyopathies?

Management of patients depends on the specific condition. Strategies are broadly divided into treatment of symptoms, prevention of disease progression, and reduction in the risk of stroke and sudden death; some treatments span more than one of these categories. Given the relative rarity of inherited cardiomyopathies, the recommendations from professional bodies for therapeutic interventions and risk stratification have been based on multicentre prospective and retrospective cohort observations. Small case series underpin recommendations for less well proved treatments.

Reducing sudden death

The risk of sudden death as a result of fatal arrhythmias can be reduced by lifestyle changes tailored to removing triggers. For example, participating in competitive sport is universally discouraged. On the basis of randomised trials, drugs such as β blockers and angiotensin converting enzyme inhibitors are commonly used to reduced the risk of death in patients with dilated cardiomyopathy, but drugs have not been shown to be useful in reducing the risk of sudden death in patients with arrhythmogenic right ventricular cardiomyopathy or hypertrophic cardiomyopathy.[5 6 18]

Implantable cardioverter defibrillators are the only intervention that has been shown to reduce sudden death in most patients with an inherited cardiomyopathy. Longitudinal observational and multicentre randomised studies have shown that a previous cardiac arrest or haemodynamically compromising ventricular arrhythmia puts people with cardiomyopathy at high risk of recurrence.[5] Such patients should be considered for a secondary prevention implantable defibrillator.[5] Implantable defibrillators may also be offered for primary prevention to those who are at sufficiently high risk of sudden death. Risk is determined by the severity of left ventricular systolic dysfunction and conduction disease for patients with dilated cardiomyopathy, a risk scoring system for those with hypertrophic cardiomyopathy, and severity of disease and symptoms in patients with arrhythmogenic right ventricular cardiomyopathy.[5 11 19]

Management of progression of disease and symptoms

Symptoms of heart failure, including dyspnoea, may be reduced by achieving euvolaemia with diuretics, although we advise caution in hypertrophic cardiomyopathy because of the predominance of diastolic dysfunction. For patients with dilated cardiomyopathy, the findings of multiple large randomised controlled trials support treatment with β blockers, angiotensin converting enzyme inhibitors, angiotensin II receptor blockers, and spironolactone, in addition to cardiac resynchronisation with biventricular pacing, all of which are aimed at slowing progression of disease and reducing mortality.[20] The effectiveness of these treatments in the other cardiomyopathies is less certain, although they are recommended by international guidelines for all patients with left ventricular systolic dysfunction as a result of end stage disease.[20 21]

In patients with hypertrophic cardiomyopathy, chest pain caused by ischaemia may be ameliorated by β blockers or verapamil. Symptoms secondary to outflow tract obstruction may be reduced by the addition of disopyramide.[6] Invasive procedures such as septal alcohol ablation and surgical myomectomy may reduce the outflow tract gradient and reduce symptoms.[11 22] In patients with arrhythmogenic right ventricular cardiomyopathy, symptomatic ventricular arrhythmias may be reduced by sotalol and amiodarone.[18 23] Furthermore, radiofrequency ablation can be a useful adjunct in refractory arrhythmias, although recurrence as a result of progressive disease is a problem.[23 24] A minority of patients with severe symptomatic disease, usually as a result of heart failure, receive heart transplants.[25]

Patients with hypertrophic cardiomyopathy and dilated cardiomyopathy are at increased risk of atrial fibrillation, which is important to recognise because of the concomitant thromboembolic risk.[26]

What is the role of genetic mutation analysis?

Diagnosis

Because genetic testing is less than 100% sensitive, it is recommended only after confirmation of the clinical diagnosis, and even then usually in a limited number of genes that cause hypertrophic cardiomyopathy and arrhythmogenic right ventricular cardiomyopathy.[27] Most inherited cardiomyopathies show a mendelian autosomal dominant inheritance pattern, although less common recessive forms have been described, and dilated cardiomyopathy can also be inherited in an X linked pattern.[9 28] To date, more than 20 genes have been implicated in hypertrophic cardiomyopathy, detectable in 60% of families,[8] whereas mutations in seven genes identify almost half of those affected by arrhythmogenic right

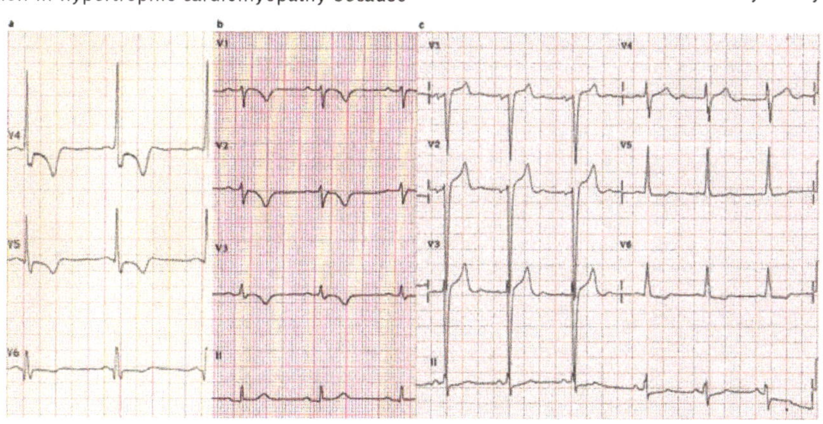

Examples of electrocardiographs from patients with inherited cardiomyopathy. (A) Lateral precordial leads of a patient with hypertrophic cardiomyopathy showing Q wave (V6), ST depression, and T wave inversion associated with large voltage QRS complexes. (B) Right precordial leads of a patient with arrhythmogenic right ventricular cardiomyopathy showing epsilon wave (V2), QRS prolongation, and T wave inversion. (C) Precordial leads of a patient with dilated cardiomyopathy showing incomplete left bundle branch block and electrocardiographic left atrial enlargement

ventricular cardiomyopathy.[2] Dilated cardiomyopathy is a heterogeneous disorder, and a myriad genetic abnormalities identified account for only around 30% of familial cases.[9]

Cascade familial testing

Once a definite disease causing mutation is identified in an affected patient, the main diagnostic role for genetic testing is identification of carriers within a pedigree, a process known as "cascade testing."[27] Family members who carry the same genetic mutation may show different severities of disease, and this is known as variable penetrance. Hence, some patients may remain entirely asymptomatic, with little evidence of disease throughout their lives.[4] However, as mutation carriers, their children remain at risk of inheriting the disorder and potentially being more severely affected. Despite an autosomal dominant inheritance pattern, the clinical picture may give the appearance of "skipped" generations in a single pedigree. Mutation analysis is useful to allow accurate identification of carriers, and it may be cost effective and reassuring because non-carriers are eliminated from clinical assessment.[29]

Prediction of risk

Risk prediction still depends mainly on clinical assessment for patients with cardiomyopathy. Mutational analysis may affect risk; one specific subgroup increases the risk of sudden death—mutations in the gene encoding lamin A/C (*LMNA*), which are associated with dilated cardiomyopathy.[30] Research to assess new markers is under way.

What is the value of tracing relatives?

Assuming an autosomal dominant inheritance, all first degree blood relatives of a proband (the first identified affected member in a family) should undergo cardiogenetic evaluation because they have a 50% chance of being a disease carrier. Case finding by family evaluation can prevent future premature deaths through the timely delivery of treatments that reduce risk.[13 14] Remember that the proband may be diagnosed after cardiological investigation, which may occur incidentally or in response to symptoms or a cardiac event, or even at autopsy after sudden death.

Because of the possibility of age related expression, familial evaluation sometimes requires serial follow-up of young relatives who initially have no evidence of disease.[4 6] As the natural course of arrhythmogenic right ventricular cardiomyopathy is poorly documented and late onset hypertrophic cardiomyopathy is increasingly recognised, follow-up may be recommended into middle age or later, particularly in people who carry a disease causing mutation identified in an affected blood relative.[6 12]

ONGOING RESEARCH

Research in inherited cardiomyopathies focuses on many different areas:

- The identification of previously undescribed disease causing genes and mutations within them
- The scientific study of the molecular consequences of specific mutations and what they can tell us about the underlying mechanisms of disease
- The study of factors that modify the presentation of inherited cardiac conditions and hence explain variable expression
- The development and assessment of new methods for the diagnosis and stratification of risk
- The development of new treatments that may be tailored to the genetic diagnosis

ADDITIONAL EDUCATIONAL RESOURCES

Resources for health professionals

- National Genetics Education and Development Centre (www.geneticseducation.nhs.uk)—Aimed at educating non-specialist doctors on inherited conditions

Resources for patients

- Genetic Alliance (www.geneticalliance.org.uk)—Information on heart conditions with a genetic cause in several languages
- Cardiac Risk in the Young (www.c-r-y.org.uk)—Provides bereavement support and patient literature; it can facilitate specialist referrals in the UK where appropriate
- Cardiomyopathy Association (www.cardiomyopathy.org)—Information on hypertrophic cardiomyopathy, dilated cardiomyopathy, and arrhythmogenic right ventricular cardiomyopathy
- Arrhythmia Alliance (www.arrhythmiaalliance.org.uk)—Information on arrhythmias and devices used to treat inherited conditions, such as defibrillators and pacemakers
- British Heart Foundation (www.bhf.org.uk)—Genetic information service for UK patients, which facilitates appropriate referrals to regional NHS cardiovascular genetics clinics; it also co-sponsors patient media from several other charitable organisations

Acknowledgements: Thanks to our patient at St George's Hospital, and his family, for their personal contribution of experiences for the patient case study.

Contributors: HR contributed to the conception, drafting, revision, and approval of the article; CA contributed to analysis, revision, and approval; GSS contributed to drafting, analysis, and approval; HB contributed to analysis, revision, and approval; ERB is guarantor and contributed to conception, drafting, revision, and approval.

Funding: HR is supported by Cardiac Risk in the Young (CRY); EB is supported by the Higher Education Funding Council for England (HEFCE); CA, GS, and HB are supported by the PHG Foundation.

Competing interests: All authors have completed the ICMJE uniform disclosure form at www.icmje.org/coi_disclosure.pdf (available on request from the corresponding author) and declare: no support from any organisation for the submitted work; no financial relationships with any organisations that might have an interest in the submitted work in the previous three years; EB has received funds for research from Biotronik and Boston Scientific.

Provenance and peer review: Not commissioned; externally peer reviewed.

Patient consent obtained.

1 Burton H, Alberg C, Stewart A. Heart to heart: inherited cardiovascular conditions services—a needs assessment and service review. PHG Foundation, 2009. www.phgfoundation.org/file/4668/.

2 Marcus FI, McKenna WJ, Sherrill D, Basso C, Bauce B, Bluemke D, et al. Diagnosis of arrhythmogenic right ventricular cardiomyopathy/dysplasia: proposed modification of the task force criteria. *Circulation* 2010;121:1533-41.

3 Millat G, Bouvagnet P, Chevalier P, Dauphin C, Jouk PS, Da Costa A, et al. Prevalence and spectrum of mutations in a cohort of 192 unrelated patients with hypertrophic cardiomyopathy. *Eur J Med Genet* 2010;53:261-7.

4 Mahon NG, Murphy RT, MacRae CA, Caforio ALP, Elliott PM, McKenna WJ. Echocardiographic evaluation in asymptomatic relatives of patients with dilated cardiomyopathy reveals preclinical disease. *Ann Intern Med* 2005;143:108-15.

5 Zipes DP, Camm AJ, Borggrefe M, Buxton AE, Chaitman B, Fromer M, et al. ACC/AHA/ESC 2006 guidelines for management of patients with ventricular arrhythmias and the prevention of sudden cardiac death: a report of the American College of Cardiology/American Heart Association Task Force and the European Society of Cardiology Committee for Practice Guidelines (writing committee to develop guidelines for management of patients with ventricular arrhythmias and the prevention of sudden cardiac death) developed in collaboration with the European Heart Rhythm Association and the Heart Rhythm Society. *Europace* 2006;8:746-837.

6 Maron BJ, McKenna WJ, Danielson GK, Kappenberger LJ, Kuhn HJ, Seidman CE, et al. American College of Cardiology/European Society of Cardiology clinical expert consensus document on hypertrophic cardiomyopathy. A report of the American College of Cardiology Foundation Task Force on Clinical Expert Consensus Documents and the European Society of Cardiology Committee for Practice Guidelines. *J Am Coll Cardiol* 2003;42:1687-713.

7 Hendrix A, Borleffs CJW, Vink A, Doevendans PA, Wilde AA, van Langen IM, et al. Cardiogenetic screening of first-degree relatives after sudden cardiac death in the young: a population-based approach. *Europace* 2011;13:716-22.

8 Bos JM, Ommen SR, Ackerman MJ. Genetics of hypertrophic cardiomyopathy: one, two, or more diseases? *Curr Opin Cardiol* 2007;22:193-9.

9 Hershberger RE, Siegfried JD. Update 2011: clinical and genetic issues in familial dilated cardiomyopathy. *J Am Coll Cardiol* 2011;57:1641-9.

10 Vetter VL, Dugan N, Guo R, Mercer-Rosa L, Gleason M, Cohen M, et al. A pilot study of the feasibility of heart screening for sudden cardiac arrest in healthy children. *Am Heart J* 2011;161:1000-6.e3.

11 Maron BJ. Risk stratification and role of implantable defibrillators for prevention of sudden death in patients with hypertrophic cardiomyopathy. *Circ J* 2010;74:2271-82.

12 Pinamonti B, Dragos AM, Pyxaras SA, Merlo M, Pivetta A, Barbati G, et al. Prognostic predictors in arrhythmogenic right ventricular

cardiomyopathy: results from a 10-year registry. *Eur Heart J* 2011;32:1105-13.
13 De Noronha SV, Sharma S, Papadakis M, Desai S, Whyte G, Sheppard MN. Aetiology of sudden cardiac death in athletes in the United Kingdom: a pathological study. *Heart* 2009;95:1409-14.
14 Maron BJ, Roberts WC, Epstein SE. Sudden death in hypertrophic cardiomyopathy: a profile of 78 patients. *Circulation* 1982;65:1388-94.
15 Bowker TJ, Wood DA, Davies MJ. Sudden unexpected cardiac death: methods and results of a national pilot survey. *Int J Cardiol* 1995;52:241-50.
16 Papadakis M, Sharma S, Cox S, Sheppard MN, Panoulas VF, Behr ER. The magnitude of sudden cardiac death in the young: a death certificate-based review in England and Wales. *Europace* 2009;11:1353-8.
17 Savage DD, Seides SF, Clark CE, Henry WL, Maron BJ, Robinson FC, et al. Electrocardiographic findings in patients with obstructive and nonobstructive hypertrophic cardiomyopathy. *Circulation* 1978;58:402-8.
18 Marcus GM, Glidden DV, Polonsky B, Zareba W, Smith LM, Cannom DS, et al. Efficacy of antiarrhythmic drugs in arrhythmogenic right ventricular cardiomyopathy: a report from the North American ARVC registry. *J Am Coll Cardiol* 2009;54:609-15.
19 Garratt CJ, Elliott P, Behr E, Camm AJ, Cowan C, Cruickshank S, et al. Heart Rhythm UK position statement on clinical indications for implantable cardioverter defibrillators in adult patients with familial sudden cardiac death syndromes. *Europace* 2010;12:1156-75.
20 Dickstein K, Cohen-Solal A, Filippatos G, McMurray JJ, Ponikowski P, Poole-Wilson PA, et al. ESC guidelines for the diagnosis and treatment of acute and chronic heart failure 2008: the Task Force for the Diagnosis and Treatment of Acute and Chronic Heart Failure 2008 of the European Society of Cardiology. Developed in collaboration with the Heart Failure Association of the ESC (HFA) and endorsed by the European Society of Intensive Care Medicine (ESICM). *Eur Heart J* 2008;29:2388-442.
21 McLeod CJ, Shen WK, Rea RF, Friedman PA, Hayes DL, Wokhlu A, et al. Differential outcome of cardiac resynchronization therapy in ischemic cardiomyopathy and idiopathic dilated cardiomyopathy. *Heart Rhythm* 2011;8:377-82.
22 Ommen SR, Maron BJ, Olivotto I, Maron MS, Cecchi F, Betocchi S, et al. Long-term effects of surgical septal myectomy on survival in patients with obstructive hypertrophic cardiomyopathy. *J Am Coll Cardiol* 2005;46:470-6.
23 Wichter T, Paul TM, Eckardt L, Gerdes P, Kirchhof P, Böcker D, et al. Arrhythmogenic right ventricular cardiomyopathy. Antiarrhythmic drugs, catheter ablation, or ICD? *Herz* 2005;30:91-101.
24 Kozeluhova M, Peichl P, Cihak R, Wichterle D, Vancura V, Bytesnik J, et al. Catheter ablation of electrical storm in patients with structural heart disease. *Europace* 2011;13:109-13.
25 Maron MS, Kalsmith BM, Udelson JE, Li W, DeNofrio D. Survival after cardiac transplantation in patients with hypertrophic cardiomyopathy. *Circ Heart Fail* 2010;3:574-9.
26 Maron BJ, Olivotto I, Bellone P, Conte MR, Cecchi F, Flygenring BP, et al. Clinical profile of stroke in 900 patients with hypertrophic cardiomyopathy. *J Am Coll Cardiol* 2002;39:301-7.
27 Garratt CJ, Elliott P, Behr E, Blair E, Connelly D, Cowan C, et al. Clinical indications for genetic testing in familial sudden cardiac death syndromes: an HRUK position statement. *Heart* 2008;94:502-7.
28 Xu T, Yang Z, Vatta M, Rampazzo A, Beffagna G, Pilichou K, et al. Compound and digenic heterozygosity contributes to arrhythmogenic right ventricular cardiomyopathy. *J Am Coll Cardiol* 2010;55:587-97.
29 Wordsworth S, Leal J, Blair E, Legood R, Thomson K, Seller A, et al. DNA testing for hypertrophic cardiomyopathy: a cost-effectiveness model. *Eur Heart J* 2010;31:926-35.
30 Pasotti M, Klersy C, Pilotto A, Marziliano N, Rapezzi C, Serio A, et al. Long-term outcome and risk stratification in dilated cardiolaminopathies. *J Am Coll Cardiol* 2008;52:1250-60.

Related links

bmj.com/archive

- Renal transplantation (2011;343:d7300)
- Diagnosis and management of anal intraepithelial neoplasia and anal cancer (2011;343:d6818)
- Management of deep vein thrombosis and prevention of post-thrombotic syndrome (2011;343:d5916)
- Diagnosis and management of autism in childhood (2011;343:d6238)

CME

- Get Cleveland Clinic CME points for this article

BMJ BPP UNIVERSITY SCHOOL OF HEALTH

Resistant hypertension

Aung Myat, British Heart Foundation clinical research training fellow[1], Simon R Redwood, professor of interventional cardiology[1], Ayesha C Qureshi, specialist registrar in cardiology[2], John A Spertus, director of cardiovascular education and outcomes research[3], Bryan Williams, professor of medicine[4]

[1]British Heart Foundation Centre of Research Excellence, Cardiovascular Division, Rayne Institute, St Thomas' Hospital, King's College London, London SE1 7EH, UK

[2]London Deanery, Stewart House, London WC1B 5DN, UK

[3]Mid America Heart Institute, University of Missouri-Kansas City, Kansas City, MO 64111, USA

[4]Institute of Cardiovascular Science, University College London, London WC1E 6BT, UK

Correspondence to: B Williams bryan.williams@ucl.ac.uk

Cite this as: *BMJ* 2012;345:e7473

‹DOI› 10.1136/bmj.e7473
http://www.bmj.com/content/345/bmj.e7473

The disease burden attributable to arterial hypertension is substantial, accounting for or contributing to 62% of all strokes and 49% of all cases of heart disease, culminating in an estimated 7.1 million deaths a year; equivalent to 13% of total worldwide deaths.[1] Although most cases of hypertension can be effectively treated with lifestyle changes or drugs, or both, hidden within this population lies a cohort at the extreme end of the cardiovascular risk spectrum—those with hypertension that is resistant to treatment.

The aim of this review is to assist non-specialist practitioners in the overall management of patients with resistant hypertension by presenting a comprehensive exploration of the evidence on the recognition, evaluation, and treatment of the condition.

What is resistant hypertension?

International guidelines have defined resistant hypertension as a raised blood pressure (that is, seated clinic blood pressure >140/90 mm Hg) despite treatment with at least three antihypertensive agents (one of which is usually a diuretic) at optimal or best tolerated doses. The recent National Institute for Health and Clinical Excellence (NICE) guideline (see box 1) has been the most proscriptive in formally defining resistant hypertension by suggesting that the three agents would usually be an angiotensin converting enzyme (ACE) inhibitor or an angiotensin receptor blocker plus a calcium channel blocker plus a thiazide-type diuretic (that is, A+C+D) in accordance with the NICE treatment algorithm. The NICE guidance also suggests that resistant hypertension should be diagnosed only after confirming inadequate blood pressure control despite treatment, by use of ambulatory blood pressure monitoring (that is, mean daytime blood pressure >135/85 mm Hg), thereby excluding so called white coat hypertension. The optimal target blood pressure in patients treated for resistant hypertension is widely accepted to be <140/90 mm Hg, as it is for all hypertensive patients in general, although lower targets may be appropriate for those with diabetes or chronic kidney disease.

SOURCES AND SELECTION CRITERIA

Using the term "resistant hypertension", we searched the PubMed, Embase, and Cochrane databases for articles from a publication date of January 2000 to June 2012. Further articles were then identified from the reference lists of the articles found in the database search. We restricted our search to those written in the English language, studies on humans, and published work only. Priority was given to systematic reviews, meta-analyses, and clinical guidelines.

SUMMARY POINTS

- Resistant hypertension is defined as high blood pressure that remains uncontrolled despite treatment with at least three antihypertensive agents (one of which is usually a diuretic) at best tolerated doses. A diagnosis of true resistant hypertension should be made only after a thorough assessment to exclude apparent or pseudo-resistant hypertension
- Post hoc analyses of large scale trials of antihypertensive drugs plus retrospective cross sectional observational studies point to a prevalence of resistant hypertension of 10-20% of the general hypertensive population
- Patients with resistant hypertension are almost 50% more likely to experience an adverse cardiovascular event compared with patients with blood pressure controlled by three or fewer antihypertensive agents
- Studies indicate that 5-10% of resistant hypertension patients have an underlying secondary cause for their elevated blood pressure—a prevalence significantly greater than that of the general hypertensive population
- No clinical trials have compared the effectiveness of specific drug regimens for the treatment of resistant hypertension. The best available evidence supports the use of low dose spironolactone as the preferred fourth drug if the patient's blood potassium level is ≤4.5 mmol/L. With higher blood potassium levels, intensification of thiazide-like diuretic therapy should be considered
- Renal sympathetic denervation therapy, as a device based intervention, could potentially stimulate a paradigm shift in the management of resistant hypertension

Who gets resistant hypertension?

Data derived from retrospective, cross sectional population studies of hypertension control in Spain and the United States indicate a resistant hypertension prevalence of between 7.6% and 8.9%.[2 3] In the recent Health Survey for England, 20% of hypertensive patients had uncontrolled blood pressure despite the administration of at least three drugs, making it reasonable to assume the population with resistant hypertension is around 0.5-1 million individuals in England alone.[4] Post hoc analysis of data from large clinical trials of antihypertensive therapy (such as ALLHAT, ASCOT, ACCOMPLISH, LIFE, INVEST, and CONVINCE[5 6 7 8 9 10]) suggests that the prevalence of resistant hypertension could be as high as 35%. However, these highly selected populations tend to be older and contain higher risk individuals with greater cardiovascular comorbidity than the general hypertensive population.[5 6 7 8 9 10] Amalgamation of the earlier clinical trial data with the more contemporaneous observational findings suggests a resistant hypertension prevalence of 10-20% of the hypertensive population.[11]

A US study found that, within a median of 1.5 years after initiation of antihypertensive therapy, about 1 in 50 of the patients developed resistant hypertension (either uncontrolled hypertension with ≥3 antihypertensive drugs or controlled hypertension with ≥4 antihypertensives).[12] This represents an incidence of 1.9% of resistant hypertension in the 205 750 hypertensive patients who began drug therapy. Among those taking three or more medications for at least one month (n=24 499), the prevalence of resistant hypertension was 16.2%. The results were further strengthened by exclusion of patients with pseudo-resistant hypertension and inclusion of a large and ethnically diverse population.[12] The analysis also revealed that patients with resistant hypertension were almost 50% more likely to experience an adverse cardiovascular event over a median follow-up of 3.8 years compared with patients with blood pressure controlled by means of three or fewer antihypertensive drugs.[12] This increased risk was largely

BOX 1: NATIONAL AND INTERNATIONAL HYPERTENSION GUIDELINES

- NICE Clinical Guideline 127. Hypertension—The clinical management of primary hypertension in adults. 2011.
- Commissioned by the National Institute for Health and Clinical Excellence (NICE) in the UK and produced in partnership with the British Hypertension Society, this 325 page document is pragmatic, evidence based, and the most contemporaneous set of guidelines currently available. There is a detailed section on resistant hypertension with related evidence to recommendation statements on pages 245-7. The document can be downloaded from http://guidance.nice.org.uk/CG127.
- Calhoun DA, Jones D, Textor S, Goff DC, Murphy TP, Toto RD, et al. Resistant hypertension: diagnosis, evaluation, and treatment—a scientific statement from the American Heart Association Professional Education Committee of the Council for High Blood Pressure Research. *Hypertension* 2008;51:1403-19
- A position statement focused on the management of resistant hypertension. Provides in-depth coverage on patient evaluation and treatment recommendations.
- The Task Force for the Management of Arterial Hypertension of the European Society of Hypertension (ESH) and of the European Society of Cardiology (ESC). 2007 Guidelines for the management of arterial hypertension. *Eur Heart J* 2007;28:1462-536.
- Resistant hypertension is given a modicum of coverage on pages 1506-7. A reappraisal of the European guidelines on hypertension management was published in 2009 (*J Hypertens* 2009;27:2121-58) to take account of publication of several large randomised trials, but there was no further guidance on the care of patients with resistant hypertension.
- Chobanian AV, Bakris GL, Black HR, Cushman WC, Green LA, Izzo JL Jr, et al. Seventh report of the Joint National Committee on Prevention, Detection, Evaluation, and Treatment of High Blood Pressure. *Hypertension* 2003;42:1206-52.
- Issued by the US National Heart Lung and Blood Institute, these guidelines are now being updated. A section on the definition of resistant hypertension can be found on page 1230 of the document. The eighth report is currently in progress (see www.nhlbi.nih.gov/guidelines/hypertension/jnc8/index.htm for further information).

BOX 2: TYPICAL CHARACTERISTICS OF PATIENTS WITH RESISTANT HYPERTENSION[13 14 15]

- Older age; especially >75 years
- High baseline blood pressure and chronicity of uncontrolled hypertension
- Target organ damage (left ventricular hypertrophy, chronic kidney disease)
- Diabetes
- Obesity
- Atherosclerotic vascular disease
- Aortic stiffening
- Sex (women)
- Ethnicity (black)
- Excessive dietary sodium

BOX 3: FACTORS ASSOCIATED WITH PSEUDO-RESISTANT HYPERTENSION

These factors should be considered, looked for, and eliminated before a diagnosis of true resistant hypertension can be made.

Factors associated with the patient

- White coat effect
- Severely calcified or arteriosclerotic arteries that are poorly compressible on palpation, giving rise to cuff related artefact (especially in elderly patients)
- Poor patient concordance to treatment:
- Side effects of antihypertensive medication
- Complicated dosing regimens
- Inadequate patient education
- Memory or psychiatric issues or poor cognition (especially in elderly patients)
- Difficult relationship between patient and doctor
- Costs of drugs (in some healthcare systems)

Factors associated with the physician

- Poor office blood pressure measurement technique
- Clinical inertia
- Inadequate doses of antihypertensive drugs
- Inappropriate choice of antihypertensive combinations
- Poor communication and lack of desire to invest in patient education

caused by the development of chronic kidney disease. However, the precise long term prognosis of patients with resistant hypertension is still to be determined.

Certain patient characteristics have been associated with an increased likelihood of developing treatment resistant hypertension (see box 2).[13 14 15] Many of these characteristics are associated with adverse cardiovascular outcomes and underscore the need for effective treatment of resistant hypertension.

How is resistant hypertension diagnosed?

Apparent or pseudo-resistant hypertension

Before a patient can be labelled as having treatment resistant hypertension, apparent or pseudo-resistant hypertension must be excluded. This is inadequate blood pressure control in a patient receiving appropriate treatment who does not actually have resistant hypertension. Most often, pseudo-resistant hypertension arises from (*a*) poor office blood pressure measurement technique (see supplementary boxes on bmj.com), (*b*) the "white coat" effect, (*c*) poor patient concordance with prescribed therapy, or (*d*) a suboptimal antihypertensive regimen (see box 3).

Medical professionals must also recognise and accept that "clinical inertia" has an important role to play in the suboptimal management of hypertension, particularly when patients require multiple drugs. The term clinical inertia can encompass a poor knowledge of clinical guidelines, a misguided acceptance of elevated blood pressure, or an underestimation of cardiovascular disease risk, all of which can lead to suboptimal blood pressure treatment.[16] It is of prime importance to consider patient and physician factors and eliminate them, before establishing a definitive diagnosis of resistant hypertension.

What is the best method for assessing blood pressure?

In a retrospective analysis of records in a Spanish registry, up to 40% of the patients defined as having resistant hypertension according to office blood pressure recordings were later found to manifest a white coat effect when evaluated by ambulatory blood pressure monitoring.[2] This highlights how common the white coat effect (that is, a persistently elevated office blood pressure but a normal home blood pressure—see supplementary boxes on bmj.com) can be. It also emphasises the importance of using ambulatory blood pressure monitoring to confirm resistant hypertension as recommended by the recent NICE guidance. A white coat effect should be suspected in any individual with persistently elevated office blood pressure readings but no signs of target organ damage or signs or symptoms of overtreatment such as postural hypotension, dizziness, or syncope.[17]

What lifestyle factors contribute to resistant hypertension?

Once a diagnosis of true resistant hypertension has been established, the next step is to evaluate the patient for potentially modifiable contributing factors (see box 4).

Obesity is a common feature of patients with resistant hypertension, partly due to an association with sodium retention, enhanced sympathetic nervous system activity, and activation of the renin-angiotensin-aldosterone system (RAAS). There is also an increased likelihood of pseudo-resistant hypertension in obese patients if too small a cuff is applied to a large arm. The HYDRA study of 45 125 primary care patients in Germany found that obese individuals (body mass index >40) had a 5.3-fold greater probability of requiring three antihypertensive drugs and a 3.2-fold greater probability of requiring four antihypertensive drugs to achieve blood pressure control compared with individuals with a normal body mass index (<25).[18]

The relationship between the prevalence of hypertension, alcohol consumption, and blood pressure is linear.[19] Moderate alcohol consumption does not generally elevate blood pressure levels, but heavy alcohol consumption (>21 units/week for men, >14 units/week for women where 1 unit = 8 g or 10 ml of alcohol or a half pint of beer, glass of wine, or shot of spirits), including binge drinking, is associated with raised blood pressure, an increased risk of stroke, and an overall poorer prognosis. Trials of structured interventions to reduce alcohol intake have resulted in significant falls in both systolic and diastolic blood pressures.[20]

Patients must be asked about the potential use of prescribed and recreational exogenous substances (see box 4) and, where possible, the offending agents stopped, minimised, or substituted appropriately. The effects of these agents can be highly variable and unpredictable, with most patients showing minimal effects whereas others experience substantial elevations in blood pressure. Where there is doubt with regard to which agents should be modified, a specialist opinion may be warranted.

Excessive dietary salt intake is a well recognised risk factor for resistant hypertension. Indeed most patients with resistant hypertension tend to consume more salt than the general population, often exceeding 10 g/day.[21] Excess salt directly increases blood pressure and also blunts the action of all antihypertensive agents in general. The effect is magnified in individuals who are particularly salt sensitive (elderly patients, black patients, and those with chronic kidney disease—see box 2). It is therefore important to review an individual's salt intake, provide dietary advice, and recommend a salt intake <6 g/day (refer to section 11.1.8 page 185 of NICE Clinical Guideline 127 on hypertension—see box 1).

BOX 4: FACTORS CONTRIBUTING TO RESISTANT HYPERTENSION

Lifestyle factors
- Obesity
- Excess alcohol intake
- Excess dietary sodium
- Cocaine and amphetamines misuse

Drug related causes
- Non-steroidal anti-inflammatory drugs
- Contraceptive hormones—Combined oral contraceptives are more often associated with elevated blood pressure, whereas menopausal hormone therapy has minimal effects on blood pressure
- Adrenal steroid hormones
- Sympathomimetic agents (nasal decongestants, diet pills)
- Erythropoeitin, ciclosporin, and tacrolimus
- Liquorice (suppresses the metabolism of cortisol)
- Herbal supplements (ephedra, bitter orange, etc)

Volume overload
- Progressive renal insufficiency
- High salt intake
- Inadequate diuretic therapy

Secondary causes of resistant hypertension and their pertinent features
- Primary hyperaldosteronism—Hypokalaemia, fatigue, low renin levels despite drug treatment that would be expected to elevate renin levels (that is, ACE inhibitor or angiotensin receptor blocker plus a calcium channel blocker and diuretic), usually raised aldosterone levels but elevation may not be extreme
- Renal artery stenosis—Carotid, abdominal, or femoral bruits; history of flash pulmonary oedema; young females (fibromuscular dysplasia), history of atherosclerotic disease
- Renal parenchymal disease—Albuminuria or microscopic haematuria, biochemical disturbances, nocturia, oedema
- Obstructive sleep apnoea—Obesity, short neck, daytime somnolence, snoring, frequent night time awakenings, witnessed apnoea
- Phaeochromocytoma—Episodic palpitations, headaches, sweating
- Thyroid diseases—Eye signs, weight loss or gain, heat or cold intolerance, heart failure, tachycardia, bradycardia, anxiety or fatigue. Hyperthyroidism usually increases systolic blood pressure, whereas hypothyroidism usually increases diastolic blood pressure
- Cushing's syndrome—Centripetal obesity, moon facies, abdominal striae, interscapular fat deposition
- Coarctation of the aorta—Radio-radial or radio-femoral delay, diminished femoral pulses, rib notching on chest radiograph
- Intracranial tumours—Early morning headache, family history

BOX 5: BIOCHEMICAL EVALUATION FOR PATIENTS WITH SUSPECTED RESISTANT HYPERTENSION

Preliminary biochemical tests should be conducted before specialist referral. These can help to delineate a potential secondary cause of resistant hypertension unearthed by the patient's history and physical examination, signal the development of renal dysfunction, and help to monitor response and side effects of antihypertensive agents.
- Urea and electrolytes
- Estimated glomerular filtration rate
- Plasma glucose
- Plasma renin or aldosterone levels
- 24 hour urinary metanephrines or normetanephrines (for phaeochromocytoma)
- Urine analysis—microalbuminuria and macroalbuminuria, haematuria

What are the secondary causes of resistant hypertension?

Potentially remediable secondary causes of resistant hypertension are listed in box 4. The prevalence of secondary hypertension is greater in people with resistant hypertension compared with the general hypertensive population, with studies indicating that 5-10% of patients with resistant hypertension have an underlying secondary cause[22] [23]—the most common being hyperaldosteronism, chronic kidney disease (which may either be the cause or adverse sequel of chronic, poorly controlled hypertension), renal artery stenosis, and obstructive sleep apnoea. It is important for the non-specialist to be able to recognise the signs and symptoms that may suggest an underlying disease process. This should include a focused history, thorough physical examination, biochemical evaluation, non-invasive imaging (such as renal ultrasound), and subsequent onward referral to a specialist hypertension clinic if necessary (see boxes 4 and 5).

What target organ damage is seen in resistant hypertension?

Target organ damage refers to left ventricular hypertrophy, hypertensive retinopathy, and renal disease (that is, persistently elevated urinary albumin excretion rate, haematuria, or renal impairment). Electrocardiography and ideally echocardiography should be performed, along with fundoscopy, urine analysis, renal biochemistry, and, if available, renal imaging. Evidence of target organ damage will help to support a diagnosis of poorly controlled hypertension and may influence decisions about an appropriate treatment target.

How is concordance with treatment assessed?

An important consideration in patients with resistant hypertension is their concordance with treatment. This is especially important in view of the fact that hypertension is largely asymptomatic and is treated with multiple drugs.

Increasingly, "directly observed therapy" clinics are used in specialist centres, where patients are asked to consume their drugs at the clinic and blood pressure is then monitored either by ambulatory blood pressure monitoring or home blood pressure monitoring over the following 6–24 hours to confirm whether there is a response to a witnessed consumption of medication. Urine testing of drug metabolites is also being introduced in specialist clinics to confirm concordance before considering further evaluation and treatment.

What treatments are available for resistant hypertension?

Non-pharmacologic intervention

The aetiology of true resistant hypertension is almost always multifactorial, and a comprehensive management strategy should therefore include recognition and reversal of contributory lifestyle factors. Thus, weight loss; regular exercise; a high fibre, low fat, low salt diet; and moderation of alcohol and caffeine intake should be encouraged, alongside the cessation or down-titration of interfering exogenous substances. Screening for secondary causes should be dictated by the initial clinical and biochemical evaluation, with appropriate investigations, treatment, and specialist referral made when needed (see box 6). A concerted effort should be made to maximise patient concordance with therapy, and, to assist this, interventions should range from promoting patient education, motivation, and "ownership" of their management programme to increasing the frequency of clinic visits, using a multidisciplinary team approach, advocating home blood pressure monitoring as a means of monitoring therapeutic response, and setting realistic goals in achieving blood pressure targets.

Drug intervention

Patients defined as having resistant hypertension will already be receiving or have received at least three antihypertensive drugs. NICE has recommended that this combination should ideally include drugs with potentially synergistic actions—that is, an ACE inhibitor or angiotensin receptor blocker plus a calcium channel blocker plus a thiazide-type diuretic (A+C+D). There is implied consensus with this recommendation in other guidelines (see box 1), but this has not always been explicitly stated in this stepwise fashion. The next question is what to add as the fourth agent to treat resistant hypertension.

To date, there have been no clinical trials that have specifically compared the various treatment options available. Moreover, it is unlikely that any one class of drug (in addition to A+C+D) will be ideal for every case of resistant hypertension.[24] What is clear is that dual RAAS blockade—that is, the combination of an ACE inhibitor and an angiotensin receptor blocker—is not recommended because of a lack of evidence in resistant hypertension, and in light of the "no added value" and increased risk of adverse events seen in high risk patients enrolled in the ONTARGET trial.[25] The best available, albeit weak, evidence (as reviewed in the recent NICE Clinical Guideline 127) is observational and supports the use of low dose spironolactone (that is, 25 mg once daily, increasing to 50 mg once daily) as the preferred fourth agent if the blood potassium concentration is ≤4.5 mmol/L.[w1-w7] Spironolactone blocks the action of aldosterone at the mineralocorticoid receptor, thereby stimulating natriuresis and alleviating fluid overload. It can also overcome the phenomenon of "aldosterone rebound" seen with chronic RAAS antagonism, where aldosterone escapes blockade and levels return to baseline.[w8] In resistant hypertension patients, spironolactone has also been shown to induce the regression of left ventricular hypertrophy irrespective of aldosterone status and reduce intra-cardiac volumes in those patients with hyperaldosteronism.[w3]

The main adverse effect associated with spironolactone use is breast tenderness and gynaecomastia. This is related to both dose and duration of therapy and can take many months or even years to develop. It is usually reversible when the drug is stopped. If the blood pressure response to spironolactone has been effective but the drug is stopped because of gynaecomastia, amiloride or eplerenone can be considered as a substitute. Both these drugs, however, are not as potent as spironolactone and so may require doses above the usual range prescribed. Hyperkalaemia is a risk when using any of these potassium sparing diuretics, especially in those patients with resistant hypertension who are already taking an ACE inhibitor or angiotensin receptor blocker (which is usually the case in these patients) and in individuals with chronic kidney disease or diabetes. Potassium levels should be monitored within two weeks of drug initiation. Subsequent monitoring will largely depend on the index result and whether dose adjustment has been necessary. Furthermore, hyponatraemia may also develop with long term use, especially in elderly patients and when potassium sparing diuretics are combined with pre-existing diuretic therapy.

Alternatively, if the blood potassium level is >4.5 mmol/L, intensification of thiazide-like diuretic therapy (that is, doubling of the dose of the existing thiazide-like diuretic) should be considered. If blood pressure remains poorly controlled despite further diuretic therapy, there is the option of adding an α or β blocker, but this guidance remains empirical in nature in the absence of robust clinical trial evidence.

Centrally acting α agonists (methyldopa and clonidine) or direct vasodilators (hydralazine and minoxidil) are further options. The potential roles of other agents such as endothelin receptor antagonists have yet to be clearly defined.[24 w9] Whatever the final combination of treatments, a patient with resistant hypertension is likely to be receiving at least four antihypertensive drugs daily, and some guidelines have recommended use of fixed combination therapies to reduce the number of tablets—there is some evidence that this may also improve adherence to treatment.[w10]

BOX 6: WHEN SHOULD PATIENTS BE REFERRED TO A SPECIALIST?

- Referral to the appropriate specialist is warranted when the history, examination, and initial screening tests suggest a secondary cause of resistant hypertension—refer to the clinical evaluation algorithm in the supplementary material on bmj.com
- Individuals under 40 years old, especially those who do not match the typical criteria seen in box 2
- Difficulty in interpretation of office and ambulatory or home blood pressure measurements
- Difficulty in differentiating pseudo-resistant from true resistant hypertension
- Difficulty in controlling blood pressure despite an assessment of adherence to treatment, modification of lifestyle factors, and appropriate intensification of combination therapy over a six month period
- Difficulty in finding a well tolerated drug regimen
- Those who have evidence of target organ damage or clinical manifestations of cardiovascular disease
- For consideration of device therapy to control blood pressure when all drug interventions have been exhausted

BOX 7: EDUCATIONAL RESOURCES ON DEVICE THERAPY FOR RESISTANT HYPERTENSION

- Joint UK Societies' Consensus Statement on Renal Denervation for Resistant Hypertension. www.bcs.com/documents/The_Joint_UK_Societies_Consensus_on_Renal_Denervation_for_resistant_hypertension.pdf
- NICE guidance. Percutaneous transluminal radiofrequency sympathetic denervation of the renal artery for resistant hypertension (IPG418). http://guidance.nice.org.uk/IPG418
- Lohmeier TE, Iliescu R. Chronic lowering of blood pressure by carotid baroreflex activation. *Hypertension* 2011;57:880-6, http://hyper.ahajournals.org/content/57/5/880.long. A comprehensive review on carotid baroreflex activation therapy
- British Hypertension Society. www.bhsoc.org/default.stm
- European Society of Hypertension. www.eshonline.org/. The society has also issued a position paper on renal denervation, published in the *Journal of Hypertension* (2012;30:837-41)
- American Society of Hypertension. www.ash-us.org/

FUTURE PERSPECTIVES

- A prospective epidemiological study is required to delineate the true prevalence, incidence, and prognostic implications of resistant hypertension, and consensus between national and international professional bodies is required on a universal definition of resistant hypertension to allow robust comparisons between future studies.

Unanswered questions

- Is there one class of drug that is commonly the most effective in resistant hypertension?
- What patient characteristics, if any, define which drug is likely to be the most effective?
- What are the ideal constituents of multidrug regimens in resistant hypertension? A prospective randomised controlled trial of different drug combinations is required
- Is there a role for routine plasma renin measurements to stratify drug treatment for resistant hypertension, and would this be cost effective? Is there a role for renin profiling in the management of resistant hypertension?
- Is there clinical benefit from chronotherapy (when one antihypertensive agent is taken at night rather than all being taken together in the morning)?
- What is the future role of device therapies in resistant hypertension management? Do they have an additive effect to antihypertensive drugs?
- What strategies are most effective in supporting adherence to drug regimens and lifestyle factors?
- Are there system based or team based strategies that can organise the health system to better identify, monitor, and treat resistant hypertension?

Ongoing research

- Studies of the effect of continuous positive airways pressure in patients with resistant hypertension secondary to obstructive sleep apnoea (ClinicalTrials.gov Identifiers: NCT01508754 and NCT00929175)
- The BHS PATHWAY studies supported by the British Heart Foundation and the National Institute of Health Research Clinical Research Network. PATHWAY 2 focuses on resistant hypertension and is evaluating whether low dose spironolactone is usually the most effective step 4 treatment for resistant hypertension, in comparison with doxazosin or bisoprolol. The participants with resistant hypertension are well characterised and already treated according to NICE guidance with A+C+D. This study will also formally evaluate the value of plasma renin profiling in determining treatment responses in resistant hypertension (refer to www.bhsoc.org/clinical_research.stm).
- The Resistant Arterial Hypertension Cohort Study (RAHyCo) (ClinicalTrials.gov Identifier NCT01083017) is investigating the epidemiology of resistant hypertension and evaluating the efficacy and feasibility of a standardised treatment regimen (including randomisation of two doses of chlortalidone). It is also studying two interventions in a group of non-compliant patients, and will study environmental and genetic variables of individuals with resistant hypertension within a family design. It plans to enrol 200 patients and is due to complete in April 2018.

EDUCATIONAL RESOURCES FOR PATIENTS

- Blood Pressure Association. www.bloodpressureuk.org/Home
- British Heart Foundation. www.bhf.org.uk/heart-health/conditions/high-blood-pressure.aspx
- Patient.co.uk. www.patient.co.uk/health/High-Blood-Pressure-(Hypertension).htm
- American Heart Association. www.heart.org/HEARTORG/Conditions/HighBloodPressure/High-Blood-Pressure_UCM_002020_SubHomePage.jsp
- Hypertension Education Foundation. www.hypertensionfoundation.org/patients.cfm

Device therapy

Interest is growing in device therapy for resistant hypertension, with the objective of improving blood pressure control without resorting to further medication. Two techniques have recently been evaluated: percutaneous transluminal radiofrequency sympathetic denervation of the renal arteries[w11-w14] and carotid baroreflex activation.[w15 w16] The former has generated the most interest, with several devices in development. Briefly, the Symplicity HTN-1 and HTN-2 trials have shown substantial blood pressure reductions in response to renal denervation, in the order of 30/15 mm Hg, maintained beyond two years on extended follow-up of the original study cohorts.[w12 w13] It should be noted, however, that, although renal denervation resulted in improved blood pressure control, the patients continued to take antihypertensive drugs, albeit at a reduced number or dose in some patients. A key point is that renal denervation is not a "cure" for resistant hypertension. Further renal denervation therapy trials are ongoing, with devices at various stages of development.[w17]

To date, there have been no safety concerns with renal denervation, in particular no evidence of significant renal artery stenosis or thrombosis in up to two years of follow-up.[w13] There is consensus that renal denervation procedures should be undertaken only in specialist centres with multidisciplinary specialist expertise in the assessment and treatment of complex hypertension (see box 7). The place of such therapies in the more routine treatment of resistant hypertension will ultimately be determined by longer term efficacy and safety data and cost effectiveness analyses.

What is the future of resistant hypertension treatment?

The BHS Collaborative Research Working Party has initiated the Prevention And Treatment of resistant Hypertension With Algorithm guided therapY (PATHWAY) studies (see "Future perspectives" box), that will specifically address the most effective way to treat resistant hypertension. These, along with other studies, should answer some of the fundamental questions still outstanding. The results are eagerly awaited and will directly inform future treatment guidelines for resistant hypertension.

Contributors: AM wrote the original draft manuscript and was involved in its conception and design. SRR and ACQ were involved in drafting the article and formulating its conception and design. JAS and BW were involved in conception and design and revising the manuscript critically for important intellectual content. All authors gave final approval of the version to be published.

Funding: AM acknowledges financial support from the Department of Health via the National Institute for Health Research comprehensive Biomedical Research Centre award to Guy's and St Thomas' NHS Foundation Trust in partnership with King's College London and King's College Hospital NHS Foundation Trust along with a British Heart Foundation Clinical Research Training Fellowship (Grant Number FS/11/70/28917). BW is an NIHR senior investigator and is supported by the University College London Hospitals NIHR Biomedical Research Centre.

Competing interests: All authors have completed the ICMJE uniform disclosure form at www.icmje.org/coi_disclosure.pdf (available on request from the corresponding author) and declare: no support from any organisation for the submitted work; ACQ has received research funding from Boston Scientific and travel and educational grants from Boston Scientific, Biosensors, Eli-Lilly, Medtronic, and Servier, and was a full time employee of Cordis (Johnson and Johnson) from April 2011 to November 2012; BW has received honoraria for lectures at conferences from Novartis, Boehringer Ingelheim, and Pfizer; no other relationships or activities that could appear to have influenced the submitted work.

Provenance and peer review: Not commissioned; externally peer reviewed.

1 World Health Organization. *Global status report on noncommunicable diseases 2010* . WHO, 2011.
2 De la Sierra A, Segura J, Banegas JR, Gorostidi M, de la Cruz JJ, Armario P, et al. Clinical features of 8295 patients with resistant hypertension classified on the basis of ambulatory blood pressure monitoring. *Hypertension* 2011;57:898-902.
3 Persell SD. Prevalence of resistant hypertension in the United States, 2003-2008. *Hypertension* 2011;57:1076-80.
4 Falaschetti E, Chaudhury M, Mindell J, Poulter N. Continued improvement in hypertension management in England: results from the Health Survey for England 2006. *Hypertension* 2009;53:480-6.
5 The ALLHAT Officers. Major outcomes in high-risk hypertensive patients randomized to angiotensin-converting enzyme inhibitor or calcium channel blocker vs diuretic. *JAMA* 2002;288:2981-97.
6 Gupta AK, Nasothimiou EG, Chang CL, Sever PS, Dahlöf B, Poulter NR. Baseline predictors of resistant hypertension in the Anglo-Scandinavian Cardiac Outcome Trial (ASCOT): a risk score to identify those at high-risk. *J Hypertens* 2011;29:2004-13.
7 Jamerson K, Weber M, Bakris G, Dahlof B, Pitt B, Shi V, et al. Benazepril plus amlodipine or hydrochlorothiazide for hypertension in high-risk patients. *N Engl J Med* 2008;359:2417-28.
8 Dahlöf B, Devereux R, Kjeldsen S, Julius S, Beevers G, de Faire U, et al. Cardiovascular morbidity and mortality in the Losartan Intervention for Endpoint reduction in hypertension study (LIFE): a randomised trial against atenolol. *Lancet* 2002;359:995-1003.
9 Pepine C, Handberg E, Cooper-DeHoff R, Marks R, Kowey P, Messerli F, et al. A calcium antagonist vs a non-calcium antagonist hypertension strategy for patients with coronary artery disease. The International Verapamil-Trandolapril Study (INVEST): a randomized controlled trial. *JAMA* 2003;290:2805-16.
10 Black HR, Elliott WJ, Grandits G, Grambsch P, Lucente T, White WB, et al. Principal results of the Controlled Onset Verapamil Investigation of Cardiovascular End Points (CONVINCE) trial. *JAMA* 2003;289:2073-82.
11 Pimenta E, Calhoun DA. Resistant hypertension: incidence, prevalence, and prognosis. *Circulation* 2012;125:1594-6.
12 Daugherty SL, Powers JD, Magid DJ, Tavel HM, Masoudi FA, Margolis KL, et al. Incidence and prognosis of resistant hypertension in hypertensive patients. *Circulation* 2012;125:1635-42.
13 Lloyd-Jones DM, Evans JC, Larson MG, O'Donnell CJ, Roccella EJ, Levy D. Differential control of systolic and diastolic blood pressure: factors associated with lack of blood pressure control in the community. *Hypertension* 2000;36:594-9.
14 Cushman WC, Ford CE, Cutler JA, Margolis KL, Davis BR, Grimm RH, et al. Success and predictors of blood pressure control in diverse North American settings: the antihypertensive and lipid-lowering treatment to prevent heart attack trial (ALLHAT). *J Clin Hypertens (Greenwich)* 2002;4:393-404.
15 Williams B. The aorta and resistant hypertension. *J Am Coll Cardiol* 2009;53:452-4.
16 Oliveria SA, Lapuerta P, McCarthy BD, L'Italien GJ, Berlowitz DR, Asch SM. Physician-related barriers to the effective management of uncontrolled hypertension. *Arch Intern Med* 2002;162:413-20.
17 Fagard RH. Resistant hypertension. *Heart* 2012;98:254-61.
18 Sharma A, Wittchen H, Kirch W, Pittrow D, Ritz E, Goke B, et al. High prevalence and poor control of hypertension in primary care: cross-sectional study. *J Hypertens* 2004;22:479-86.
19 Puddey I, Beilin LJ, Rakic V. Alcohol, hypertension and the cardiovascular system: a critical appraisal. *Addiction Biology* 1997;2:159-70.
20 Cushman W, Cutler J, Hanna E, Bingham S, Follman D, Harford T, et al. Prevention and Treatment of Hypertension Study (PATHS): effects of an alcohol treatment program on blood pressure. *Arch Intern Med* 1998;158:1197-207.
21 Nishizaka MK, Pratt-Ubunama M, Zaman MA, Cofield S, Calhoun DA. Validity of plasma aldosterone-to-renin activity ratio in African American and white subjects with resistant hypertension. *AJH* 2005;18:805-12.
22 Yakovlevitch M, Black HR. Resistant hypertension in a tertiary care clinic. *Arch Intern Med* 1991;151:1786-92.
23 Garg JP, Elliott WJ, Folker A, Izhar M, Black HR. Resistant hypertension revisited: a comparison of two university-based cohorts. *AJH* 2005;18(5 Pt 1):619-26.
24 Williams B. Resistant hypertension: an unmet treatment need. *Lancet* 2009;374:1396-8.
25 THE ONTARGET Investigators. Telmisartan, ramipril, or both in patients at high risk for vascular events. *N Engl J Med* 2008;358:1547-59.

Related links

bmj.com/archive

- Childhood constipation (2012;345:e7309)
- Preparing young travellers for low resource destinations (2012;345:e7179)
- Management of chronic rhinosinusitis (2012;345:e7054)
- Salivary gland swellings (2012;345:e6794)
- Management of anal fistula (2012;345:e6705)
- Plantar fasciitis (2012;345:e6603)

bmj.com

- Cardiovascular medicine updates from BMJ Group

BMJ BPP UNIVERSITY SCHOOL OF HEALTH

Pulmonary hypertension: diagnosis and management

David G Kiely, consultant respiratory physician[1], Charlie A Elliot, consultant respiratory physician[1], Ian Sabroe, consultant respiratory physician[1,2], Robin Condliffe, consultant respiratory physician [1]

[1]National Pulmonary Hypertension Service (Sheffield), Pulmonary Vascular Disease Unit, Royal Hallamshire Hospital, Sheffield Teaching Hospitals NHS Foundation Trust, Sheffield S10 2JF, UK

[2]Academic Unit of Respiratory Medicine, Department of Infection and Immunity, Faculty of Medicine, Dentistry and Health, Medical School, University of Sheffield, Sheffield, UK

Correspondence to: D G Kiely david.kiely@sth.nhs.uk

Cite this as: *BMJ* 2013;346: f2028

‹DOI› 10.1136/bmj.f2028
http://www.bmj.com/content/346/bmj.f2028

Pulmonary hypertension was previously considered a rare untreatable condition. The past two decades have seen major changes in our understanding of the spectrum of disease affecting the pulmonary circulation. More than 30 randomised controlled trials (RCTs) of treatments have been performed, and surgery for patients with chronic thromboembolic pulmonary hypertension has been developed. Advances in imaging have enabled more detailed patient assessment, but pulmonary hypertension continues to be a life shortening condition, and there is often a delay of around two years from onset of symptoms to diagnosis.[1] This article focuses on adult pulmonary hypertension in primary and secondary care, its diagnosis, and management.

What is pulmonary hypertension and how common is it?

Pulmonary hypertension is defined at cardiac catheterisation as a mean pulmonary artery pressure of 25 mm Hg or more. The initial clinical classification in 1973 arose from a World Health Organization sponsored international meeting after an epidemic related to use of the appetite suppressant, aminorex fumarate.[2] It defined primary pulmonary hypertension (now termed idiopathic pulmonary arterial hypertension) as being characterised by vasculopathy of the pulmonary arteries. Better understanding of disease mechanisms led to subsequent classification of conditions with shared clinical and pathophysiological characteristics:

- Group 1: Pulmonary arterial hypertension (PAH), which can be idiopathic (IPAH) or associated with other conditions, notably systemic sclerosis and congenital heart disease
- Group 2: Pulmonary hypertension owing to left heart disease (PH-LHD)
- Group 3: Pulmonary hypertension owing to lung disease or hypoxia (PH-Lung), or both
- Group 4: Chronic thromboembolic pulmonary hypertension (CTEPH)
- Group 5: Unclear or multifactorial mechanisms (fig 1).[3]

Many mechanisms can lead to elevation of pulmonary pressures. In PAH, progressive narrowing of the pulmonary arterial bed results from an imbalance of vasoactive mediators, including prostacyclin, nitric oxide, and endothelin-1. This leads to an increased right ventricular afterload, right heart failure, and premature death. Between 11% and 40% of patients with IPAH and 70% of patients with a family history of PAH carry a mutation in the gene encoding bone morphogenetic receptor-2 (*BMPR2*); however, penetrance is low—carriers have a 20% lifetime risk of developing pulmonary hypertension.[4,5] Therefore, "multiple hits" are probably needed for the development of PAH. In PH-LHD, raised left atrial pressures result in secondary elevation of pulmonary pressure. In PH-Lung, raised pulmonary arterial pressures result from mechanisms such as vascular destruction and hypoxic vasoconstriction. In CTEPH, mechanical obstruction of the pulmonary vascular bed is the primary process.

Incidences are estimated to be 1-3.3 per million per year for IPAH and 1.75-3.7 per million per year for CTEPH; the prevalence of PAH is estimated at 15-52 per million.[6,7,8,9,10] Pulmonary hypertension is more common in severe respiratory and cardiac disease, occurring in 18-50% of patients assessed for transplantation or lung volume reduction surgery, and in 7-83% of those with diastolic heart failure.[11,12,13,14]

Who gets pulmonary hypertension and why is classification important?

IPAH is rare and primary care doctors may never encounter a case. By contrast, the prevalence of PAH is high in certain patient groups, such as those with systemic sclerosis (9%), portal hypertension (2-6%), congenital heart disease (5-10%), and HIV (0.5%).[15,16,17,18,19,20] Between 0.5% and 4% of patients develop CTEPH after acute pulmonary embolism; patients at increased risk include those presenting with large, recurrent, or unprovoked clots.[21,22] Classification is crucial in determining treatment and prognosis.[9] Specific treatments exist for PAH and CTEPH. By contrast, in PH-LHD and PH-Lung, treatment is best directed at the underlying condition, and currently PAH specific treatments are not recommended. Distinguishing between IPAH and PH-LHD due to diastolic dysfunction in the setting of normal left ventricular systolic function may be challenging (table 1).

Median survival in untreated IPAH is 2.8 years, but more recent registries have observed overall median survival of

SOURCES AND SELECTION CRITERIA

This review is based on our personal experience, personal archives of references, and a PubMed search using terms including pulmonary hypertension, chronic thromboembolic disease, and prognosis. We consulted international guidelines from the European Society of Cardiology, European Respiratory Society, and American College of Chest Physicians.

SUMMARY POINTS

- Pulmonary hypertension has many causes so prognoses and treatments vary
- The condition is diagnosed by systematically evaluating the breathless patient and screening patients at high risk
- Patients at high risk of severe and treatable pulmonary hypertension include those with systemic sclerosis, portal hypertension, congenital heart disease, and previous pulmonary embolism
- Specialist centres provide access to tailored investigative and treatment pathways and support networks for patients
- Patients with severe pulmonary hypertension can deteriorate rapidly—do not delay referral to perform specialist investigations
- Only selected patients with pulmonary arterial hypertension and chronic thromboembolic pulmonary hypertension benefit from interventions directed at pulmonary vasculature; for most patients treatment is aimed at the underlying condition

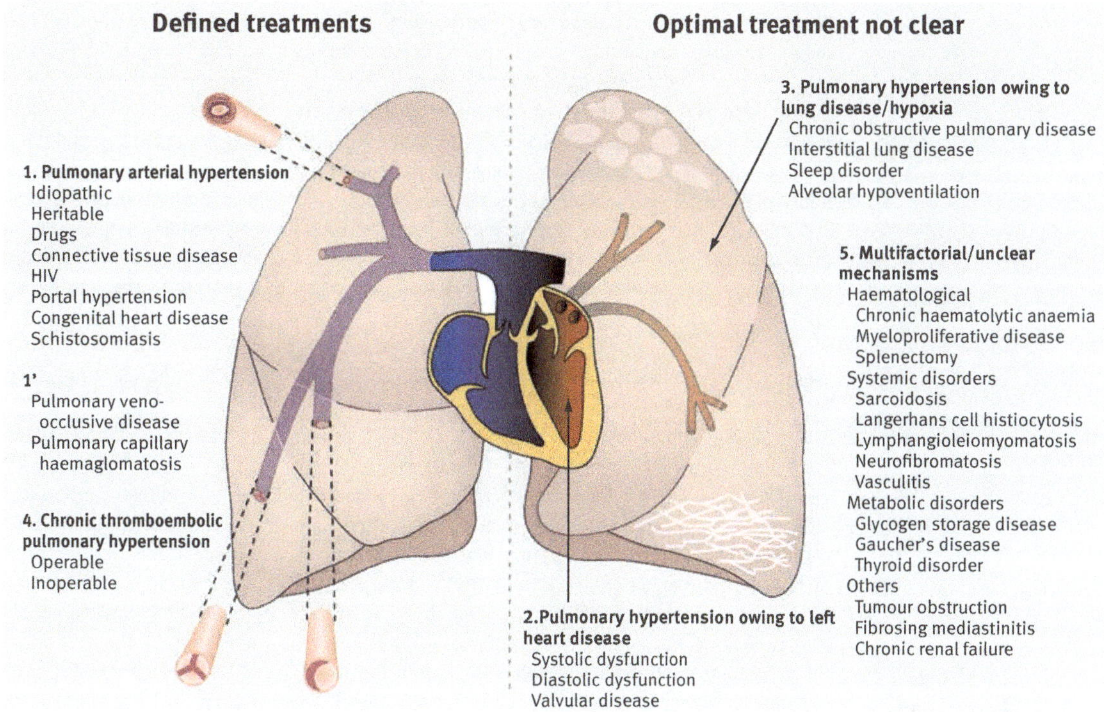

Fig 1 Classification of adult pulmonary hypertension. The condition can be caused by narrowing of the pulmonary arterial tree as a result of vasculopathy (group 1) or webs and stenoses of chronic thromboembolic disease (group 4). Optimal treatments are generally defined for groups 1 and 4. More commonly, it is associated with left heart disease (group 2) or lung disease (group 3), and optimal treatments are unclear. Several conditions associated with pulmonary hypertension have multifactorial or unclear mechanisms (group 5). *Chronic haemolytic anaemia will probably be in group 5 in next classification update

Table 1 Pulmonary hypertension in patients with normal left ventricular systolic function: features useful in discriminating between idiopathic pulmonary arterial hypertension and pulmonary hypertension caused by left ventricular diastolic dysfunction

Factor	Idiopathic pulmonary arterial hypertension	Diastolic dysfunction
Age	Younger	Older[9]
Comorbidities	None	Essential hypertension, atrial fibrillation, diabetes[76]
Electrocardiography	Right axis deviation, right ventricular hypertrophy, ST depression inferiorly and anteriorly	Left axis deviation, left ventricular hypertrophy, ST depression laterally
Echocardiography		
Left atrial size	Normal	Large[76]
Mitral flow and tissue Doppler	Normal	E/E′ >15*[77]
Cardiac magnetic resonance imaging		
Morphology	Ventricular mass index† often raised	Ventricular mass index† often normal[37]
Septal position	Systolic eccentricity index‡ often raised	Systolic eccentricity index‡ often normal[37]
Function	Right ventricular function often moderately or severely impaired	Right ventricular function often normal or mildly impaired[37]
Right heart catheter:	Pulmonary arterial wedge pressure normal	Pulmonary arterial wedge pressure raised[43]

**Ratio of mitral peak velocity of early filling (E) to early diastolic mitral annular velocity (E′); †Ratio of right ventricular mass to left ventricular mass; ‡Ratio of maximal short axis left ventricular diameters parallel and perpendicular to interventricular septum.*

at least five years.[9 23] In the past, the mean age at diagnosis in IPAH was 35 years; current five year survival in this younger age group is now about 75%.[10] PAH associated with systemic sclerosis carries a worse prognosis than IPAH, whereas the opposite is true for congenital heart disease.[9] The development of pulmonary hypertension in cardiac and respiratory disease has a negative impact on prognosis, which depends on the underlying cause and severity of pulmonary hypertension.

What are the symptoms and signs of pulmonary hypertension?

PAH most commonly presents with progressive breathlessness.[24] As right ventricular dysfunction develops patients can experience exertional dizziness and syncope. Oedema and ascites occur late in the disease. Anginal chest pain may occur due to exertional myocardial hypoperfusion in the setting of right ventricular hypertrophy, left main coronary artery compression by the pulmonary artery, or ischaemic heart disease.[25] Patients are prone to tachyarrythmias, most commonly atrial flutter, which can cause sudden decompensation.[26] Haemoptysis, although uncommon, can occur in Eisenmenger's syndrome and CTEPH, where bronchial arteries may be enlarged. Signs suggestive of pulmonary hypertension include a loud pulmonary second heart sound, systolic murmur of tricuspid regurgitation, raised jugular venous pressure, peripheral oedema and ascites, but these signs may be subtle or absent in early disease. Look for signs of associated conditions (such as connective tissue disease or liver disease).

When should I suspect pulmonary hypertension?

Pulmonary hypertension is diagnosed by systematically evaluating the breathless patient and screening high risk groups. Unexplained progressive exertional breathlessness in the absence of symptoms or signs of respiratory or left heart disease is suggestive. Screening protocols exist for high risk groups. Rheumatology centres screen patients with systemic sclerosis annually, and potential liver transplant recipients are routinely investigated for portopulmonary hypertension. Persistent breathlessness after pulmonary embolism should alert the doctor to the possibility of CTEPH.

What investigations should I perform if pulmonary hypertension is suspected?

Electrocardiography, chest radiography, and pulmonary function tests may identify an alternative cause of breathlessness (fig 2). Evidence of right heart strain on electrocardiography and prominent pulmonary arteries or cardiomegaly on chest radiography were seen in 80-90% of cases in a large IPAH registry.[24] In clinical practice, however, a normal electrocardiograph and chest radiograph cannot exclude the diagnosis. A reduction in gas transfer (lung capacity to "transfer" an inhaled gas into the blood) and mildly deranged spirometry both occur in IPAH.[27] If pulmonary hypertension is still suspected, echocardiography should be performed.[28] Figure 3 describes the estimation and interpretation of systolic pulmonary artery pressure, together with other echocardiographic features suggesting the presence of pulmonary hypertension. Importantly, pulmonary hypertension is defined by mean pulmonary artery pressure (measured at right heart catheterisation) not systolic pulmonary artery pressure (estimated by echocardiography). In addition, systolic estimates are less accurate in respiratory disease and during intercurrent illness.[14]

How is pulmonary hypertension assessed in a specialist unit?

If initial investigations suggest that pulmonary hypertension is possible, further tests are needed to confirm the diagnosis and to establish cause and severity. In the United Kingdom, a network of specialist centres was commissioned in 2001 to standardise and improve care (box 1). If severe disease is suspected, do not delay referral to a specialist centre, although imaging to exclude thromboembolic disease may be considered. If the degree of pulmonary hypertension seems to be disproportionate to the underlying cardiorespiratory disease, or if diagnostic doubt exists, discussion with a specialist centre is recommended. In these groups it is also important to exclude coexisting thromboembolic disease as a cause of pulmonary hypertension. Accurate classification and assessment of disease severity (fig 2) requires integration of clinical, physiological, and radiological data. This is central to further management (fig 4).

BOX 1 UK DESIGNATED PULMONARY HYPERTENSION CENTRES FOR ADULTS AND CHILDREN

Nationwide
- UK national centres: www.pulmonaryhypertensioncentres.co.uk

Glasgow
- Golden Jubilee Hospital: www.spvu.co.uk

Newcastle
- Freeman Hospital: www.newcastle-hospitals.org.uk

Sheffield
- Royal Hallamshire Hospital: www.thoracic.group.shef.ac.uk

Cambridge
- Papworth Hospital: www.papworthhospital.nhs.uk

London
- Royal Brompton Hospital: www.rbht.nhs.uk
- Hammersmith Hospital: www.pulmonary-hypertension.org.uk
- Royal Free Hospital: www.royalfree.nhs.uk
- Great Ormond Street (children): www.gosh.nhs.uk

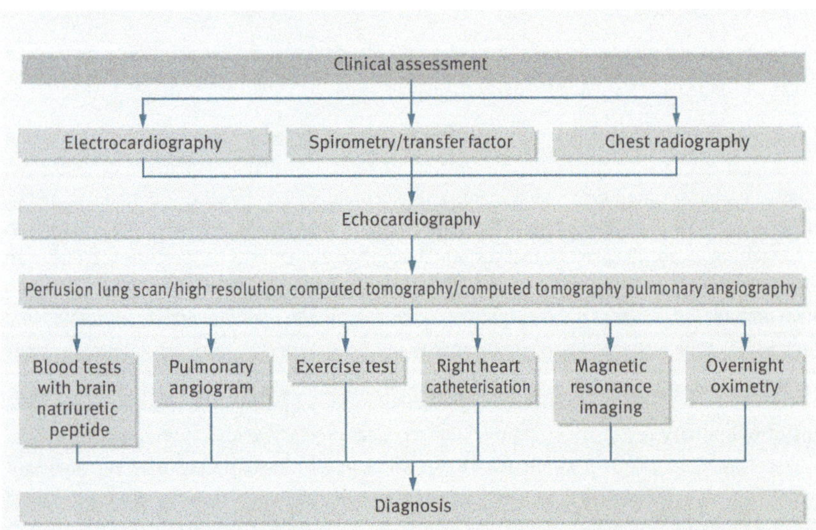

Fig 2 Diagnostic pathway for patients with suspected pulmonary hypertension

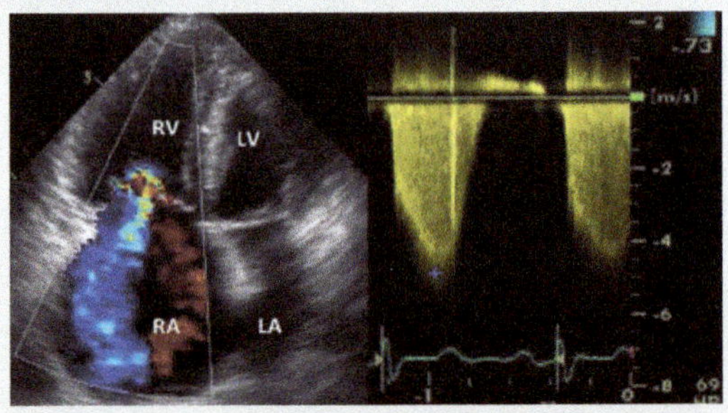

Estimation of systolic pulmonary arterial pressure (sPAP)
Maximal tricuspid regurgitant jet velocity (V) measured using continuous wave Doppler
RV systolic pressure (RVSP) calculated using equation: $RVSP = 4V^2$
sPAP = RVSP + right atrial pressure (RAP)
RAP estimated at 5 mm Hg unless size of interventricular septum suggests higher
In this example $sPAP = 4 \times (4.8)^2 + RAP = 92$ mm Hg + RAP

Other features suggestive of pulmonary hypertension
Dilated right sided chambers
Reduced RV function
RV hypertrophy
Enlarged pulmonary artery
Abnormal interventricular septal motion

Likelihood of pulmonary hypertension
Pulmonary hypertension unlikely
sPAP ≤36 mm Hg* with no other features of pulmonary hypertension
Pulmonary hypertension possible
sPAP ≤36 mm Hg* + other features of pulmonary hypertension
sPAP 37-50 mm Hg*
Pulmonary hypertension likely
sPAP >50 mm Hg*

*including 5 mm Hg RAP

Fig 3 Echocardiographic assessment of pulmonary hypertension. RA=right atrium; RV=right ventricle; LA=left atrium; LV=left ventricle

Blood, exercise testing, and overnight oximetry

Immunological and HIV testing may identify a cause of pulmonary hypertension. Brain natriuretic peptide (BNP) and N-terminal-pro-BNP have prognostic importance. Lower levels at baseline and improvement during follow-up are associated with better outcomes.[29 30] The six minute walk test has been extensively evaluated. It provides functional and prognostic information and can be used to monitor treatment response.[31 32] Cardiopulmonary exercise testing in selected patients gives more detailed physiological and prognostic information.[33] Overnight oximetry is performed if sleep disordered breathing is a suspected cause.

Imaging

Isotope perfusion lung scanning has high sensitivity for CTEPH and a normal scan excludes the diagnosis, whereas increased renal isotope uptake may identify right to left shunts and explain hypoxaemia.[34 35] High resolution computed tomography and computed tomography pulmonary angiography visualise the pulmonary arterial tree and provide a wealth of additional diagnostic information (fig 5). Direct features of chronic thromboembolic disease include occlusions, stenoses, and intraluminal webs (fig 1), whereas indirect signs include a mosaic perfusion pattern. These signs can be subtle and may be missed by a non-specialist radiologist. Magnetic resonance imaging provides a radiation-free method of quantitatively assessing cardiac structure and function, prognosis, and response to treatment.[36 37] Magnetic resonance pulmonary angiography can supplement computed tomography pulmonary angiography in the assessment of CTEPH operability, and magnetic resonance perfusion imaging is as sensitive as isotope perfusion lung scanning.[38 39] Pulmonary angiography is not commonly used in the UK to select CTEPH patients for pulmonary endarterectomy, but is used widely in other centres throughout the world to assess for surgical accessibility.

Right heart catheterisation

If non-invasive investigations support a diagnosis of pulmonary hypertension, right heart catheterisation is needed to confirm the diagnosis by directly measuring pulmonary pressure. It also allows measurement of cardiac output and estimation of left atrial pressure using pulmonary arterial wedge pressure. Haemodynamic parameters (such as right atrial pressure, cardiac index, and pulmonary vascular resistance) and pulmonary artery saturations have important prognostic value. Raised pulmonary arterial wedge pressure is suggestive of PH-LHD. Changes in oxygen saturations between right sided cardiac chambers may suggest an intracardiac shunt. Vasoreactivity testing, usually using inhaled nitric oxide, can identify patients with IPAH who may respond to long term high dose calcium channel blockers. A positive response is defined as a reduction in mean pulmonary artery pressure of at least

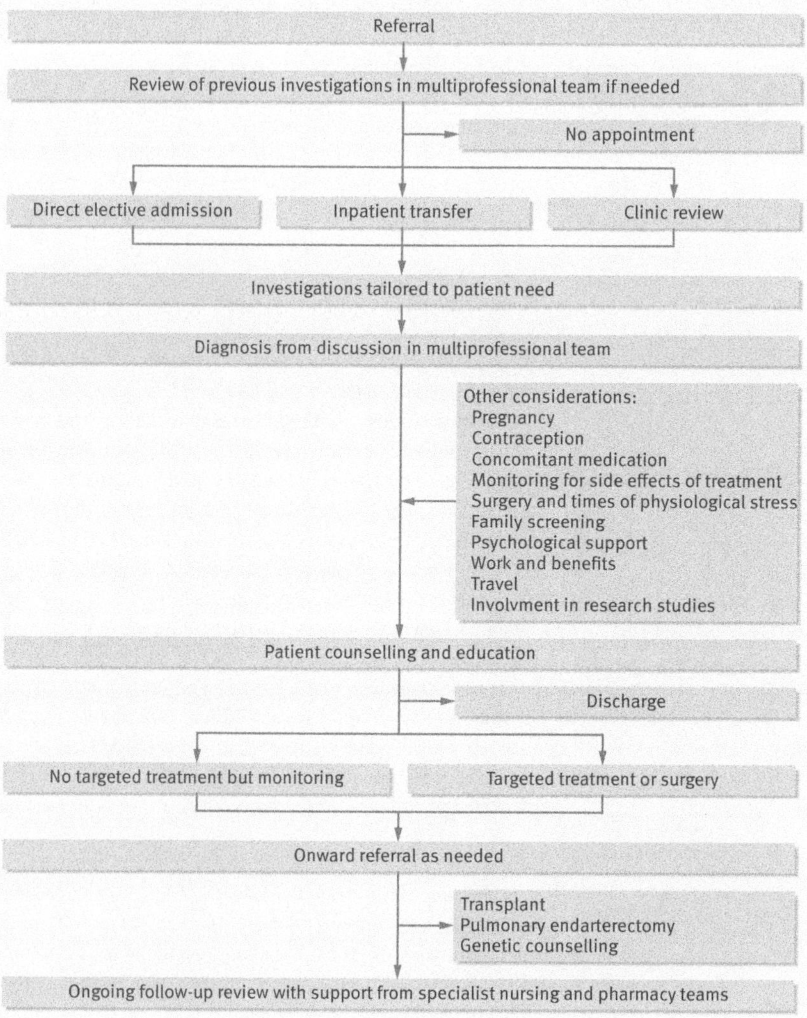

Fig 4 Overview of patient pathway at a specialist centre

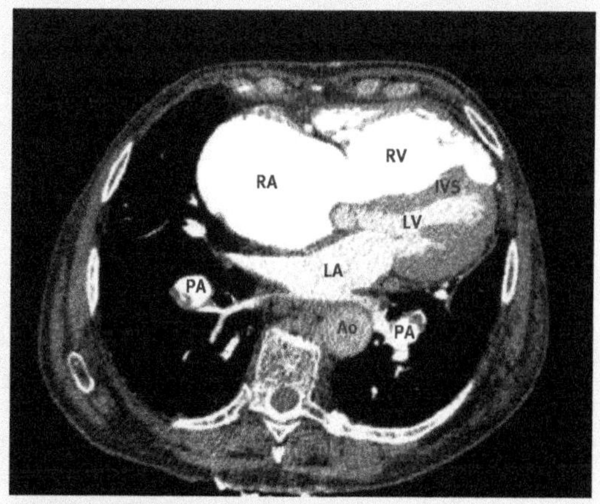

Features on this image
- Dilation of right sided chambers
- Flattening/posterior bowing of interventricular septum
- Presence of chronic thromboembolic disease in both lower lobe pulmonary arteries
- Normal sized left atrium

Other features that may be demonstrated using computed tomography pulmonary angiography
- Pulmonary artery: ascending aorta >1 suggestive of pulmonary hypertension
- Right ventricular hypertrophy
- Underlying lung disease
- Dilated left atrium and normal right ventricle in pulmonary hypertension of the left heart
- Mosaic parenchymal perfusion in CTEPH
- Congenital heart disease
  - Anomalous pulmonary venous drainage
  - Patent ductus arteriosus
- Bronchial artery hypertrophy in Eisenmenger's syndrome and CTEPH
- Dilated oesophagus in systemic sclerosis
- Splenomegaly in porto-pulmonary hypertension

Fig 5 Computed tomography assessment of pulmonary hypertension. RA=right atrium; RV=right ventricle, LA=left atrium; LV=left ventricle; IVS, interventricular septum; PA, pulmonary artery; Ao, aorta; CTEPH=chronic thromboembolic pulmonary hypertension

10 mm Hg, to less than 40 mm Hg, without a fall in cardiac output.[40]

What treatments are available for pulmonary hypertension?

Supportive treatment

Patients with CTEPH require anticoagulants because of the central role of thromboembolic disease. Although anticoagulation is recommended in IPAH, its role in PAH associated with other conditions is less clear.[41 42] Diuretics are often needed to treat heart failure. Digoxin and long term oxygen therapy may be considered, but there is no evidence from RCTs on their use. Annual flu vaccination is recommended.[43] Pregnancy is poorly tolerated despite changing practices,[44] and a recent systematic review found that maternal mortality remains high (17-33%).[45] Women are counselled about the high risks and are offered effective contraception; termination is recommended if pregnancy occurs.[43] Progesterone-only contraceptives—oral desogestrel, intramuscular medroxyprogesterone, and etonogestrel implants—avoid the prothrombotic effects of combined oral contraceptives. The levonorgestrel releasing coil is effective, but poor tolerance of potential vasovagal episodes mandates insertion in hospital. Emergency hormonal contraception is safe after unprotected intercourse. Non-obstetric surgical intervention also poses risks and its indication requires careful evaluation.

Specific medical treatment (table 2)

High dose calcium channel blockade

About 10% of patients with IPAH have a positive response to vasoreactivity testing at right heart catheterisation. Observational studies suggest that half of these patients exhibit long term clinical responses to high dose calcium channel blockade (such as diltiazem titrated to 480-720 mg/day or nifedipine titrated to 60-120 mg/day), with near normalisation of prognosis.[46 47] No evidence exists for this treatment in other forms of PAH, and because of the potential negative inotropic effect, treatment should not be started without a positive acute vasoreactive test.

Prostanoids

Prostacyclin is a vasodilator with antiproliferative effects. Infused continuously through an indwelling central line, it was the first PAH specific drug shown to be efficacious in a small RCT, demonstrating improvements in exercise capacity, haemodynamics, and, uniquely, survival.[48] It has a half life of about six minutes, is unstable at room temperature, and intravenous administration has an associated risk of line infection. Alternative routes of administration were therefore developed. A larger RCT found that nebulised iloprost (half life about 30 minutes) improved exercise capacity and haemodynamics when given seven times a day.[49] Because of its superior stability, iloprost is also given intravenously in some centres. Treprostinil (half life about four hours) was shown, in a very large RCT, to significantly improve exercise capacity when given by continuous subcutaneous infusion.[50] Further RCTs also showed significant improvements in exercise capacity when it was given by nebulised and intravenous routes.[51 52] Oral prostanoids have also been assessed with large RCTs, but results have generally been disappointing, and studies are ongoing.[53 54 55 56]

Endothelin receptor antagonists

Endothelin is a potent vasoconstrictor of vascular smooth muscle. Two oral endothelin receptor antagonists are currently licensed, bosentan and ambrisentan, on the basis of well conducted RCTs showing improved exercise capacity and time to clinical worsening.[57 58] Bosentan causes reversible abnormalities in liver function tests in 5-10% of patients, so monthly monitoring is needed.[59]

Phophodiesterase-5 inhibitors

Nitric oxide acts via cyclic GMP to increase pulmonary vascular relaxation and reduce cellular proliferation and is degraded by phophodiesterase-5. Two oral phophodiesterase-5 inhibitors (sildenafil and tadalafil) improved exercise and functional capacity in large well conducted RCTs.[60 61] These drugs have important interactions with nitrates, so concomitant use is contraindicated.

Treatment approach

Guidelines suggest starting oral treatment for patients with PAH in WHO functional classes II and III, and considering parenteral prostanoids in suitable patients in class IV or those with poor prognostic markers in class III (box 2).[43] If response to treatment is suboptimal, switching or adding further drugs is suggested.[43] Sequential addition of drugs to achieve predefined treatment goals in six minute walk distance, maximal oxygen capacity, and peak systolic blood pressure was associated with improved outcome compared with patients whose treatment had been escalated in a non-standardised manner.[62] Several RCTs of combination therapy are ongoing. Assessment of the patient's ability to use complex prostanoid therapy and adherence to treatment require the support of experienced healthcare professionals.

Chronic thromboembolic pulmonary hypertension

About two thirds of patients with CTEPH are candidates for pulmonary endarterectomy. This operation offers the best prospect of substantial improvement in symptoms, haemodynamics, and long term survival, as shown by a recent UK observational study.[8] Surgical eligibility criteria are not clearly established, and suitable candidates are identified after assessment at specialist surgical centres

Table 2 Licensed drugs for treating pulmonary hypertension

Drug	Randomised controlled trial	Administration	Important or common side effects	Important complications
Prostanoid				
Epoprostenol	Barst and colleagues[48]	Intravenous	Nausea, headache, leg pain, jaw pain, flushing, diarrhoea	Line infection
Iloprost	AIR[49]	Nebuliser; intravenous	As for eposprostenol but less severe when nebulised	Line infection with intravenous administration
Treprostinil	Simonneau and colleagues[50]	Subcutaneous	As for eposprostenol; infusion site pain for subcutaneous administration	
	TRIUMPH[51]	Nebuliser; intravenous		
	TRUST[52]			
Endothelin receptor antagonists				
Bosentan	BREATHE-1[57]	Oral		Abnormal liver function tests in 10% of patients; teratogenecity
Ambrisentan	ARIES-1 and 2[58]	Oral	Peripheral oedema	
Phosphodiesterase-5 inhibitors				
Sildenafil	SUPER-1[60]			
Tadalafil	PHIRST[61]	Oralt	Headache, indigestion, nasal stuffiness, blurred vision, visual colour change	Non-arteritic ischaemic optic neuropathy

(Papworth Hospital in the UK). Perioperative mortality in large volume centres is now less than 5%. In inoperable cases PAH specific drugs are often used, although evidence is suboptimal. Do not delay referral for surgery for trials of medical therapy, although such treatment can be used to support patients with severe CTEPH as a "bridge" to surgery.

Other non-medical treatments

Lung transplantation (usually double lung), which has overall five year survival of around 50%, is indicated in severe PAH or inoperable CTEPH if medical management fails.[63] Atrial septostomy decompresses the pressure loaded heart and may be useful in patients with severe PAH who have intractable syncope but not severe hypoxaemia, or as a bridge to transplantation.[64] Supervised exercise training improves exercise capacity, but effects on haemodynamics and prognosis are unclear.[65]

BOX 2 WHO FUNCTIONAL CLASSES

- Class I: Patients with pulmonary hypertension but in whom ordinary physical activity does not cause undue symptoms
- Class II: Patients with pulmonary hypertension resulting in slight limitation of physical activity. They are comfortable at rest but ordinary physical activity causes undue dyspnoea or fatigue, chest pain, or near syncope
- Class III: Patients with pulmonary hypertension resulting in marked limitation of physical activity. They are comfortable at rest but less than ordinary activity causes undue dyspnoea or fatigue, chest pain, or near syncope
- Class IV: Patients with pulmonary hypertension who cannot carry out any physical activity without symptoms. These patients manifest signs of right heart failure. Dyspnoea or fatigue may be present at rest. Discomfort is increased by any physical activity

TIPS FOR NON-SPECIALISTS

- Consider pulmonary hypertension as a cause of progressive unexplained breathlessness
- Echocardiography is the most useful non-invasive test for investigating pulmonary hypertension but estimates systolic, not mean, pulmonary artery pressure
- Computed tomography pulmonary angiography is useful for assessing suspected pulmonary hypertension and also allows estimation of cardiac chamber size
- A large left atrium suggests that pulmonary hypertension is more likely to be caused by left heart disease
- Pulmonary hypertension should not be empirically treated until a clear diagnosis is established
- If a patient has suspected severe pulmonary hypertension remember that the differential diagnosis is wide and outlook has improved considerably over the past 10 years

ADDITIONAL EDUCATIONAL RESOURCES

Resources for healthcare professionals

- European Society of Cardiology (www.escardio.org/guidelines)—Guidelines for the management of pulmonary hypertension
- Pulmonary Hypertension Association UK (www.paheducation.co.uk)—elearning course for healthcare professionals developed to educate non-specialist healthcare professionals including general practitioners, nurses, and clinicians about pulmonary hypertension and its management
- Pulmonary Hypertension Online University (www.phaonlineuniv.org)—Specialist internet resource for continuing medical education
- Pulmonary Vascular Research Institute (www.pvri.info)—Independent medical research organisation devoted to increasing the awareness and knowledge of pulmonary vascular diseases and to facilitating advances in the treatment of affected people worldwide

Resources for patients

- UK Pulmonary Hypertension Patients Association (www.phassociation.uk.com)—Supports adults and children with pulmonary hypertension and their families
- PHA Europe (www.phaeurope.org)—Information for patients with pulmonary hypertension as well as their family and friends
- UK Raynaud's and Scleroderma Association (www.raynauds.org.uk)—Supports patients with Raynaud's syndrome and scleroderma
- The Sommerville Foundation (www.thesf.org.uk)—Supports young people and adults born with a heart condition (congenital)

What challenges are on the horizon?

Despite progress in the management of PAH, it remains a life shortening condition. Understanding disease mechanisms and developing new treatments is a focus of international collaboration. Recent data have shown efficacy for drugs targeting existing pathways, such as macitentan (endothelin receptor antagonist)[66] and riociguat (nitric oxide pathway via soluble guanylate cyclase stimulation).[67 68] Selexipag,[69] a prostacyclin receptor agonist, is also under investigation. Despite promising effects on pulmonary haemodynamics the tyrosine kinase inhibitor, imatinib, has recently been withdrawn from licensing application, partly because of safety concerns.[70] Studies with stem cell therapy are ongoing.[71] The role of mechanical treatments, such as cardiac resynchronisation and right ventricular assist devices, in PAH are of interest.[72 73] The optimal treatment of PH-LHD and PH-Lung is unclear and drugs are being studied in phase III trials. Pulmonary artery balloon angioplasty is being investigated in patients with CTEPH who are not amenable to pulmonary endarterectomy.[74] Future availability of generic oral drugs for pulmonary hypertension may lead to inappropriate prescribing in PH-LHD and PH-Lung. It may also increase late referral to specialist centres and delays in escalation of treatment.

Improved diagnostics and treatments provide increasingly complex choices for patients and healthcare professionals in this rare illness. The delivery of care through specialist centres is increasingly advocated worldwide as a cost effective way to deliver high quality care.[43] Education on disease trajectory, provision of psychological support, and access to social and end of life care are championed by patients and their representative organisations, and they are key to improving the quality of life for patients with pulmonary hypertension.[75]

We thank Heather Allen for her help with fig 1.

Contributors: DGK, CAE, IS, and RC conceived and designed the article and approved the final manuscript. DGK is guarantor.

Competing interests: All authors have completed the ICMJE uniform disclosure form at www.icmje.org/coi_disclosure.pdf (available on request from the corresponding author) and declare: no support from any organisation for the submitted work; DGK has received speaker fees, attended advisory boards, and received funding to attend meetings from Actelion, Bayer, Pfizer, United Therapeutics, Lily, and GSK; CAE has received speaker fees and attended advisory boards for Actelion, Bayer, and GSK; IS has received travel funding from Actelion and GSK; RC has received speaker fees from Actelion and GSK and has attended advisory boards for Actelion, Bayer, and GSK. The department has received funding for research and education through unrestricted grants from Actelion, Bayer, and Pfizer.

Provenance and peer review: Commissioned; externally peer reviewed.

1 Badesch DB, Raskob GE, Elliott CG, Krichman AM, Farber HW, Frost AE, et al. Pulmonary arterial hypertension: baseline characteristics from the REVEAL registry. *Chest* 2010;137:376-87.
2 Hatano S, Strasser T. Primary pulmonary hypertension. Report on a WHO meeting. October 15-17, 1973, WHO, 1975.
3 Simonneau G, Robbins IM, Beghetti M, Channick RN, Delcroix M, Denton CP, et al. Updated clinical classification of pulmonary hypertension. *J Am Coll Cardiol* 2009;54:S43-54.
4 Thomson JR, Machado RD, Pauciulo MW, Morgan NV, Humbert M, Elliott GC, et al. Sporadic primary pulmonary hypertension is associated with germline mutations of the gene encoding BMPR-II, a receptor member of the TGF-beta family. *J Med Genet* 2000;37:741-5.
5 Fessel JP, Loyd JE, Austin ED. The genetics of pulmonary arterial hypertension in the post-BMPR2 era. *Pulmon Circ* 2011;1:305-19.
6 Humbert M, Sitbon O, Chaouat A, Bertocchi M, Habib G, Gressin V, et al. Pulmonary arterial hypertension in France: results from a national registry. *Am J Respir Crit Care Med* 2006;173:1023-30.
7 Peacock AJ, Murphy NF, McMurray JJ, Caballero L, Stewart S. An epidemiological study of pulmonary arterial hypertension. *Eur Respir J* 2007;30:104-9.
8 Condliffe R, Kiely DG, Gibbs JS, Corris PA, Peacock AJ, Jenkins DP, et al. Improved outcomes in medically and surgically treated chronic

thromboembolic pulmonary hypertension. *Am J Respir Crit Care Med* 2008;177:1122-7.
9 Hurdman J, Condliffe R, Elliot CA, Davies C, Hill C, Wild JM, et al. ASPIRE registry: assessing the spectrum of pulmonary hypertension identified at a referral centre. *Eur Respir J* 2012;39:945-55.
10 Ling Y, Johnson MK, Kiely DG, Condliffe R, Elliot CA, Gibbs JS, et al. Changing demographics, epidemiology, and survival of incident pulmonary arterial hypertension: results from the pulmonary hypertension registry of the United Kingdom and Ireland. *Am J Respir Crit Care Med* 2012;186:790-6.
11 Thabut G, Dauriat G, Stern JB, Logeart D, Lévy A, Marrash-Chahla R, et al. Pulmonary hemodynamics in advanced COPD candidates for lung volume reduction surgery or lung transplantation. *Chest* 2005;127:1531-56.
12 Lam CS, Roger VL, Rodeheffer RJ, Borlaug BA, Enders FT, Redfield MM, et al. Pulmonary hypertension in heart failure with preserved ejection fraction: a community-based study. *J Am Coll Cardiol* 2009;53:1119-26.
13 Damy T, Goode KM, Kallvikbacka-Bennett A, Lewinter C, Hobkirk J, Nikitin NP, et al. Determinants and prognostic value of pulmonary arterial pressure in patients with chronic heart failure. *Eur Heart J* 2010;31:2280-90.
14 Arcasoy SM, Christie JD, Ferrari VA, Sutton MS, Zisman DA, Blumenthal NP, et al. Echocardiographic assessment of pulmonary hypertension in patients with advanced lung disease. *Am J Respir Crit Care Med* 2003;167:735-40.
15 Avouac J, Airo P, Meune C, Beretta L, Dieude P, Caramaschi P, et al. Prevalence of pulmonary hypertension in systemic sclerosis in European Caucasians and metaanalysis of 5 studies. *J Rheumatol* 2010;37:2290-8.
16 Hadengue A, Benhayoun MK, Lebrec D, Benhamou JP. Pulmonary hypertension complicating portal hypertension: prevalence and relation to splanchnic hemodynamics. *Gastroenterology* 1991;100:520-8.
17 Castro M, Krowka MJ, Schroeder DR, Beck KC, Plevak DJ, Rettke SR, et al. Frequency and clinical implications of increased pulmonary artery pressures in liver transplant patients. *Mayo Clin Proc* 1996;71:543-51.
18 Colle IO, Moreau R, Godinho E, Belghiti J, Ettori F, Cohen-Solal A, et al. Diagnosis of portopulmonary hypertension in candidates for liver transplantation: a prospective study. *Hepatology* 2003;37:401-9.
19 Gatzoulis MA, Alonso-Gonzalez R, Beghetti M. Pulmonary arterial hypertension in paediatric and adult patients with congenital heart disease. *Eur Respir Rev* 2009;18:154-61.
20 Sitbon O, Lascoux-Combe C, Delfraissy JF, Yeni PG, Raffi F, De Zuttere D, et al. Prevalence of HIV-related pulmonary arterial hypertension in the current antiretroviral therapy era. *Am J Respir Crit Care Med* 2008;177:108-3.
21 Klok FA, van Kralingen KW, van Dijk AP, Heyning FH, Vliegen HW, Huisman MV. Prospective cardiopulmonary screening program to detect chronic thromboembolic pulmonary hypertension in patients after acute pulmonary embolism. *Haematologica* 2010;95:970-5.
22 Pengo V, Lensing AW, Prins MH, Marchiori A, Davidson BL, Tiozzo F, et al. Incidence of chronic thromboembolic pulmonary hypertension after pulmonary embolism. *N Engl J Med* 2004;350:2257-64.
23 D'Alonzo GE, Barst RJ, Ayres SM, Bergofsky EH, Brundage BH, Detre KM, et al. Survival in patients with primary pulmonary hypertension. Results from a national prospective registry. *Ann Intern Med* 1991;115:343-9.
24 Rich S, Dantzker DR, Ayres SM, Bergofsky EH, Brundage BH, Detre KM, et al. Primary pulmonary hypertension. A national prospective study. *Ann Intern Med* 1987;107:216-23.
25 Bonderman D, Fleischmann D, Prokop M, Klepetko W, Lang IM. Images in cardiovascular medicine. Left main coronary artery compression by the pulmonary trunk in pulmonary hypertension. *Circulation* 2002;105:265.
26 Tongers J, Schwerdtfeger B, Klein G, Kempf T, Schaefer A, Knapp JM, et al. Incidence and clinical relevance of supraventricular tachyarrhythmias in pulmonary hypertension. *Am Heart J* 2007;153:127-32.
27 Sun XG, Hansen JE, Oudiz RJ, Wasserman K. Pulmonary function in primary pulmonary hypertension. *J Am Coll Cardiol* 2003;41:1028-35.
28 Howard LS, Grapsa J, Dawson D, Bellamy M, Chambers JB, Masani ND, et al. Echocardiographic assessment of pulmonary hypertension: standard operating procedure. *Eur Respir Rev* 2012;21:239-48.
29 Nagaya N, Nishikimi T, Uematsu M, Satoh T, Kyotani S, Sakamaki F, et al. Plasma brain natriuretic peptide as a prognostic indicator in patients with primary pulmonary hypertension. *Circulation* 2000;102:865-70.
30 Nickel N, Golpon H, Greer M, Knudsen L, Olsson K, Westerkamp V, et al. The prognostic impact of follow-up assessments in patients with idiopathic pulmonary arterial hypertension. *Eur Respir J* 2012;39:589-96.
31 Miyamoto S, Nagaya N, Satoh T, Kyotani S, Sakamaki F, Fujita M, et al. Clinical correlates and prognostic significance of six-minute walk test in patients with primary pulmonary hypertension. Comparison with cardiopulmonary exercise testing. *Am J Respir Crit Care Med* 2000;161:487-92.
32 Paciocco G, Martinez FJ, Bossone E, Pielsticker E, Gillespie B, Rubenfire M. Oxygen desaturation on the six-minute walk test and mortality in untreated primary pulmonary hypertension. *Eur Respir J* 2001;17:647-52.
33 Wensel R, Opitz CF, Anker SD, Winkler J, Hoffken G, Kleber FX, et al. Assessment of survival in patients with primary pulmonary hypertension: importance of cardiopulmonary exercise testing. *Circulation* 2002;106:319-24.
34 Worsley DF, Palevsky HI, Alavi A. Ventilation-perfusion lung scanning in the evaluation of pulmonary hypertension. *J Nucl Med* 1994;35:793-6.
35 Tunariu N, Gibbs SJ, Win Z, Gin-Sing W, Graham A, Gishen P, et al. Ventilation-perfusion scintigraphy is more sensitive than multidetector CTPA in detecting chronic thromboembolic pulmonary disease as a treatable cause of pulmonary hypertension. *J Nucl Med* 2007;48:680-4.
36 Van de Veerdonk MC, Kind T, Marcus JT, Mauritz GJ, Heymans MW, Bogaard HJ, et al. Progressive right ventricular dysfunction in patients with pulmonary arterial hypertension responding to therapy. *J Am Coll Cardiol* 2011;58:2511-9.
37 Swift AJ, Rajaram S, Condliffe R, Capener D, Hurdman J, Elliot CA, et al. Diagnostic accuracy of cardiovascular magnetic resonance imaging of right ventricular morphology and function in the assessment of suspected pulmonary hypertension results from the ASPIRE registry. *J Cardiovasc Magn Reson* 2012;14:40.
38 Rajaram S, Swift AJ, Capener D, Telfer A, Davies C, Hill C, et al. Diagnostic accuracy of contrast-enhanced MR angiography and unenhanced proton MR imaging compared with CT pulmonary angiography in chronic thromboembolic pulmonary hypertension. *Eur Radiol* 2012;22:310-7.
39 Rajaram S, Swift AJ, Telfer A, Hurdman J, Marshall H, Lorenz E, et al. 3D contrast-enhanced lung perfusion MRI is an effective screening tool for chronic thromboembolic pulmonary hypertension: results from the ASPIRE Registry. *Thorax* 2013; published online 24 Jan.
40 Barst RJ, McGoon M, Torbicki A, Sitbon O, Krowka MJ, Olschewski H, et al. Diagnosis and differential assessment of pulmonary arterial hypertension. *J Am Coll Cardiol* 2004;43:40S-7S.
41 Frank H, Mlczoch J, Huber K, Schuster E, Gurtner HP, Kneussl M. The effect of anticoagulant therapy in primary and anorectic drug-induced pulmonary hypertension. *Chest* 1997;112:714-21.
42 Johnson SR, Mehta S, Granton JT. Anticoagulation in pulmonary arterial hypertension: a qualitative systematic review. *Eur Respir J* 2006;28:999-1004.
43 Galie N, Hoeper MM, Humbert M, Torbicki A, Vachiery JL, Barbera JA, et al. Guidelines for the diagnosis and treatment of pulmonary hypertension. *Eur Respir J* 2009;34:1219-63.
44 Kiely DG, Condliffe R, Webster V, Mills GH, Wrench I, Gandhi SV, et al. Improved survival in pregnancy and pulmonary hypertension using a multiprofessional approach. *BJOG* 2010;117:565-74.
45 Bedard E, Dimopoulos K, Gatzoulis MA. Has there been any progress made on pregnancy outcomes among women with pulmonary arterial hypertension? *Eur Heart J* 2009;30:256-65.
46 Rich S, Kaufmann E, Levy PS. The effect of high doses of calcium-channel blockers on survival in primary pulmonary hypertension. *N Engl J Med* 1992;327:76-81.
47 Sitbon O, Humbert M, Jais X, Ioos V, Hamid AM, Provencher S, et al. Long-term response to calcium channel blockers in idiopathic pulmonary arterial hypertension. *Circulation* 2005;111:3105-11.
48 Barst RJ, Rubin LJ, Long WA, McGoon MD, Rich S, Badesch DB, et al. A comparison of continuous intravenous epoprostenol (prostacyclin) with conventional therapy for primary pulmonary hypertension. The Primary Pulmonary Hypertension Study Group. *N Engl J Med* 1996;334:296-302.
49 Olschewski H, Simonneau G, Galie N, Higenbottam T, Naeije R, Rubin LJ, et al. Inhaled iloprost for severe pulmonary hypertension. *N Engl J Med* 2002;347:322-9.
50 Simonneau G, Barst RJ, Galie N, Naeije R, Rich S, Bourge RC, et al. Continuous subcutaneous infusion of treprostinil, a prostacyclin analogue, in patients with pulmonary arterial hypertension: a double-blind, randomized, placebo-controlled trial. *Am J Respir Crit Care Med* 2002;165:800-4.
51 McLaughlin VV, Benza RL, Rubin LJ, Channick RN, Voswinckel R, Tapson VF, et al. Addition of inhaled treprostinil to oral therapy for pulmonary arterial hypertension: a randomized controlled clinical trial. *J Am Coll Cardiol* 2010;55:1915-22.
52 Hiremath J, Thanikachalam S, Parikh K, Shanmugasundaram S, Bangera S, Shapiro L, et al. Exercise improvement and plasma biomarker changes with intravenous treprostinil therapy for pulmonary arterial hypertension: a placebo-controlled trial. *J Heart Lung Transplant* 2010;29:137-49.
53 Barst RJ, McGoon M, McLaughlin V, Tapson V, Rich S, Rubin L, et al. Beraprost therapy for pulmonary arterial hypertension. *J Am Coll Cardiol* 2003;41:2119-25.
54 Tapson VF, Torres F, Kermeen F, Keogh AM, Allen RP, Frantz RP, et al. Oral treprostinil for the treatment of pulmonary arterial hypertension in patients on background endothelin receptor antagonist and/or phosphodiesterase type 5 inhibitor therapy (the FREEDOM-C study): a randomized controlled trial. *Chest* 2012;142:1383-90.
55 Jing ZC, Parikh K, Pulido T, Jeres-Sanchez C, White RJ, Allen R, et al. Efficacy and safety of oral treprostinil monotherapy for the treatment of pulmonary arterial hypertension: a randomised controlled trial. *Circulation* 2013;127:624-33.
56 Tapson V, Jing ZC, Xu KF, Pan L, Feldman J, Kiely DG, et al. Oral treprostinil for the treatment of pulmonary arterial hypertension in patients on background endothelin receptor antagonist and/or phosphodiesterase type 5 inhibitor therapy (the FREEDOM-C2 Study): a randomized controlled trial. *Chest* 2013 [forthcoming].

57 Rubin LJ, Badesch DB, Barst RJ, Galie N, Black CM, Keogh A, et al. Bosentan therapy for pulmonary arterial hypertension. *N Engl J Med* 2002;346:896-903.

58 Galie N, Olschewski H, Oudiz RJ, Torres F, Frost A, Ghofrani HA, et al. Ambrisentan for the treatment of pulmonary arterial hypertension: results of the ambrisentan in pulmonary arterial hypertension, randomized, double-blind, placebo-controlled, multicenter, efficacy (ARIES) study 1 and 2. *Circulation* 2008;117:3010-9.

59 Humbert M, Segal ES, Kiely DG, Carlsen J, Schwierin B, Hoeper MM. Results of European post-marketing surveillance of bosentan in pulmonary hypertension. *Eur Respir J* 2007;30:338-44.

60 Galie N, Ghofrani HA, Torbicki A, Barst RJ, Rubin LJ, Badesch D, et al. Sildenafil citrate therapy for pulmonary arterial hypertension. *N Engl J Med* 2005;353:2148-57.

61 Galie N, Brundage BH, Ghofrani HA, Oudiz RJ, Simonneau G, Safdar Z, et al. Tadalafil therapy for pulmonary arterial hypertension. *Circulation* 2009;119:2894-903.

62 Hoeper MM, Markevych I, Spiekerkoetter E, Welte T, Niedermeyer J. Goal-oriented treatment and combination therapy for pulmonary arterial hypertension. *Eur Respir J* 2005;26:858-63.

63 Christie JD, Edwards LB, Kucheryavaya AY, Benden C, Dipchand AI, Dobbels F, et al. The registry of the International Society for Heart and Lung Transplantation: 29th adult lung and heart-lung transplant report—2012. *J Heart Lung Transplant* 2012.

64 Sandoval J, Gaspar J, Pena H, Santos LE, Cordova J, Del Valle K, et al. Effect of atrial septostomy on the survival of patients with severe pulmonary arterial hypertension. *Eur Respir J* 38:1343-8.

65 Mereles D, Ehlken N, Kreuscher S, Ghofrani S, Hoeper MM, Halank M, et al. Exercise and respiratory training improve exercise capacity and quality of life in patients with severe chronic pulmonary hypertension. *Circulation* 2006;114:1482-9.

66 Rubin LJ, Pulido T, Channick R, Delcroix M, Galie N, Ghofrani HA, et al. Effect of macitentan on morbidity and mortality in pulmonary arterial hypertension (PAH): results from the SERAPHIN trial. *Chest* 2012;142:1026A.

67 Ghofrani HA, Galie N, Grimminger F, Humbert M, Keogh A, Langleben D, et al. Riociguat for the treatment of pulmonary arterial hypertension: a randomized, double-blind, placebo-controlled study (PATENT-1). *Chest* 2012;142:1027.

68 Ghofrani HA, Grimminger F, Hoeper M, Kim N, Mayer E, Neuser D, et al. Riociguat for the treatment of inoperable chronic thromboembolic pulmonary hypertension: a randomized, double-blind, placebo-controlled study (CHEST-1). *Chest* 2012;142:1023A.

69 Simonneau G, Torbicki A, Hoeper MM, Delcroix M, Karlocai K, Galie N, et al. Selexipag, an oral, selective IP receptor agonist for the treatment of pulmonary arterial hypertension. *Eur Respir J* 2012;40:874-80.

70 Hoeper MM, Barst RJ, Bourge RC, Feldman J, Frost AE, Galie N, et al. Imatinib mesylate as add-on therapy for pulmonary arterial hypertension: results of the randomized IMPRES study. *Circulation* 2013;127:1128-38.

71 Stewart DJ, Zhao YD, Courtman DW. Cell therapy for pulmonary hypertension: what is the true potential of endothelial progenitor cells? *Circulation* 2004;109:e172-3.

72 Kalogeropoulos AP, Vega JD, Smith AL, Georgiopoulou VV. Pulmonary hypertension and right ventricular function in advanced heart failure. *Congest Heart Fail* 2011;17:189-98.

73 Keogh AM, Mayer E, Benza RL, Corris P, Dartevelle PG, Frost AE, et al. Interventional and surgical modalities of treatment in pulmonary hypertension. *J Am Coll Cardiol* 2009;54:S67-77.

74 Mizoguchi H, Ogawa A, Munemasa M, Mikouchi H, Ito H, Matsubara H. Refined balloon pulmonary angioplasty for inoperable patients with chronic thromboembolic pulmonary hypertension. *Circ Cardiovasc Interv* 2012;5:748-55.

75 Armstrong I, Rochnia N, Harries C, Bundock S, Yorke J. The trajectory to diagnosis with pulmonary arterial hypertension: a qualitative study. *BMJ Open* 2012;2:e000806.

76 Guazzi M, Galie N. Pulmonary hypertension in left heart disease. *Eur Respir Rev* 2012;21:338-46.

77 Paulus WJ, Tschope C, Sanderson JE, Rusconi C, Flachskampf FA, Rademakers FE, et al. How to diagnose diastolic heart failure: a consensus statement on the diagnosis of heart failure with normal left ventricular ejection fraction by the heart failure and echocardiography associations of the European Society of Cardiology. *Eur Heart J* 2007;28:2539-50.

Related links

bmj.com

- Respiratory medicine updates from BMJ Group

bmj.com/archive

- Leukaemia update. Part 2: managing patients with leukaemia in the community (2013;346:f1932)
- Leukaemia update. Part 1: diagnosis and management (2013;346:f1660)
- Outpatient parenteral antimicrobial therapy (2013;346:f1585)
- Diagnosis and management of carotid atherosclerosis (2013;346:f1485)
- Achilles tendon disorders (2013;346:f1262)
- Malignant and premalignant lesions of the penis (2013;346:f1149)
- Postpartum management of hypertension (2013;346:f894)

BMJ BPP UNIVERSITY SCHOOL OF HEALTH

Difficult to treat asthma in adults

Graeme P Currie, consultant chest physician[1], J Graham Douglas, consultant chest physician[1], Liam G Heaney, consultant chest physician[2]

[1]Aberdeen Royal Infirmary, Aberdeen AB25 2ZN

[2]Belfast City Hospital, Belfast BT9 7AB

Correspondence to: G P Currie Graeme.currie@nhs.net

Cite this as: *BMJ* 2009;338:b494

‹DOI› 10.1136/bmj.b494 http://www.bmj.com/content/338/bmj.b494

References numbered w1 to w25 are on bmj.com, labelled as extra

There is no universally accepted definition of difficult asthma. However, it is reasonable to consider it present when people have persistent symptoms and frequent exacerbations, despite being treated at steps 4 or 5 of the British Thoracic Society and Scottish Intercollegiate Guideline Network (BTS/SIGN) guidelines (fig 1).[1] Such patients typically receive high dose inhaled steroids (≥800 μg beclometasone equivalent), a long acting β2 agonist, plus add-on treatment. The prevalence of difficult asthma is uncertain, but it may account for 5-10% of adults with asthma.[2] Morbidity and health costs are disproportionately high in these patients,[w1] and they are at greater risk of fatal and near fatal exacerbations.[w2] In addition, frequent, intermittent, or continuous courses of oral prednisolone (plus regular high dose inhaled steroids) increase the risk of steroid related adverse effects.

Why are some people with asthma difficult to treat?

Several key questions must be considered before prescribing add-on treatments and higher doses of inhaled or oral steroids to patients with difficult to treat asthma.

Do they really have asthma?

To answer this question, the patient's history and objective support for a diagnosis of asthma need to be reviewed (boxes 1 and 2). In patients with airflow obstruction, bronchodilator reversibility to 400 μg of inhaled salbutamol should be performed. In patients without airflow obstruction, other objective ways of confirming the diagnosis—such as exercise testing, measuring exhaled nitric oxide, and bronchial challenge testing—may be necessary.[1] According to BTS-SIGN guidelines, the diagnosis should be reconsidered in patients with persistent symptoms who do not show airway hyper-responsiveness to bronchoconstrictor stimuli such as methacholine (or in the future mannitol).[1] [w3] Box 2 outlines other tests that may help establish whether asthma is present. Not all tests will be needed in each patient—this will depend on the clinical situation.

Do coexisting conditions exacerbate the asthma?

Asthma often occurs alongside other conditions. In two case series, coexisting disorders with asthma-like symptoms were found in 19%[3] and 34%[4] of patients with difficult asthma (fig 2). If coexisting conditions are correctly identified and managed, it may be possible to improve symptom control without escalating treatment. Moreover, bronchiectasis, gastro-oesophageal reflux disease, rhinosinusitis, and psychological disorders are more common in people with frequent versus infrequent severe exacerbations of asthma.[w4] Vocal cord dysfunction (paradoxical adduction during inspiration) is an important disorder that can mimic or coexist with asthma.[w5] [w6] It may masquerade as wheeze and breathlessness, with episodes beginning and remitting abruptly (unrelated to treatment). Its prevalence is uncertain, and diagnosis requires a high index of suspicion and direct visualisation of the vocal cords when symptomatic.[w7]

What aggravating factors might be considered?

Psychological factors

Difficult to control asthma often causes considerable psychological stress, especially if a life threatening episode has occurred; psychological factors (especially anxiety) may also worsen asthma control. Adverse psychological factors are associated with hospital admission with acute asthma,[w8] [w9] and psychosocial morbidity has also been linked to fatal and near fatal episodes of asthma.[1] In a study where sequential patients referred to a difficult asthma service were assessed by a psychiatrist, 32 out of 65 had an ICD-10 (international classification of diseases, 10th revision)

SOURCES AND SELECTION CRITERIA

All authors performed a comprehensive search of articles published up to January 2009 using PubMed and Medline. Keywords and phrases used were "asthma", "exacerbations", "symptoms", "difficult asthma", "lung function", "diagnosis", "bronchial hyper-responsiveness", "nitric oxide", "sputum eosinophils", "treatment", "monitoring", "inhaled steroids", "long acting β2 agonists", "leukotriene receptor antagonists", "bronchial thermoplasty", "immunoglobulin E therapy", and "tumour necrosis factor".

SUMMARY POINTS

- Difficult asthma is present when patients using treatment at steps 4 or 5 of the British Thoracic Society and Scottish Intercollegiate Guideline Network guidelines remain symptomatic and have exacerbations
- Determine whether the patient truly has asthma, whether prescribed treatment is being taken, and whether an alternative or coexisting diagnosis or aggravating factors exist
- After taking a detailed history and examination, further directed investigations may be needed
- Assessment and further management should ideally take place within a multidisciplinary clinic setting

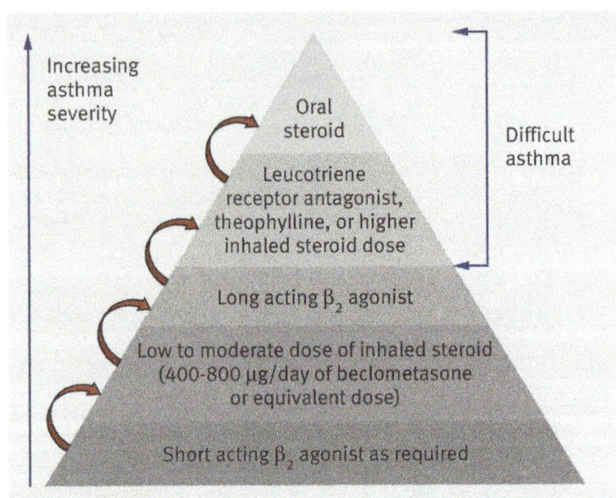

Fig 1 Simplified diagram of the pharmacological management of chronic asthma in adults[1] [w1]

psychiatric diagnosis (usually depression).[4] In the same study, the hospital anxiety and depression scale (HADS) had a good negative predictive value for depression. In a cohort of 56 patients, 33 had a psychiatric component to their asthma, and in 10 this was thought to be "major."[3] It is unclear whether psychological morbidity negatively affects difficult asthma, and whether treating concomitant psychiatric morbidity improves asthma control. Although patients often identify acute stress and depression as triggers, psychological factors may cause poor adherence to treatment, rather than have a direct effect on asthma severity.

BOX 1 IMPORTANT CLINICAL ASPECTS TO COVER IN PATIENTS WITH DIFFICULT ASTHMA

History
- Details of original diagnosis: "who, when, and how," previous demonstration of airflow obstruction, documented response to treatment
- Morbidity: length of history, severity of symptoms, exacerbating factors, frequency of exacerbations, previous admissions to intensive care with abnormal airway inflation pressures
- Presence of other respiratory symptoms (sputum production, chest pain, haemoptysis)
- Smoking history
- Family history of respiratory disorders
- Past and present occupation
- Potential aggravating medical conditions (features of rhinosinusitis, nasal polyps, depression or anxiety, gastro-oesophageal reflux disease, relation to menstrual cycle)
- Drugs (β blockers, aspirin, non-steroidal anti-inflammatory drugs, angiotensin converting enzyme inhibitors)
- Adherence to treatment
- Psychosocial circumstances

Examination
- Respiratory system: look for signs that may or may not be consistent with asthma
- Cardiovascular system: look for signs that may indicate an alternative diagnosis
- Body mass index: obesity is associated with difficult to control asthma, and uncertainty may arise in differentiating between breathlessness caused by obesity and that caused by asthma

BOX 2 INVESTIGATIONS THAT MAY BE NEEDED IN PATIENTS WITH DIFFICULT ASTHMA

Blood tests
- Blood eosinophil count
- Total serum IgE and allergen skin prick testing (or radioallergosorbent test) especially to *Aspergillus*
- Blood theophylline or prednisolone concentrations (where appropriate) to support adherence
- Other blood tests depending on clinical features (α1 antitrypsin, angiotensin converting enzyme, immunoglobulins and functional antibody testing, antineutrophil cytoplasmic antibody, *Aspergillus* serology)

Pulmonary function
- Spirometry
- Airflow obstruction present: test for bronchodilator reversibility
- Airflow obstruction absent: consider exercise test, bronchial challenge test (using inhaled methacholine or mannitol), exhaled nitric oxide (raised in eosinophilic airway inflammation), sputum eosinophil count
- Flow volume loop, lung volumes, and transfer factor to identify features not consistent with asthma (where appropriate)

Radiography
- Chest radiography
- High resolution computed tomography of thorax (to look for bronchiectasis or interstitial lung disease)
- Computed tomography of sinuses (to look for sinus disease after nasal endoscopy or a trial of nasal steroids)

Other tests (as clinically indicated)
- Nasal endoscopy (to look for polyps and features of rhinosinusitis)
- Bronchoscopy (to look for tumours or foreign bodies)
- Laryngoscopy during symptomatic episodes (to look for vocal cord dysfunction)
- Echocardiogram (where wheeze may be caused by "cardiac asthma")
- Psychiatric assessment
- Cardiopulmonary exercise testing

Upper airway disease

The upper and lower airways have a direct anatomical connection, share a similar epithelial lining, and release similar inflammatory mediators. Asthma and allergic rhinitis represent a continuation of the same inflammatory process so it is not surprising that they commonly coexist.[6] Indeed, treating allergic airway inflammation in the nose can improve markers of asthma control.[w10-w13] The allergic rhinitis and its impact upon asthma (ARIA) guidelines emphasise the importance of identifying symptoms of asthma in people with rhinitis and vice versa. [7] Management strategies for allergic rhinitis consist of allergen avoidance, immunotherapy, intranasal steroids, and systemic or topical antihistamines.[7]

Gastro-oesophageal reflux disease

The incidence of gastro-oesophageal reflux disease is higher in patients with asthma than in the general population, although its relation to difficult asthma is not clear.[w14 w15] A systematic review of 12 studies found no convincing evidence to support improved asthma control with treatment for gastro-oesophageal reflux disease,[8] and in difficult asthma, identification and treatment of the disease failed to improve control.[w16]

Adverse drug effects

Non-steroidal anti-inflammatory drugs, β blockers (including eye drops), and aspirin can exacerbate asthma. Indeed, aspirin sensitive asthma may exist in up to 20% of people with asthma.[9] Chronic cough caused by angiotensin converting enzyme inhibitors may also mimic less well controlled asthma.

Allergy

Increased sensitisation to aeroallergens has been associated with greater airway hyper-responsiveness,[10 w17] and sensitisation to fungal allergens has been linked to life threatening asthma.[w18] However, little evidence exists to suggest that reducing exposure to house dust mite and

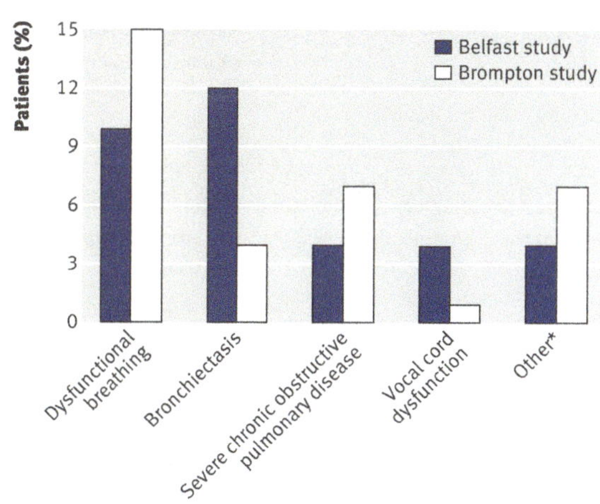

*** Other:** Chronic bronchitis, IgA deficiency, cystic fibrosis, obliterative bronchiolitis, cardiomyopathy, pulmonary hypertension, hypereosinophilia, extrinsic allergic alveolitis, respiratory muscle incoordination, obstructive sleep apnoea

Fig 2 The frequency and type of coexistent diagnoses in two studies of patients with difficult asthma. Adapted, with permission, from Heaney and Robinson[5]

other ubiquitous allergens reduces symptom scores and exacerbations or improves peak expiratory flow.[11]

Occupational factors

Many patients with difficult asthma may have stopped work because of symptoms. Because occupational asthma may account for as much as 10-15% of adult onset disease,[1] questioning patients about occupational exposure to airway irritants may uncover a trigger. Those who are better on days away from work or when on holiday should be investigated for occupational asthma.

Cigarette smoking

Cigarette smoking is associated with persistent asthma, an accelerated decline in lung function, and higher mortality after admission with an episode of near fatal asthma.[w19-w21] People who currently smoke or previously smoked have reduced airway sensitivity to the effects of inhaled steroids compared with non-smokers.[12 13]

Obesity

Accumulating data associate obesity with persistent asthma and asthma related visits to the emergency department, and obese women seem to have an increased risk of having asthma.[14] Although the association between asthma and obesity is not fully understood, weight loss should be encouraged.

Are patients taking their treatment?

In a cross sectional observational study of non-adherence in difficult asthma (n=182), 34% of people were collecting less than 50% of their prescriptions for inhaled combination therapy.[w22] In a case series, 50% of patients prescribed oral steroids were found to be non-adherent when assessed by plasma prednisolone and cortisol concentrations.[3] Thus, despite persistent symptoms, many patients choose not to take their prescribed treatment and reasons for this need to be explored (box 3).

BOX 3 POTENTIAL REASONS FOR PATIENTS NOT ADHERING TO TREATMENT

- Treatment considered unnecessary, ineffective, or dangerous
- Lack of immediate effect after taking inhaled steroids
- Poor understanding of the treatment regimen
- Poor inhaler technique
- Resentment about the need for treatment
- Economic restriction on access to health care and drugs
- Demographic factors such as sex and ethnicity
- Forgetfulness and stress
- Secondary gain from persistent symptoms

Should you refer a patient with difficult asthma?

Patients who are refractory to guideline based treatment should be referred to a specialised clinic. This is important if the diagnosis is in doubt or when excessive amounts of drugs, especially oral steroids, are used. Ideally, referring doctors should have access to a multidisciplinary clinic where experienced personnel (respiratory physicians, psychologists, and specialist nurses) have the necessary tools (such as bronchial challenge test kits and fibreoptic nasoendoscopy) and infrastructure available for assessment. However, a UK postal questionnaire sent to more than 600 consultant members of the BTS (50% response rate) found that only 23% of responding respiratory physicians had a dedicated difficult asthma clinic in their hospital.[15]

What new approaches are available?

Anti-immunoglobulin E

Many people with asthma are atopic, with the consequence that aeroallergens interact with IgE and cause the release of inflammatory mediators.[w23] Omalizumab is a humanised monoclonal antibody that can be given subcutaneously; its dose is determined by baseline IgE and body weight. Omalizumab cannot be given if the total IgE is more than 700 IU/l, which effectively excludes highly atopic patients. A randomised controlled trial evaluated the addition of omalizumab in people with severe asthma who had persistent symptoms despite using inhaled steroids and long acting $\beta 2$ agonists.[16] The clinically significant asthma exacerbation rate was 0.68 with omalizumab and 0.91 with placebo over 28 weeks (P=0.042), and compared with placebo, active treatment significantly reduced severe asthma exacerbation rates (0.24 *v* 0.48; P=0.002) and emergency visit rates (0.24 *v* 0.43; P=0.038). The National Institute for Health and Clinical Excellence advises that omalizumab should be considered only for patients who have had at least two severe exacerbations requiring hospital admission within the previous year, whereas the Scottish Medicines Consortium advises its restriction to patients requiring maintenance oral steroids when all other treatments have failed.

Other biological treatments

Tumour necrosis factor α is thought to have a role in some chronic inflammatory conditions. Despite initial promise, however, a randomised double blind study evaluating etanercept (a tumour necrosis factor antagonist) over 12 weeks found no significant improvement in major outcomes in patients with steroid dependent asthma.[17] Moreover, a trial of 24 weeks' treatment with gomilumab (a humanised monoclonal antibody against tumour necrosis factor) also found no important differences in asthma outcome. The trial

Asthma control test[20]

Questions and answers	Score 1	2	3	4	5
Question 1	How much of the time did your asthma keep you from getting as much done at work, school, or home?				
Answers	All the time	Most of the time	Some of the time	A little of the time	None of the time
Question 2	How often have you had shortness of breath?				
Answers	More than once a day	Once a day	3-6 times a week	Once or twice a week	Not at all
Question 3	How often did your asthma symptoms wake you up at night or earlier than usual in the morning?				
Answers	≥4 nights a week	2-3 nights a week	Once a week	Once or twice	Not at all
Question 4	How often have you used your rescue inhaler or nebulised drug?				
Answers	≥3 times a day	1-2 times a day	2-3 times a week	At least once a week	Not at all
Question 5	How would you rate your asthma control?				
Answers	Not at all controlled	Poorly controlled	Somewhat controlled	Well controlled	Completely controlled

The five questions refer to the past 4 weeks. A total score of 25 indicates perfect control; 20-24 indicates that asthma may be well controlled, although further advice should be obtained; and <20 indicates that further recommendations regarding management should be made by a nurse or doctor.

was stopped early because of the significantly increased numbers of infections and incidence of malignancies in the active treatment arm.[18] Whether other biological agents such as anti-interleukin 13 antibody or anti-neutrophilic strategies such as anti-CXCR1/R2 will be beneficial in refractory asthma remains to be seen.

Other drugs

Various drugs such as ciclosporin, methotrexate, gold, and subcutaneous terbutaline have been tried with various degrees of success in difficult asthma. These agents are not in widespread use but may be considered under specialist supervision.

Bronchial thermoplasty

An increase in airway smooth muscle mass is thought to be an important factor in severe or fatal asthma.[w24 w25] Bronchial thermoplasty—where controlled thermal energy is delivered to the airway wall during several bronchoscopy procedures—results in prolonged reduction of smooth muscle mass. In people with moderate to severe asthma, this procedure reduces symptoms, use of relievers, and exacerbations, and it improves quality of life and lung function.[19] Larger long term studies are needed to evaluate this new technique fully.

How should patients with difficult asthma be monitored?

It is unclear how best to monitor patients in the community, although regular follow-up by doctors and nurses trained in asthma management may be beneficial. This also provides an opportunity to assess inhaler technique and switch to a more efficient device if necessary or one that the patient can use more easily. Non-specific questions tend to underestimate symptoms,[20] but asthma control can be assessed by well validated questions, such as those in the asthma control test (table).

It is difficult to assess adherence to inhaled drugs, although surrogate markers such as prescription filling of maintenance inhalers may be helpful. Direct measurements such as plasma theophylline concentrations or plasma prednisolone and cortisol measurements can provide supportive evidence.

In the future it may be increasingly important to monitor disease activity—and thereby titrate treatment—using surrogate inflammatory biomarkers; examples of these include airway hyper-responsiveness (using indirect challenge tests such as mannitol), induced sputum eosinophil counts, and exhaled nitric oxide.[21] Indeed, asthma control may be improved when a surrogate inflammatory biomarker is incorporated into algorithms (along with conventional measures of asthma control) by which treatment is altered.[22 23 24] However, in one study, the use of exhaled nitric oxide as an indicator of asthma control resulted in higher doses of inhaled steroids being used, without a clinically important reduction in symptoms.[25]

Conclusions

Managing asthma that is refractory to usual treatment requires a systematic approach to ensure a correct diagnosis, identify coexisting disorders, tailor treatment, and evaluate adherence. The BTS has established UK registries of adults and children with difficult to control asthma to standardise and optimise assessment protocols across UK centres. In the future, this may facilitate research into severe asthma phenotypes and disease mechanisms in an attempt to define best practice.

Contributors: GPC had the original idea for the manuscript and wrote it along with JGD and LGH; GPC is guarantor.

Competing interests: GPC has received funding and honorariums from AstraZeneca, Merck Sharp and Dohme, and GlaxoSmithKline; JGD from GlaxoSmithKline, AstraZeneca, and Novartis; and LGH from AstraZeneca, Merck Sharp and Dohme, Novartis, and GlaxoSmithKline for attending postgraduate educational meetings and giving talks.

Provenance and peer review: Commissioned; externally peer reviewed.

1 British Thoracic Society and Scottish Intercollegiate Guideline Network. British guideline on the management of asthma. *Thorax* 2008;63(suppl 4):iv1-121.
2 Barnes PJ, Woolcock AJ. Difficult asthma. *Eur Respir J* 1998;12:1209-18.
3 Robinson DS, Campbell DA, Durham SR, Pfeffer J, Barnes PJ, Chung KF. Systematic assessment of difficult-to-treat asthma. *Eur Respir J* 2003;22:478-83.
4 Heaney LG, Conway E, Kelly C, Johnston BT, English C, Stevenson M, et al. Predictors of therapy resistant asthma: outcome of a systematic evaluation protocol. *Thorax* 2003;58:561-6.
5 Heaney LG, Robinson DS. Severe asthma treatment: need for characterising patients. *Lancet* 2005;365:974-6.
6 Corren J. Allergic rhinitis and asthma: how important is the link? *J Allergy Clin Immunol* 1997;99:S781-6.
7 Bousquet J, Van Cauwenberge P, Khaltaev N. Allergic rhinitis and its impact on asthma. *J Allergy Clin Immunol* 2001;108:S147-334.
8 Coughlan JL, Gibson PG, Henry RL. Medical treatment for reflux oesophagitis does not consistently improve asthma control: a systematic review. *Thorax* 2001;56:198-204.
9 Jenkins C, Costello J, Hodge L. Systematic review of prevalence of aspirin induced asthma and its implications for clinical practice. *BMJ* 2004;328:434.
10 Currie GP, Jackson CM, Lee DK, Lipworth BJ. Allergen sensitization and bronchial hyper-responsiveness to adenosine monophosphate in asthmatic patients. *Clin Exp Allergy* 2003;33:1405-8.
11 Woodcock A, Forster L, Matthews E, Martin J, Letley L, Vickers M, et al. Control of exposure to mite allergen and allergen-impermeable bed covers for adults with asthma. *N Engl J Med* 2003;349:225-36.
12 Tomlinson JE, McMahon AD, Chaudhuri R, Thompson JM, Wood SF, Thomson NC. Efficacy of low and high dose inhaled corticosteroid in smokers versus non-smokers with mild asthma. *Thorax* 2005;60:282-7.
13 Thomson NC, Chaudhuri R, Livingston E. Asthma and cigarette smoking. *Eur Respir J* 2004;24:822-33.
14 Sin DD, Sutherland ER. Obesity and the lung: 4. Obesity and asthma. *Thorax* 2008;63:1018-23.
15 Roberts NJ, Robinson DS, Partridge MR. How is difficult asthma managed? *Eur Respir J* 2006;28:968-73.
16 Humbert M, Beasley R, Ayres J, Slavin R, Hebert J, Bousquet J, et al. Benefits of omalizumab as add-on therapy in patients with severe persistent asthma who are inadequately controlled despite best available therapy (GINA 2002 step 4 treatment): INNOVATE. *Allergy* 2005;60:309-16.

ADDITIONAL EDUCATIONAL RESOURCES

Additional educational resources for healthcare professionals

- British Thoracic Society (www.brit-thoracic.org.uk)—The main UK respiratory society for clinicians
- Lung and Asthma Information Agency (www.laia.ac.uk)—Gives epidemiological data on asthma, allergy, and other respiratory conditions
- National Heart, Lung, and Blood Institute (www.nhlbi.nih.gov/health/public/lung/index.htm)—Gives information on lung diseases such as asthma
- Oasys and Occupational Asthma (www.occupationalasthma.com/)—Provides information on occupational asthma
- Dendrite Clinical Systems Ltd (http://host.e-dendrite.com/csp/asthma/FrontPages/asthmafront.csp)—British Thoracic Society difficult asthma registry

Additional educational resources for patients

- Asthma UK (www.asthma.org.uk)—A leading UK asthma charity organisation
- British Lung Foundation (www.lunguk.org)—A leading UK charity helping those with respiratory disorders
- ASH (www.ash.org.uk)—A public health charity dedicated to limiting harm caused by smoking

TIPS FOR NON-SPECIALISTS

- Always check that the diagnosis of asthma is correct
- Consider further tests to help confirm the diagnosis; refer to a specialist if the diagnosis remains questionable
- Always ask about adherence to treatment
- Assess inhaler technique at every opportunity
- Always encourage smoking cessation and weight reduction

17 Morjaria JB, Chauhan AJ, Babu KS, Polosa R, Davies DE, Holgate ST. The role of a soluble TNFalpha receptor fusion protein (etanercept) in corticosteroid refractory asthma: a double blind, randomised, placebo controlled trial. *Thorax* 2008;63:584-91.

18 Wenzel SE, Barnes PJ, Bleecker ER, Bousquet J, Busse W, Dahlen SE, et al. A randomized, double-blind, placebo-controlled study of TNF-{alpha} blockade in severe persistent asthma. *Am J Respir Crit Care Med* 2009 Jan 8 (Epub ahead of print).

19 Cox G, Thomson NC, Rubin AS, Niven RM, Corris PA, Siersted HC, et al. Asthma control during the year after bronchial thermoplasty. *N Engl J Med* 2007;356:1327-37.

20 Nathan RA, Sorkness CA, Kosinski M, Schatz M, Li JT, Marcus P, et al. Development of the asthma control test: a survey for assessing asthma control. *J Allergy Clin Immunol* 2004;113:59-65.

21 Currie GP, Fardon TC, Lee DK. The role of measuring airway hyperresponsiveness and inflammatory biomarkers in asthma. *Ther Clin Risk Manag* 2005;1:83-92.

22 Smith AD, Cowan JO, Brassett KP, Herbison GP, Taylor DR. Use of exhaled nitric oxide measurements to guide treatment in chronic asthma. *N Engl J Med* 2005;352:2163-73.

23 Green RH, Brightling CE, McKenna S, Hargadon B, Parker D, Bradding P, et al. Asthma exacerbations and sputum eosinophil counts: a randomised controlled trial. *Lancet* 2002;360:1715-21.

24 Sont JK, Willems LN, Bel EH, van Krieken JH, Vandenbroucke JP, Sterk PJ. Clinical control and histopathologic outcome of asthma when using airway hyperresponsiveness as an additional guide to long-term treatment. The AMPUL Study Group. *Am J Respir Crit Care Med* 1999;159:1043-51.

25 Szefler SJ, Mitchell H, Sorkness CA, Gergen PJ, O'Connor GT, Morgan WJ, et al. Management of asthma based on exhaled nitric oxide in addition to guideline-based treatment for inner-city adolescents and young adults: a randomised controlled trial. *Lancet* 2008;372:1065-72.

BMJ BPP UNIVERSITY SCHOOL OF HEALTH

Management and prevention of exacerbations of COPD

Shawn D Aaron, professor, University of Ottawa

[1]Ottawa Hospital Research Institute, Ottawa, ON, Canada, K1H 8L6

Correspondence to: S D Aaron saaron@ohri.ca

Cite this as: *BMJ* 2014;349:g5237

‹DOI› 10.1136/bmj.g5237
http://www.bmj.com/content/349/bmj.g5237

Patients with chronic obstructive pulmonary disease (COPD) are prone to acute respiratory exacerbations, which can develop suddenly or subacutely over the course of several days. Exacerbations have a detrimental effect on patients' health status and increase the burden on the healthcare system. Initial treatment is unsuccessful in 24-27% of patients, who have a relapse or a second exacerbation within 30 days of the initial event. No obvious benefit has been seen in recent clinical trials of anti-tumour necrosis factor therapy, anti-leukotriene therapy, intensive chest physiotherapy, or early inpatient pulmonary rehabilitation for treatment of exacerbations. By contrast, clinical trials of prevention rather than acute treatment have shown promising results. Long acting β agonist (LABA) or long acting anti-muscarinic (LAMA) bronchodilators and inhaled corticosteroid-LABA combinations prevent exacerbations in patients at risk, with relative risk reductions averaging 14-27% for each of these drugs relative to placebo. Triple therapy with inhaled corticosteroid-LABA plus LAMA may provide additional benefit, although study results to date are heterogeneous and more studies are needed. Pneumonia is an important complication of treatment with inhaled corticosteroid-LABA products, and the risk of pneumonia seems to be doubled in patients with COPD who use fluticasone. The addition of azithromycin to usual COPD therapy prevents exacerbations, although it may prolong the Q-T interval and increase the risk of death from cardiovascular disease in patients prone to arrhythmia. New potential drugs—including mitogen activated protein kinase inhibitors, phosphodiesterase 3 inhibitors, and monoclonal antibodies to the interleukin 1 receptor—offer additional hope for treatments that may prevent exacerbations in the future.

Introduction

Acute exacerbations of chronic obstructive pulmonary disease (COPD) are characterized clinically by worsening dyspnea, cough, sputum production, and airflow obstruction.[1] Such exacerbations are associated with short term and long term reductions in quality of life and lung function, as well as increased risk of death.[2 3] Owing to the considerable impact of these exacerbations on patients' health status, their frequency is now recognized as a key component of the characterization of patients with COPD, and the prevention and treatment of exacerbations has become a primary goal of treatment.[4]

SOURCES AND SELECTION CRITERIA

We searched the Cochrane Airways Group register of clinical trials and Medline from 1990 to October 2013 and November 2013, respectively. Search terms included: chronic obstructive pulmonary disease (COPD), or chronic bronchitis, or emphysema, or exacerbations of COPD, and therapy or prevention. Controlled clinical trials and systematic reviews with meta-analyses of interventions or drugs to prevent or treat acute exacerbations of chronic obstructive pulmonary disease were selected for potential inclusion in this article. We excluded observational studies and non-randomized trials.

This article aims to review recent evidence, mostly from randomized controlled trials (RCTs), on new drug and non-drug based therapies for the prevention and treatment of COPD exacerbations. Research in this area—both industry driven and academic—has increased greatly over the past decade, and new studies and drugs are rapidly emerging. Results of recent clinical trials suggest that substantial gains have been made in developing new strategies to prevent such exacerbations. However, studies evaluating new therapies for the acute treatment of COPD exacerbations have not been so successful.

Definition of an exacerbation of COPD

Exacerbations of COPD are characterized by a sustained worsening of respiratory symptoms from the usual stable state beyond normal day to day variations.[5] Typical symptoms associated with exacerbations include worsening of dyspnea and cough, as well as increased sputum volume and sputum purulence.[1] Exacerbations range in severity from transient reductions in functional status to fatal events.

Definitions of exacerbations vary between clinical studies. Studies that use home based symptom diaries or other symptom monitoring tools—such as the COPD assessment test or the exacerbations of chronic pulmonary disease tool scales—may use symptom based definitions that rely on a sustained worsening of respiratory symptoms for two consecutive days.[6 7] Studies in COPD cohorts suggest that many of these symptom based events may go unreported and untreated.[8 9] Most clinical trials that evaluate drugs to prevent exacerbations use event based definitions of exacerbation, which require an increase in both symptoms and the use of healthcare resources.[10 11 12] Recent pivotal clinical trials define moderate exacerbations as those that require treatment with systemic glucocorticoids or antibiotics (or both) and severe exacerbations as those that require hospital admission.[13 14 15]

To investigate whether the use of different definitions of COPD exacerbations affected the results of clinical trials, the INSPIRE study compared the incidence of exacerbations using both symptom based definitions and treatment based ones.[16] In this long term study, three COPD exacerbations were detected per patient year when a symptom based definition was used compared with about 1.5 exacerbations per patient year when a treatment based definition was used. Thus about 50% of symptom defined COPD exacerbations are not treated by physicians, and these exacerbations are unlikely to be counted as exacerbation events in most clinical trials.

Causes of COPD exacerbations

COPD exacerbations are caused by complex interactions between the host, respiratory viruses, and airway bacteria, which lead to an increase in the inflammatory burden within the airway.[17] Studies suggest that airway neutrophils, as well as systemic and local mediators of inflammation,

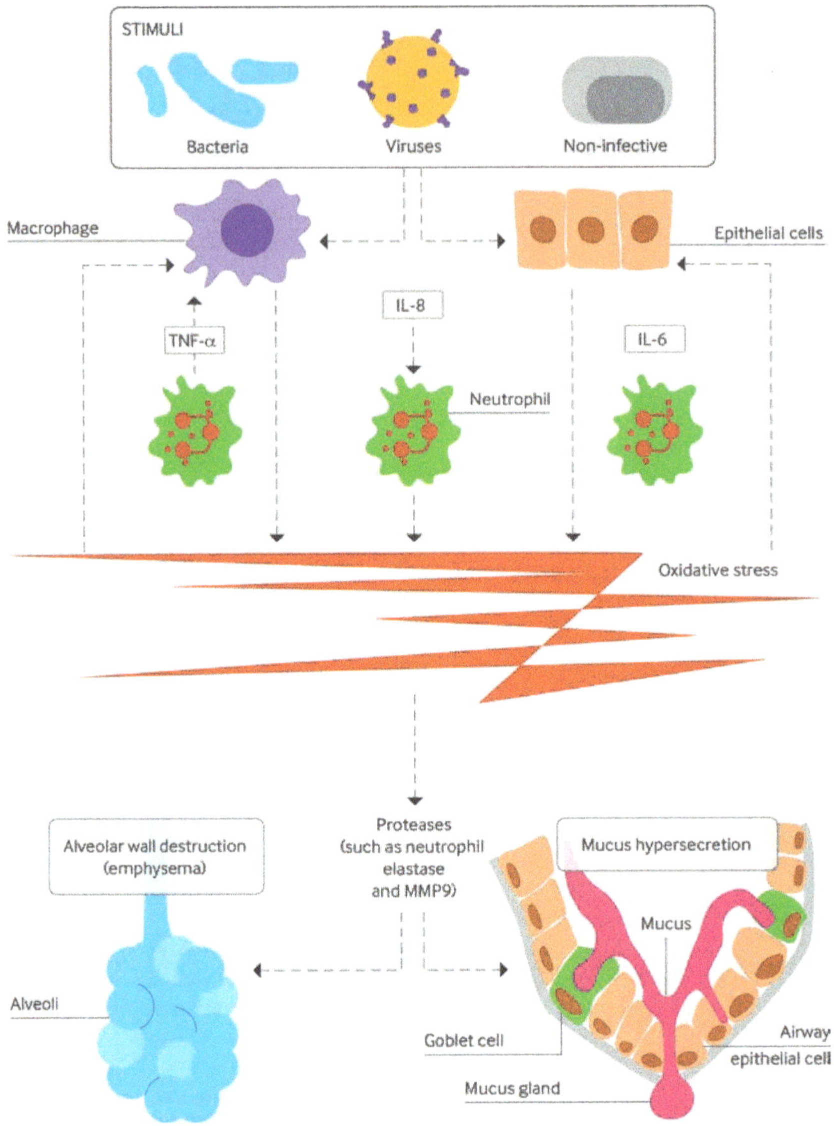

Fig 1 Mechanism for acute exacerbations in chronic obstructive pulmonary disease (COPD). Triggers of COPD exacerbations include infectious agents such as bacteria and viruses and non-infectious agents such as air pollution. These stimuli activate airway epithelial cells and macrophages to release inflammatory cytokines including tumor necrosis factor α (TNF-α), interleukin 6 (IL-6), and IL-8. These cytokines lead to neutrophil recruitment and the release of reactive oxidant species and proteases from activated neutrophils, which magnify the inflammatory process[20]

such as interleukin 8 and tumor necrosis factor α (TNF-α) increase during COPD exacerbations compared with the stable state.[18] Migration and activation of neutrophils within the airway leads to the release of proteases and reactive oxygen species; this further damages the airway epithelium and leads to worsening of airway inflammation and airflow limitation (fig 1). A minority of exacerbations are associated with airway and sputum eosinophilia.[19]

COPD exacerbations are accompanied by changes in airway physiology that induce dyspnea.[21] A clinical study suggested that patients experience acute worsening of airflow obstruction accompanied by acute lung hyperinflation at the time of a moderate exacerbations.[22] At recovery, 60 days after the onset of the exacerbation, inspiratory capacity and forced expiratory volume in one second (FEV1) increased by 18% compared with values during the exacerbation, and air trapping (residual volume) decreased by 11%. Improvements in dyspnea after acute exacerbations significantly correlated with a reduction in lung hyperinflation and consequent increase in expiratory flow rates. This suggests that dyspnea during an acute exacerbation is probably partially mediated by the dynamic hyperinflation that occurs in response to the airflow limitation associated with these events (fig 2).[22]

In general, viral and bacterial infections are the most important triggers of exacerbation.[23 24 25] Studies suggest that exacerbations are often associated with the isolation of new strains of airway bacteria, with an accompanying host inflammatory response to these new strains.[23 26] Respiratory bacteria and viruses often act in combination.[27] Recent studies of experimentally induced rhinovirus infection in patients with COPD suggest that bacterial infection of the airways often follows acute rhinovirus infection, and that infection with both viruses and bacteria can exert a synergistic inflammatory effect.[28]

Coinfection with viruses and bacteria has been detected in 25% of exacerbations and is associated with more severe functional impairment and longer hospital stays.[29] Molecular techniques, including multiplex polymerase chain reaction, provide greater sensitivity to detect acute viral respiratory tract infections that cause exacerbations. However, a specific infectious or environmental cause cannot be identified in about a third of severe exacerbations.[30]

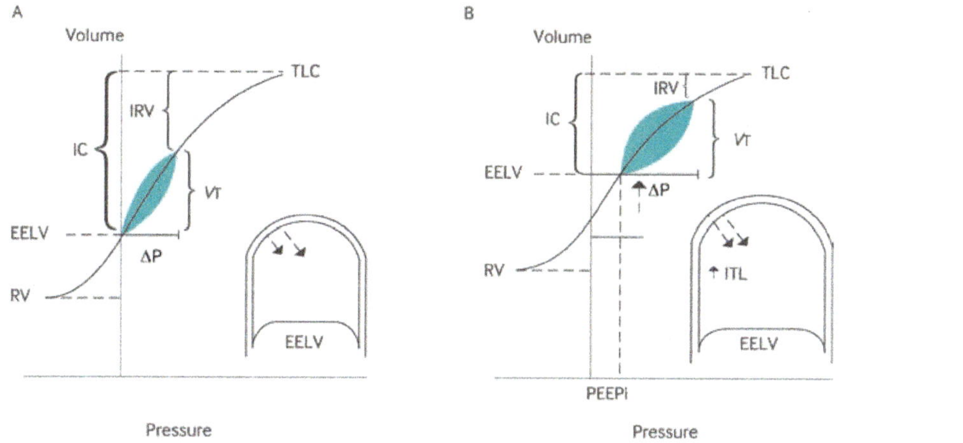

Fig 2 Schematic diagram of the pathophysiologic effects of an exacerbation of chronic obstructive pulmonary disease (COPD). Pressure-volume plots are shown during (A) stable COPD and (B) an exacerbation. During exacerbation, worsening airflow obstruction leads to dynamic hyperinflation, with increased end expiratory lung volume (EELV) and air trapping manifested as an increased residual volume (RV). Corresponding reductions occur in inspiratory capacity (IC) and inspiratory reserve volume (IRV). As a result, tidal breathing is shifted to the right on the pressure-volume curve, closer to total lung capacity (TLC), resulting in unfavorable overall compliance of the respiratory system. Increased mechanical pressures must be generated by the respiratory muscles to maintain tidal volume (VT). At EELV during an exacerbation, intrapulmonary pressures do not return to zero, as a result of the development of intrinsic positive end expiratory pressure (PEEPi), which imposes further increased inspiratory threshold loading (ITL) on the inspiratory muscles (inset). ΔP=change in pleural pressure. Reproduced, with permission, from Bafadhel and colleagues[19]

Recent investigations using cluster analysis suggest that exacerbations can be grouped into four categories: bacterial, viral, predominantly eosinophilic, and a "pauci-inflammatory" category associated with limited changes in the inflammatory profile.[19] Each of these clusters is associated with a biomarker, suggesting that biomarkers may become useful for categorizing the cause of an exacerbation.

Natural course of exacerbations: onset and recovery

A recent prospective cohort of 212 patients with COPD was monitored using daily symptom diaries for a median of 2.8 years to characterize the time course of the onset of COPD exacerbations.[31] Patients recorded 4439 episodes of worsening respiratory symptoms from baseline; 55% of these events resolved spontaneously and 45% resulted in an exacerbation. In 56% of COPD exacerbations the onset was sudden and the exacerbation threshold was crossed on the same day that respiratory symptoms began. By contrast, in 44% of exacerbations the onset of symptoms was gradual (median duration from symptom onset to exacerbation: four days; fig 3). Patients with sudden onset exacerbations had more intense symptoms but a shorter median recovery time back to baseline health status (11 *v* 13 days; P<0.001). The study concluded that COPD exacerbations exhibit two distinct patterns—sudden and gradual onset—and that sudden exacerbations are associated with increased peak respiratory symptoms but shorter exacerbation recovery times.[31]

Previous data have suggested that the median duration of recovery time after an acute exacerbation is 7-10 days for lung function as measured by peak expiratory flow, although there is wide variation, and a minority (<10%) of patients never recover to their pre-exacerbation lung function.[32] Symptoms may take longer to recover than peak expiratory flow, and the median duration of symptom recovery back to previous baseline is 11-13 days.[31 33]

About a quarter of inpatients treated for an acute COPD exacerbation do not respond to initial treatment and experience an adverse outcome, defined as either death, intubation, or need for readmission or intensification of

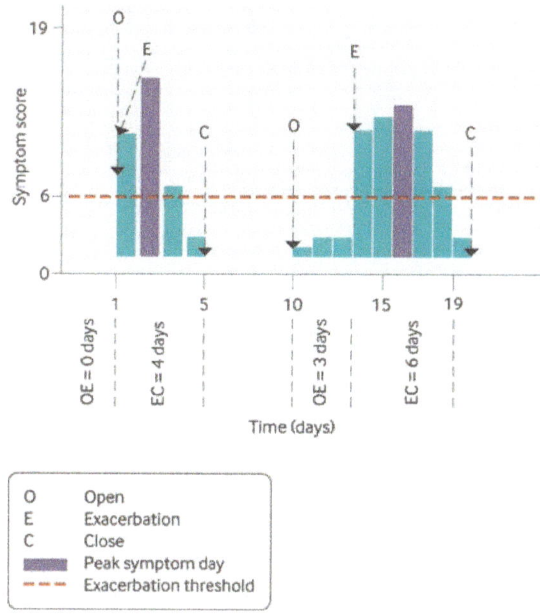

Fig 3 Time course and calculation of the onset and duration of exacerbation intervals: a sudden onset exacerbation is shown on the left, a gradual onset exacerbation on the right. The opening event (O) was defined as the first day of worsening of respiratory symptoms above usual baseline values. An exacerbation (E) was defined as the first of two or more consecutive days during which the patient recorded two or more new or worsening symptoms, at least one of which was a major symptom (a daily symptom score of ≥6 points for two consecutive days (indicated by the dotted line)). A closing (C) was defined as the first of five consecutive days during which symptoms had returned to their usual baseline levels. For sudden onset exacerbations the OE interval is 0 days, indicating that the exacerbation occurs on the first day of worsening of respiratory symptoms. About 55% of exacerbations are sudden onset. The EC represents the duration of the exacerbation—the time from the onset of the exacerbation to recovery back to baseline. Reproduced, with permission, from Papi and colleagues[29]

drug therapy. Similarly, studies suggest that a quarter of outpatients treated for an acute exacerbation either relapse (defined as an unscheduled visit to a physician or the emergency department because of worsening dyspnea) or have a second exacerbation within 30 days of the initial presentation.[33] Many of these patients require readmission to hospital.[33]

In 2010 in the United States, there were 606000 hospital admissions for COPD and 126000 patients (21%) required readmission within 30 days.[33] Clinical trials indicate that about 27% of outpatients treated with combined antibiotic and corticosteroid therapy relapse within 30 days.[34] Treatment failure rates in inpatients with an exacerbation average 24% at 30 days and rise to 36-37% by 90 days.[35 36] A recent systematic review found that there was not enough evidence to recommend specific interventions to reduce the risk of readmission in patients who have been treated in hospital for an acute exacerbation.[37]

COPD exacerbations and mortality

A prospective five year cohort study of 304 Spanish men with COPD found that the frequency of exacerbations is independently associated with mortality.[38] When a service based definition of COPD exacerbation (need for emergency department treatment) was used, patients with three or more exacerbations had a survival rate of 30% at five years, whereas those without an exacerbation had a survival rate of 80% (hazard ratio 4.13, 95% confidence interval 1.80 to 9.41). Survival was also influenced by the severity of the exacerbation—exacerbations that necessitated hospital admission or readmission were associated with the poorest survival.[38]

Patients who are admitted for an exacerbation have an in-hospital mortality of about 10%. Patients with an exacerbation and hypercapnic respiratory failure have a two year mortality rate of about 50%.[39] A recent study of 1824 European patients with COPD documented a 45% four year mortality rate after discharge from hospital in those admitted with an exacerbation.[40]

Incidence of COPD exacerbations across GOLD categories of severity

The severity of airflow limitation is traditionally classified using the Global Initiative for Chronic Obstructive Lung Disease (GOLD) spirometric grading system, which uses specific spirometric cut-off points for simplicity.[4] Although this classification system correlates poorly with health related quality of life,[41] numerous studies suggest that the risk of COPD exacerbations, hospital admission, and death from COPD increase with worsening of GOLD spirometric stage.[42 43 44]

A recent longitudinal cohort study enrolled 2138 patients with COPD whose post-bronchodilator FEV1 was less than 80% of predicted.[42] Patients were followed prospectively for three years, and the rate of moderate exacerbations that needed treatment with systemic steroids or antibiotics (or both) and severe exacerbations that required hospital admission was recorded. The study found a mean incidence of 1.21 exacerbations per patient year among the entire cohort and that incidence was associated with GOLD stage of airflow obstruction at baseline. Patients with GOLD stage II COPD (FEV1 50-80% of predicted) had 0.85 exacerbations per patient year that needed treatment with systemic steroids or antibiotics (or both). However, this figure was 1.34 for those with GOLD stage III COPD (FEV1 30-50% of predicted) and 2.00 for those with the most severe GOLD stage IV COPD (FEV1 <30% of predicted).[42]

Exacerbations become more frequent and severe as the severity of COPD increases. However, a distinct group of patients seems to be susceptible to exacerbations, irrespective of disease severity, and these susceptible patients typically experience two or more moderate or severe exacerbations a year.[42] This susceptibility phenotype is relatively stable over time and occurs across all severities of airflow obstruction, suggesting that these patients are prone to exacerbations, perhaps as a result of intrinsic susceptibility to particular triggers, such as respiratory infections or pollutants.[45]

Treatment of acute exacerbations

Corticosteroids

Standard treatment for acute COPD exacerbations includes treatment with bronchodilators, antibiotics, and corticosteroids.[46] Clinical trials have shown that the addition of oral or intravenous corticosteroids to antibiotics significantly decreases treatment failure rates in inpatients with COPD exacerbations[35] and prevents relapse in outpatients with an exacerbation.[34] A recent RCT suggested that, in patients presenting to the emergency department with acute exacerbations of COPD (most of whom were admitted), a five day treatment course with 40 mg of prednisone daily was non-inferior to a 14 day treatment course.[36] Patients treated with five days of prednisone had similar rates of re-exacerbation within six months of follow-up but had significantly reduced exposure to glucocorticoids.[36]

Another recent randomised controlled trial investigated whether blood eosinophilia could be used as a biomarker to predict response to oral corticosteroids in patients with a COPD exacerbation.[47] Serum eosinophilia of ≥2% occurs in about 50% of patients who present with a COPD exacerbation.[47 48] People in the biomarker directed arm of the study were treated with prednisone for two weeks if their serum eosinophil count was ≥2%, whereas those whose eosinophil count was <2% received placebo. Both groups received antibiotics. Patients with eosinophil counts <2% in the biomarker directed treatment arm (who were treated with placebo) had a greater improvement in quality of life than those in the other arm, who were given prednisone (mean difference in chronic respiratory questionnaire score 0.45; P=0.04). Similarly, treatment failure rates were lower in those with serum eosinophils <2% who were treated with placebo rather than prednisone (15% *v* 2%; P=0.04).[47] These results suggest that a subgroup of patients with COPD exacerbations who have serum eosinophil counts <2% of their total leukocyte count at presentation may not respond to systemic steroids. However, further clinical trials are needed to confirm the results of this relatively small study.

Antibiotics

GOLD guidelines[4] and European Respiratory Society guidelines[49] advocate antibiotics for patients with acute COPD exacerbations who also have worsening dyspnoea as well as increased sputum volume and purulence, or if any two of these symptoms, particularly increased sputum purulence, worsen. These recommendations are based on older studies that demonstrated better outcomes in outpatients with COPD exacerbations treated with broad spectrum antibiotics such as trimethoprim-sulfamethoxazole, doxycycline, or amoxicillin.[1] In addition, a clinical trial in patients with severe exacerbations, who needed mechanical ventilation, showed that ofloxacin significantly reduced mortality associated with severe exacerbations.[50]

Two recently published RCTs assessed the use of antibiotics in COPD exacerbations. The first study of 223 inpatients with COPD exacerbations compared the addition of seven days of doxycycline or placebo with treatment with systemic corticosteroids.[51] It found no significant difference in the primary endpoint of clinical success (61% *v* 53%; P=0.32), clinical cure, or lung function at day 30.[51] By contrast, the other RCT studied 310 outpatients with mild to moderate exacerbations, most of whom were not treated with concomitant oral steroids.[20] Amoxicillin-clavulinic acid significantly increased clinical cure rates at the end of treatment (days 9-11) compared with placebo (74% *v* 60%; difference 14.2%, 3.7% to 24.3%). Treatment with amoxicillin-clavulinic acid was also associated with a prolonged time to next exacerbation compared with placebo.[20]

Non-invasive ventilation

Non-invasive ventilation using pressure cycled bilevel positive airway pressure has been studied in several RCTs. It decreases respiratory rate and work of breathing, improves acute respiratory acidosis, and decreases the requirement for intubation and invasive ventilation in patients with COPD exacerbations and respiratory failure.[52] A decrease in the need for invasive ventilation with this treatment has also translated into lower rates of ventilator associated pneumonia, shorter hospital stays, and reduced mortality.[53] GOLD guidelines recommend that patients with severe dyspnea, increased work of breathing, and respiratory acidosis (pH ≤7.35 or arterial carbon dioxide pressure >45 mm Hg, or both) should be considered for this treatment, provided they are conscious and able to protect their airway and deal with respiratory secretions.[4]

New potential treatments for COPD exacerbations

Novel anti-inflammatory drugs

Several RCTs of novel drugs for the treatment of COPD exacerbations have been published recently. A trial from Canada evaluated the TNF-α antagonist etanercept as an anti-inflammatory treatment for this condition.[48] The investigators randomized 81 patients with a COPD exacerbation to treatment with prednisone (40 mg/day for 10 days) or etanercept 50 mg given subcutaneously on the day of the exacerbation and seven days later. Both groups were treated with antibiotics (levofloxacin) plus long acting bronchodilators. No significant difference was seen in lung function at 14 days or treatment failure at 90 days (32% *v* 40%; P=0.44). A subgroup analysis suggested that prednisone was more effective than etanercept in patients who presented with serum eosinophils greater than 2%.[48]

A similar study of alternative anti-inflammatory treatment randomized 119 inpatients with an exacerbation to oral treatment with the anti-leukotriene inhibitor zileuton 600 mg four times daily or placebo. Patients were treated with 14 days of oral prednisone plus an antibiotic. The study found no significant difference in duration of hospital stay and treatment failure rates.[54]

Novel enhanced secretion clearance techniques

A recent RCT evaluated positive expiratory pressure therapy to enhance sputum clearance in 90 inpatients with a COPD exacerbation. Patients were randomized to receive this new treatment or usual care while in hospital. The addition of positive expiratory pressure therapy did not significantly improve short term outcomes, such as respiratory symptoms at day of discharge, or disease specific quality of life at eight weeks. Similarly, rates of exacerbation and admission to hospital did not differ between the two treatment groups during the six months after discharge.[55]

Early inpatient respiratory rehabilitation during an exacerbation

An RCT of 389 people evaluated early inpatient pulmonary rehabilitation begun within 48 hours of admission to hospital for an acute exacerbation and continued for six weeks after discharge. It found no significant effect of early pulmonary rehabilitation on readmission rates in the year after initial admission (hazard ratio 1.1, 0.86 to 1.43; P=0.440) compared with usual care. An increase in mortality was seen in the intervention group at one year (odds ratio 1.74, 1.05 to 2.88; P=0.031), but not during the intervention period or at six months. Physical performance and health status recovered after discharge in both groups, with no significant difference between groups at one year. The authors concluded that early rehabilitation during hospital admission for an acute exacerbation did not reduce the risk of subsequent readmission or enhance recovery of physical function after the initial event.[56]

Summary: acute management of COPD exacerbations

Despite extensive research, the medical management of COPD exacerbations has not changed substantially over the past 25 years (box). Recent studies evaluating new anti-inflammatory drugs, intensive chest physiotherapy, and early inpatient pulmonary rehabilitation have all failed to show obvious benefits. More research is needed to improve the treatment of these exacerbations and to prevent treatment failure and relapse.

Prevention of COPD exacerbations

Given the global health, social, and economic importance of this condition, the prevention of exacerbations is now recognized as a primary goal of maintenance therapy for COPD.[4] Several drug and non-drug based interventions have been studied in clinical trials, with the aim of decreasing the frequency and severity of exacerbations (table).[57]

Vaccinations

Influenza vaccine reduces the rate and severity of influenza symptoms, including respiratory ones. A meta-analysis of 11 trials, including six performed exclusively in patients with

ACUTE MANAGEMENT OF MODERATE TO SEVERE EXACERBATIONS OF CHRONIC OBSTRUCTIVE PULMONARY DISEASE

- Supplemental oxygen: titrate to keep oxygen saturation 90-94%
- Short acting β agonist and an anticholinergic bronchodilator
- Oral prednisone 40 mg daily for five days
- Add antibiotics (amoxicillin-clavulinic acid, a respiratory fluoroquinolone, or a macrolide) if the patient has at least two of the following symptoms:
- Worsening dyspnea
- Increased sputum volume
- Increased sputum purulence (particularly if this is one of the symptoms)
- Consider non-invasive ventilation for patients with increased work of breathing and respiratory acidosis (pH <7.35)

Pharmacologic treatments for the prevention of acute exacerbations of chronic obstructive pulmonary disease

Pharmacologic treatment	Clinical trial evidence to support efficacy
Influenza vaccination	Efficacy confirmed[58]
Pneumococcal vaccination	Efficacy not confirmed[59]
Long acting antimuscarinic agent bronchodilators (LAMAs)	Efficacy confirmed[60]
Long acting β agonist bronchodilators (LABAs)	Efficacy confirmed[61]
Corticosteroid-LABA combination inhalers	Efficacy confirmed[62]
Triple therapy (inhaled corticosteroid-LABA + LAMA)	Efficacy not confirmed[10 63]
LABA-LAMA combination inhalers	Efficacy not confirmed[64]
Roflumilast	Efficacy confirmed (only in subgroup of patients with chronic bronchitis phenotype)[65]
Pulsed moxifloxacin	Efficacy not confirmed[66]
Azithromycin	Efficacy confirmed[67 68]
Simvastatin	Not effective[69]
N-acetylcysteine	Efficacy not confirmed[70-72]
Vitamin D	Not effective[73]

COPD, found that, in patients with COPD, influenza vaccine significantly reduced the total number of exacerbations per patient compared with those who received placebo (weighted mean difference −0.37, −0.64 to −0.11; P=0.006).[58]

A meta-analysis of seven trials that assessed the effects of a 23 valent pneumococcal vaccine in patients with COPD found no significant effect on morbidity or mortality.[59] The reduction in likelihood of acute exacerbations of COPD from two studies of 216 people was not significant (odds ratio 0.58, 0.30 to 1.13). The pooled results from three studies of 888 people showed no significant reduction in all cause mortality up to 48 months after vaccination (0.94, 0.67 to 1.33).[59]

Long acting bronchodilators

Two classes of bronchodilators are in widespread use for COPD: long acting antimuscarinic agents (LAMAs) and long acting β agonists (LABAs). Bronchodilators clearly have a role in the prevention of COPD exacerbations. Studies suggest that dyspnea during an exacerbation is caused by acute increases in expiratory airflow limitation and air trapping, which increase levels of dyspnea when they exceed a threshold value.[21 22] By improving expiratory airflow when patients are stable, long acting bronchodilators decrease baseline air trapping and move the patient further away from the critical threshold of air trapping that is associated with a COPD exacerbation.

LAMAs

The tiotropium dry powder inhaler is the best studied LAMA.

The most recent systematic review on chronic tiotropium therapy in COPD suggests that, compared with placebo, tiotropium reduces COPD exacerbations by 22% (odds ratio 0.78, 0.70 to 0.87).[60]

Two RCTs included in the review were pivotal to the result. The first examined the role of tiotropium versus placebo added to standard treatment in decreasing exacerbations in 1829 patients treated in the US.[74] Tiotropium significantly decreased the proportion of patients who experienced one or more exacerbations during six months of treatment (27.9% *v* 32.3%; P=0.037).

The second RCT, termed the UPLIFT study, assessed the use of tiotropium in more than 5900 patients. It found a significant 14% reduction in exacerbations over four years in people treated with tiotropium compared with those who received usual care for their COPD (0.73 *v* 0.85 exacerbations per person year; relative risk 0.86, 0.81 to 0.91).[14]

Newer LAMAs are becoming available for the treatment of COPD. Tiotropium is available in an aqueous solution inhaler (tiotropium Respimat) in several countries in Europe. An RCT of more than 17000 patients with COPD compared tiotropium dry powder inhaler with tiotropium aqueous inhaler over a mean of 2.3 years. The mortality rate was non-inferior for aqueous tiotropium compared with standard dry powder inhaler tiotropium. Time to first exacerbation and rates of exacerbation over the entire study period were also equivalent.[13] These data suggest that aqueous tiotropium may have similar efficacy to dry powder tiotropium in preventing exacerbations.

Other new LAMAs include glycopyrronium bromide and aclidinium bromide. An RCT randomized 1066 patients with COPD to glycopyrronium bromide 50 µg per day or to placebo or open label tiotropium. Compared with placebo, glycopyrronium significantly reduced the risk of moderate to severe exacerbations by 34% (P=0.001). This reduction in exacerbations was comparable to that seen with open label tiotropium.[75]

A second RCT of glycopyrronium versus placebo had similar results. Glycopyrronium significantly reduced the time to first moderate or severe exacerbation of COPD by 31% compared with placebo (hazard ratio 0.69, 0.50 to 0.95; P=0.023).[76] No studies have investigated whether aclidinium bromide reduces exacerbations relative to placebo or to its active comparators.

LABAs

Clinical studies suggest that LABAs can also prevent exacerbations, although the effect size is slightly less than for LAMAs. The TORCH study suggested that salmeterol monotherapy reduces the frequency of exacerbations compared with placebo (0.97 *v* 1.13 exacerbations per year; relative risk 0.85, 0.78 to 0.93; P=0.001).[12] A meta-analysis found that, compared with placebo, LABAs (mainly salmeterol or formoterol) significantly reduced moderately severe COPD exacerbations that necessitated a course of antibiotics or oral steroids (odds ratio 0.73, 0.61 to 0.87) or hospital admission (0.73, 0.56 to 0.95).[60]

A subsequent RCT of 3444 patients with severe COPD and a history of exacerbations compared indicaterol, a new once daily LABA, to tiotropium. Tiotropium was significantly more effective at preventing exacerbations than indicaterol over one year (rate ratio 1.29 in favour of tiotropium).[77]

LABA-LAMA combinations

Several combination LABA-LAMA inhalers are in the final stages of development and should be available for general use within the next 12-24 months. Of the fixed dose combinations currently under investigation, tiotropium plus olodaterol, umeclidinium bromide plus vilanterol, aclidinium plus formoterol, and glycopyrronium plus indacaterol have the largest phase III clinical trial programs.

To date, only one published study has evaluated whether a LAMA-LABA product can prevent COPD exacerbations. The once daily fixed dose combination LABA-LAMA inhaler QVA149 contains both glycopyrronium (50 μg) and indicaterol (110 μg) in a single inhaler. An RCT in patients with severe to very severe COPD and a history of exacerbations showed that QVA149 significantly decreased the rate of moderate to severe exacerbations by 12% compared with glycopyrronium alone, although QVA149 did not significantly reduce exacerbation rates compared with open label tiotropium.[64]

Inhaled corticosteroid-LABA combinations

The largest clinical trial to date of inhaled corticosteroid-LABA combination therapy was the three year TORCH study, which randomized 6112 patients to treatment with fluticasone-salmeterol, either monocomponent, or placebo. Patients treated with fluticasone-salmeterol had an annual rate of 0.85 exacerbations per person compared with 1.13 in the placebo group (rate ratio 0.75, 0.69 to 0.81), and 0.97 in the group treated with salmeterol (0.88, 0.81 to 0.95).[12]

A meta-analysis confirmed that inhaled corticosteroid-LABA combination inhalers significantly reduce COPD exacerbations when compared with placebo (0.73, 0.69 to 0.78).[78] A second meta-analysis confirmed that they also reduced exacerbations when compared with LABA alone (0.76, 0.68 to 0.84).[62]

Triple therapy (inhaled corticosteroid-LABA plus LAMA)

An RCT randomized of 449 patients to tiotropium plus placebo, tiotropium plus salmeterol, or tiotropium plus fluticasone-salmeterol for one year. The primary endpoint was the proportion of patients who experienced a moderate or severe exacerbation over one year. Although tiotropium plus fluticasone-salmeterol did not significantly decrease exacerbations compared with tiotropium plus placebo (0.85, 0.65 to 1.11), it reduced the number of severe exacerbations that necessitated hospital admission by 47% (0.53, 0.33 to 0.86).[10]

A similar RCT that evaluated triple therapy with tiotropium plus placebo or tiotropium plus budesonide-formoterol found a 62% reduction in exacerbations (0.38, 0.25 to 0.57) and a 65% reduction in hospital admissions or emergency department visits (0.35, 0.16 to 0.78).[63] However, the study was limited by a short duration of three months, and the relatively high rate of exacerbations in the group randomized to tiotropium plus placebo may reflect the effect of inhaled steroid withdrawal.

Potential increased risk of pneumonia associated with inhaled corticosteroid containing therapies

Although inhaled corticosteroids are not indicated as monotherapy for COPD, products that contain them (corticosteroid-LABA combinations and "triple therapy" combinations) are widely used to treat chronic COPD and prevent exacerbations. Recent clinical trials, including the TORCH study, suggested that pneumonia (a listed adverse effect) was more prevalent in patients who used fluticasone or fluticasone-salmeterol combination products.[12] However, because none of the clinical trials was designed to assess the risk of pneumonia, radiographic confirmation of pneumonia was not usually obtained, and the extent to which pneumonia events may have been confused with COPD exacerbations was unclear. Increased pneumonia events were not associated with increased mortality in patients treated with inhaled corticosteroids in these clinical trials.

Recent analysis of the new inhaled corticosteroid-LABA product fluticasone furoate-vilanterol suggests an increased risk of pneumonia. These clinical trials required pneumonia to be confirmed as an adverse event on chest radiography. In an integrated analysis of two replicate one year studies in patients with COPD the number of pneumonia events per 1000 patient years was 42.3 in the vilanterol-treated group and 97.9 in the fluticasone furoate-vilanterol treated group. This suggests that treatment with fluticasone furoate in patients with COPD more than doubled the relative risk of pneumonia.[79 80] The exposure adjusted cases of fatal pneumonia were 0 in the patients treated with vilanterol but 8.8 per 1000 patient years in those treated with fluticasone furoate-vilanterol.

The risk of pneumonia may not be a class effect and may be higher with certain inhaled corticosteroid products than others. A recently published administrative database study of 163 000 patients with COPD from Quebec identified more than 20 000 serious pneumonia events during 5.4 years of follow-up. Use of inhaled corticosteroid was associated with a 69% increase in the rate of serious pneumonia (relative risk 1.69, 1.63 to 1.75). The increased risk declined gradually after inhaled corticosteroid was stopped and disappeared after six months (1.08, 0.99 to 1.17). The risk of pneumonia seemed to be higher with fluticasone (2.01, 1.93 to 2.10) than with budesonide (1.17, 1.09 to 1.26).[81]

Similarly, a meta-analysis of seven large clinical trials in which 3801 patients were on inhaled budesonide and 3241 were on control treatment found no significant difference between treatment groups in the occurrence of pneumonia as an adverse event or a serious adverse event (adjusted hazard ratio 1.05, 0.81 to 1.37).[82]

Risk factors for pneumonia in patients with COPD receiving fluticasone furoate-vilanterol include current smoking, a history of pneumonia, a body mass index less than 25, and FEV1 less than 50% of predicted. It therefore seems reasonable to consider using a budesonide containing inhaled corticosteroid-LABA combination in patients with risk factors that might predispose them to pneumonia. It is also advisable to keep doses of inhaled corticosteroid to the lowest effective dose in patients with COPD and to be vigilant in searching for pneumonia in these patients because symptoms of pneumonia can often overlap with those of an acute exacerbation.[83]

Phosphodiesterase enzyme inhibitors

Clinical trials have shown that the selective phosphodiesterase 4 inhibitor roflumilast reduces COPD exacerbations in a subpopulation of patients with symptoms of chronic bronchitis (chronic cough and sputum production) who have had at least one exacerbation within the past year. In this subgroup, two clinical trials of more than 3000 patients have shown that roflumilast reduces exacerbations by 17% compared with placebo (rate ratio 0.83, 0.75 to 0.92).[65] These effects have not been studied when the drug is added to inhaled corticosteroid-LABA combination therapy or triple therapy. The drug's gastrointestinal side effects, such as nausea, diarrhea, and weight loss, may also limit its effectiveness in some patients.

Antibiotics

Moxifloxacin is a respiratory fluoroquinolone with activity against bacteria that are associated with COPD exacerbations. One RCT randomized stable patients with COPD to oral moxifloxacin 400 mg (n=573) or placebo (n=584) once a day for five days. Treatment was repeated every eight weeks for a total of six courses. At 48 weeks, the odds ratio of having an exacerbation was not significantly lower in the moxifloxacin group in the intent to treat analysis (0.81, 0.645 to 1.008; P=0.059),[65] although it was significantly lower in the per protocol analysis (0.75, 0.565 to 0.994). Guidelines do not currently recommend pulsed antibiotic therapy to prevent exacerbations.[84]

Macrolide antibiotics have pleiotropic immunomodulatory and anti-inflammatory properties in addition to their antibiotic effects. A one year RCT of 1142 patients randomized them to 250 mg of azithromycin once daily or placebo, in addition to their usual drugs for COPD. After one year, the rates of exacerbation were 1.48 per patient year in the azithromycin group and 1.83 per patient year in the placebo group, suggesting a 17% reduction in exacerbations with daily azithromycin (rate ratio 0.83, 0.72 to 0.95).[67] Smaller studies have also shown similar reductions with azithromycin, and a recent meta-analysis of six trials found a 37% relative risk reduction (0.63, 0.45 to 0.87) in COPD exacerbations in patients taking macrolides versus placebo.[68]

Controversies related to azithromycin

Azithromycin is a potent inducer of antimicrobial resistance. In the above RCT, the incidence of macrolide resistance, as measured in nasopharyngeal flora, was significantly higher in those treated with azithromycin versus placebo (81% *v* 41%).[67] The impact of the widespread use of macrolides to prevent COPD exacerbations on bacterial flora in the wider community is hard to quantify, and there is concern that widespread outpatient use of azithromycin may induce macrolide resistance in communities.[68]

Azithromycin has very occasionally been associated with prolongation of the Q-T interval and ventricular arrhythmias.[85] A study from a Tennessee Medicaid cohort found that relative to amoxicillin, azithromycin was associated with an increased risk of death from cardiovascular disease (hazard ratio 2.49, 1.38 to 4.50; P=0.002) and death from any cause (2.02, 1.24 to 3.30; P=0.005), with an estimated 47 additional deaths from cardiovascular disease per one million courses.[86] However, a study of Danish adults aged 18-64 years found no increased risk of death with azithromycin use relative to other antibiotics. Compared with penicillin V potassium, current azithromycin use was not associated with an increased risk of cardiovascular death (rate ratio 0.93, 0.56 to 1.55).[87]

Given the uncertainties related to antibiotic resistance and potential cardiac toxicity, the most recent 2013 GOLD guidelines do not recommend once daily azithromycin to prevent COPD exacerbations.[4] Most physicians reserve azithromycin for patients with relatively severe COPD and a history of frequent exacerbations. Patients with a history of cardiac disease, specifically long Q-T syndrome or ventricular arrhythmias, should probably not receive chronic therapy with azithromycin.

Statins

A recent nested case-control study from Taiwan suggested that statin use may be associated with a reduction in COPD exacerbations.[88] A multicenter RCT of simvastatin 40 mg once daily was recently completed in the US and Canada. The primary aim of this study was to investigate whether simvastatin prevented COPD exacerbations. The study recruited 885 patients and followed them for a mean of 640 days. Exacerbation rates in the simvastatin and placebo groups were similar (1.36 (standard deviation 1.61) per year *v* 1.39 (1.73) per year; P=0.539). Median days to first exacerbation were similar (223 *v* 231 days; P=0.342). These results suggest that simvastatin 40 mg daily does not affect exacerbation rates or time to first exacerbation in patients with COPD.[69]

Mucolytics

Data on the use of mucolytics, such as N-acetylcysteine, to prevent COPD exacerbations are contradictory. A large European clinical trial enrolled 523 patients with COPD and randomly assigned them to 600 mg daily N-acetylcysteine or placebo. Patients were followed for three years. The number of exacerbations each year did not differ between groups (1.25 (standard deviation 1.35) *v* 1.29 (1.46); hazard ratio 0.99, 0.89 to 1.10; P=0.85).[77]

After publication of this study, a smaller trial from Hong Kong randomized 120 patients with COPD to one year of treatment with N-acetylcysteine 600 mg twice daily or placebo. At one year the frequency of exacerbations was reduced in the N-acetylcysteine group versus the placebo group (0.96 *v* 1.71 exacerbations per year; P=0.019).[71]

Finally, a third larger RCT randomized 1006 Chinese patients with moderate to severe COPD to treatment with N-acetylcysteine 600 mg twice daily or placebo for one year. After one year, there were 497 acute exacerbations in 482 patients in the N-acetylcysteine group (1.16 exacerbations per patient year) and 641 acute exacerbations in 482 patients in the placebo group (1.49 exacerbations per patient year; risk ratio 0.78, 0.67 to 0.90; P=0.0011).[72]

The therapeutic effects of N-acetylcysteine may be dose dependent, so that although 600 mg once daily was ineffective in the European study, 1200 mg daily was effective in the two later Chinese studies. However, in the last two trials all patients were ethnic Chinese, so a population effect (linked to genetic, environmental, or dietary factors) that explains the effectiveness of N-acetylcysteine in these patients cannot be excluded.[89]

In addition, only 10% of the patients in these last two trials used LAMAs and a relatively high proportion (27%) used oral theophylline, which may render the results of the study less applicable to North American and European patients, in whom LAMA use is common and theophylline use is relatively rare. Finally, the larger Chinese study has been criticized because exacerbations were assessed symptomatically by diary cards and were mostly unreported and mild in severity.

Vitamin D

An RCT of 182 patients with moderate to severe COPD and a history of exacerbations explored whether high dose vitamin D, given once monthly over 12 months, could reduce the incidence of exacerbations. The median time to first exacerbation did not differ significantly between vitamin D treated and placebo groups (hazard ratio 1.1,

0.82 to 1.56; P=0.41), and neither did exacerbation rates or hospital admissions.[73]

Disease self management for prevention of exacerbations

Several RCTs have evaluated disease self management strategies and the effects of these strategies on rates of exacerbation, emergency department visits, hospital admissions, and death. A systematic review has shown that action plans, in the absence of disease education and self management, do not reduce the use of urgent healthcare for exacerbations.[90] The provision of such action plans is therefore not recommended in the absence of a disease self management strategy.

Several large RCTs have studied the provision of education on disease self management in addition to treatment action plans. An RCT of 181 patients found that a comprehensive COPD teaching and self management program, in addition to an exacerbation action plan, decreased hospital admissions and emergency department visits for exacerbation by 40% over the one year trial period, relative to usual care.[91] A second RCT randomized 741 patients with COPD to a 90 minute education session, an exacerbation action plan, and monthly phone calls or usual care. Results were similar, showing a 41% reduction (22% to 56%) in emergency visits and hospital admissions in patients randomized to the intervention arm.[92]

However, this subject is controversial. A recent RCT of 426 patients from COPD clinics associated with Veterans' Affairs hospitals compared an educational program, written action plans, and access to a case manager by phone with usual care. The study was terminated early by the study Data Safety Monitoring Board because of excess mortality in the group randomized to disease self management. Patients randomized to disease self management and action plans were three times more likely to die during the one year study period than those randomized to usual care (hazard ratio 3.00, 1.46 to 6.17).[93] The cause of this excess mortality is unclear. Given this result, the safety of disease self management and exacerbation action plans needs further assessment before this strategy can be recommended for all patients.

Looking ahead: new drugs under development

Treatment of exacerbations

A novel p38 mitogen activated protein kinase (MAPK) inhibitor, currently named BCT197, is being developed as an oral anti-inflammatory agent by Novartis for management of acute exacerbations. A phase II trial evaluating this agent against prednisone in patients with exacerbations has been completed, but results have not yet been released.[94] Bedoradrine is a highly selective β adrenergic agent for management of exacerbations. In a phase II study in patients with an exacerbation, this agent was given by slow intravenous injection and resulted in prolonged bronchodilatation without an increase in adrenergic adverse events.[95]

Prevention of exacerbations

Several drug companies are developing triple combinations of an inhaled corticosteroid, LABA, and LAMA. GlaxoSmithKline is developing a fluticasone-vilaneterol-umeclidinium product that will be administered in a single inhaler, which is likely to undergo clinical trials to determine whether it is effective at preventing exacerbations of COPD.

The effect of roflumilast plus an inhaled corticosteroid-LABA fixed dose combination on exacerbations is being investigated in a one year randomized double blind placebo controlled phase III-IV study.[96]

Phosphodiesterase 3 is an important mediator of airway smooth muscle relaxation, as confirmed by the observation that phosphodiesterase 3 inhibitors cause bronchodilatation in people with asthma.[97] Combined phosphodiesterase 3 and 4 inhibitors, such as RPL554, could therefore relax airway smooth muscle and suppress inflammation. These drugs are currently being investigated for the treatment of COPD symptoms and for the prevention of exacerbations,[98] and may also be investigated as acute treatment of exacerbation.

Other compounds in early phase development include monoclonal antibodies directed at the interleukin 1 receptor. Medimmune-8986 is a human monoclonal antibody that inhibits the binding and activation of interleukin 1a and interleukin 1b. These cytokines are thought to be involved in the pathogenesis of exacerbation, and a trial of patients with moderate to severe COPD and a history of frequent exacerbations is due to begin shortly.[95]

MAPK inhibitors are potentially attractive agents that can inhibit inflammatory responses to cigarette smoke and respiratory viruses. Phase II studies of inhaled MAPK inhibitors, such as the Janssen product JNJ-49095397, are currently assessing short term improvements in airflow limitation and symptoms as well as longer term effects on the incidence of COPD exacerbations.[99]

Conclusion

Patients with COPD are prone to acute respiratory exacerbations, which can develop suddenly and explosively or subacutely over several days. Exacerbations become more frequent and severe as airflow obstruction related to COPD increases, although a distinct subgroup of patients seems to be susceptible to frequent exacerbations irrespective of disease severity. The median duration of recovery from exacerbations is seven to 10 days for peak flow and 11-13 days for other symptoms. Unfortunately, 24-27% of patients do not respond adequately to initial treatment for exacerbations. These patients experience either a relapse or a second exacerbation that requires additional urgent treatment within 30 days. Clinical trials exploring alternative anti-inflammatory treatments instead of corticosteroids, intensive chest physiotherapy, and early inpatient pulmonary rehabilitation for treatment of exacerbations have all failed to show obvious benefits. Treatment for exacerbations has not evolved over many years and still revolves around short acting bronchodilators, oxygen, corticosteroids, and antibiotics.

Considerable recent research has focused on preventing exacerbations in susceptible patients. Chronic treatments that have been shown to prevent and reduce rates of exacerbation include LABAs, LAMAs, and inhaled corticosteroid-LABA combinations. Triple therapy with a combination of these products may provide additional benefits. Roflumilast reduces exacerbations in patients with a chronic bronchitis phenotype, and azithromycin, when added to usual drugs for COPD, significantly reduces the risk of an exacerbation. Potential side effects of roflumilast and azithromycin may limit their effectiveness in the general COPD population. Many new potential bronchodilators and anti-inflammatory drugs are being studied in ongoing

FUTURE RESEARCH QUESTIONS

- Exacerbations of chronic obstructive pulmonary disease (COPD) are currently diagnosed on the basis of clinical criteria alone. Could a sensitive and specific blood or sputum derived diagnostic biomarker be developed?
- Do all patients with COPD exacerbations benefit from prednisone? Can a more selective anti-inflammatory treatment be developed?
- Will new anti-inflammatory drugs—such as phosphodiesterase 3 inhibitors, mitogen activated protein kinase inhibitors, statins, and triple therapy combination inhalers—be more effective than current drugs in preventing exacerbations in those at risk?

clinical trials to try to generate alternatives to treat and prevent exacerbations in susceptible patients.

Contributors: SDA was the sole author and is guarantor.

Competing interests: I have read and understood BMJ policy on declaration of interests and declare the following interests: I have served on advisory boards for Boerhinger-Ingelheim, Astra-Zeneca, and Novartis and have been paid about $10000 (£6000; €7530) for these activities in the past 24 months.

Provenance and peer review: Commissioned; externally peer reviewed.

1 Anthonisen NR, Manfreda J, Warren CPW, Hershfield ES, Harding GKM, Nelson NA. Antibiotic therapy in exacerbations of chronic obstructive pulmonary disease. *Ann Intern Med* 1987;106:196-204.
2 Aaron SD, Vandemheen K, Clinch J, Ahuja J, Brison R, Dickinson G, et al. Measurement of short-term changes in dyspnea and disease-specific quality of life following an acute COPD exacerbation. *Chest* 2002;121:688-96.
3 Seemungal TA, Donaldson GC, Paul EA, Bestall JC, Jeffries DJ, Wedzicha JA. Effect of exacerbation on quality of life in patients with chronic obstructive pulmonary disease. *Am J Respir Crit Care Med* 1998;157:1418-22.
4 Global Initiative for Chronic Obstructive Lung Disease (GOLD). Global strategy for the diagnosis, management and prevention of COPD. 2014. www.goldcopd.org/guidelines-global-strategy-for-diagnosis-management.html.
5 Rodriguez-Roisin R. Toward a consensus definition of COPD exacerbations. *Chest* 2000;117:398S-401S.
6 Mackay AJ, Donaldson GC, Patel ARC, Jones PW, Hurst JR, Wedzicha JA. Usefulness of the chronic obstructive pulmonary disease assessment test to evaluate severity of COPD exacerbations. *Am J Respir Crit Care Med* 2012;185:1218-24.
7 Leidy N, Murray L. Patient-reported outcome (PRO) measures for clinical trials of COPD: the EXACT and E-RS. *COPD* 2013;10:393-8.
8 Langsetmo L, Platt RW, Ernst P, Bourbeau J. Underreporting exacerbation of chronic obstructive pulmonary disease in a longitudinal cohort. *Am J Respir Crit Care Med* 2008;177:396-401.
9 Xu W, Collet JP, Shapiro S, Lin Y, Yang T, Wang C, et al. Negative impacts of unreported COPD exacerbations on health-related quality of life at one year. *Eur Respir J* 2010;35:1022-30.
10 Aaron SD, Vandemheen K, Fergusson D, Maltais F, Bourbeau J, Balter M, et al. Tiotropium in combination with placebo, salmeterol, or fluticasone/salmeterol for treatment of chronic obstructive pulmonary disease: a randomized trial. *Ann Intern Med* 2007;146:545-55.
11 Aaron SD, Fergusson D, Marks GB, Suissa S, Vandemheen KL, Doucette S, et al. Counting, analysing and reporting exacerbations of COPD in randomised controlled trials. *Thorax* 2008;63:122-8.
12 Calverley PM, Anderson JA, Celli B, Ferguson GT, Jenkins C, Jones PW, et al. Salmeterol and fluticasone propionate and survival in chronic obstuctive pulmonary disease. *N Engl J Med* 2007;356:775-89.
13 Wise RA, Anzueto A, Cotton D, Dahl R, Devins T, Disse B, et al. Tiotropium Respimat inhaler and the risk of death in COPD. *N Engl J Med* 2013;369:1491-501.
14 Tashkin D, Celli B, Senn S, Burkhart D, Kesten S, Menjoge SS, et al. A 4-year trial of tiotropium in chronic obstructive pulmonary disease. *N Engl J Med* 2008;359:1543-54.
15 Vogelmeier C, Hederer B, Glaab T, Schmidt H, Rutten-van Molken MPMH, Beeh KM, et al. Tiotropium versus salmeterol for the prevention of exacerbations of COPD. *N Engl J Med* 2011;364:1093-103.
16 Wedzicha JA, Calverley PM, Seemungal TA, Hagan G, Ansari Z, Stockley RA, et al. The prevention of chronic obstructive pulmonary disease exacerbations by salmeterol/fluticasone propionate or tiotropium bromide. *Am J Respir Crit Care Med* 2008;177:19-26.
17 Donaldson GC, Seemungal TAR, Patel IS, Bhowmik A, Wilkinson TMA, Hurst JR, et al. Airway and systemic inflammation and decline in lung function in patients with COPD. *Chest* 2005;128:1995-2004.
18 Aaron SD, Angel JB, Lunau M, Wright K, Fex C, Le Saux N, et al. Granulocyte inflammatory markers and airway infection during acute exacerbation of chronic obstructive pulmonary disease. *Am J Respir Crit Care Med* 2001;163:349-355.
19 Bafadhel M, McKenna S, Terry P, Mistry V, Reid C, Haldar P. Acute exacerbations of chronic obstructive pulmonary disease: identification of biologic clusters and their biomarkers. *Am J Respir Crit Care Med* 2012;184:662-71.
20 Llor C, Moragas A, Hernández S, Bayona C, Miravitlles M. Efficacy of antibiotic therapy for acute exacerbations of mild to moderate chronic obstructive pulmonary disease. *Am J Respir Crit Care Med* 2012;186:716-23.
21 O'Donnell DE, Parker CM. COPD exacerbations. 3: Pathophysiology. *Thorax* 2006;61:354-61.
22 Parker C, Voduc N, Aaron SD, Webb KA, O'Donnell DE. Physiological changes during symptom recovery from moderate exacerbations of COPD. *Eur Respir J* 2005;26:420-8.
23 Sethi S, Evans N, Brydon JB, Murphy TF. New strains of bacteria and exacerbations of chronic obstructive pulmonary disease. *N Engl J Med* 2002;347:465-71.
24 Sethi S, Murphy TF. Infection in the pathogenesis and course of chronic obstructive pulmonary disease. *N Engl J Med* 2008;359:2355-65.
25 Seemungal TAR, Harper-Owen R, Bhowmik A, Moric I, Sanderson G, Message S, et al. Respiratory viruses, symptoms, and inflammatory markers in acute exacerbations and stable chronic obstructive pulmonary disease. *Am J Respir Crit Care Med* 2001;164:1618-23.
26 Murphy TF, Brauer AL, Grant BJB, Sethi S. Moraxella catarrhalis in chronic obstructive pulmonary disease. *Am J Respir Crit Care Med* 2005;172:195-9.
27 Wilkinson TMA, Hurst JR, Perera WR, Wilks M, Donaldson GC, Wedzicha JA. Effect of interactions between lower airway bacterial and rhinoviral infection in exacerbations of COPD. *Chest J* 2006;129:317-24.
28 Molyneaux PL, Mallia P, Cox MJ, Footitt J, Willis-Owen SAG, Homola D, et al. Outgrowth of the bacterial airway microbiome after rhinovirus exacerbation of chronic obstructive pulmonary disease. *Am J Respir Crit Care Med* 2013;188:1224-31.
29 Papi A, Bellettato CM, Braccioni F, Romagnoli M, Casolari P, Caramori G, et al. Infections and airway inflammation in chronic obstructive pulmonary disease severe exacerbations. *Am J Respir Crit Care Med* 2006;173:1114-21.
30 Celli BR, Barnes PJ. Exacerbations of chronic obstructive pulmonary disease. *Eur Respir J* 2007;29:1224-38.
31 Aaron SD, Donaldson GC, Whitmore GA, Hurst JR, Ramsay T, Wedzicha JA. Time course and pattern of COPD exacerbation onset. *Thorax* 2012;67:238-43.
32 Seemungal TA, Donaldson GC, Bhowmik A, Jeffries DJ, Wedzicha JA. Time course and recovery of exacerbations in patients with chronic obstructive pulmonary disease. *Am J Respir Crit Care Med* 2000;161:1608-13.
33 Elixhauser A, Steiner C. Readmissions to US hospitals by diagnosis, 2010. Agency For Healthcare Research and Policy, 2013.
34 Aaron SD, Vandemheen K, Hebert P, Dales R, Stiell IG, Ahuja J, et al. Outpatient oral prednisone after emergency treatment of chronic obstructive pulmonary disease. *N Engl J Med* 2003;348:2618-25.
35 Niewoehner DE, Erbland ML, Deupree RH, Collins D, Gross NJ, Light RW, et al. Effect of systemic glucocorticoids on exacerbations of chronic obstructive pulmonary disease. *N Engl J Med* 1999;340:1941-7.
36 Leuppi JD, Schuetz P, Bingisser R. Short-term vs conventional glucocorticoid therapy in acute exacerbations of chronic obstructive pulmonary disease: the REDUCE randomized clinical trial. *JAMA* 2013;309:2223-31.
37 Prieto-Centurion V, Markos MA, Ramey NI, Gussin HA, Nyenhuis SM, Joo MJ, et al. Interventions to reduce rehospitalizations after chronic obstructive pulmonary disease exacerbations. A systematic review. *Ann Am Thorac Soc* 2014;11:417-24.
38 Soler-Cataluna JJ, Martinez-Garcia MA, Sanchez PR, Salcedo E, Navarro M, Ochando R. Severe acute exacerbations and mortality in patients with chronic obstructive pulmonary disease. *Thorax* 2005;60:925-31.
39 Seneff MG, Wagner DP, Wagner RP, Zimmerman JE, Knaus WA. Hospital and 1-year survival of patients admitted to intensive care units with acute exacerbations of chronic obstructive pulmonary disease. *JAMA* 1995;274:1852-7.
40 Piquet J, Chavaillon JM, David P, Martin F, Blanchon F, Roche N. High-risk patients following hospitalisation for an acute exacerbation of COPD. *Eur Respir J* 2013;42:946-55.
41 Jones P. Health status and the spiral of decline. *COPD* 2009;6:59-63.
42 Hurst JR, Vestbo J, Anzueto A, Locantore N, Mullerova H, Tal-Singer R, et al. Susceptibility to exacerbation in chronic obstructive pulmonary disease. *N Engl J Med* 2010;363:1128-38.
43 Decramer M, Celli B, Kesten S, Lystig T, Mehra S, Tashkin DP. Effect of tiotropium on outcomes in patients with moderate chronic obstructive pulmonary disease (UPLIFT): a prespecified subgroup analysis of a randomised controlled trial. *Lancet* 2009;374:1171-8.
44 Jenkins C, Jones P, Calverley P, Celli B, Anderson J, Ferguson G, et al. Efficacy of salmeterol/fluticasone propionate by GOLD stage of chronic obstructive pulmonary disease: analysis from the randomised, placebo-controlled TORCH study. *Respir Res* 2009;10:59.
45 Thomsen M, Ingebrigtsen T, Marott J. Inflammatory biomarkers and exacerbations in chronic obstructive pulmonary disease. *JAMA* 2013;309:2353-61.
46 O'Donnell DE, Aaron S, Bourbeau J, Hernandez P, Marciniuk DD, Balter M, et al. Canadian Thoracic Society recommendations for management of chronic obstructive pulmonary disease—2007 update. *Can Respir J* 2007;14:5B-32B.
47 Bafadhel M, McKenna S, Terry S, Mistry V, Pancholi M, Venge P, et al. Blood eosinophils to direct corticosteroid treatment of exacerbations of chronic obstructive pulmonary disease. A randomized, placebo-controlled trial. *Am J Respir Crit Care Med* 2012;186:48-55.

48 Aaron SD, Vandemheen KL, Maltais F, Field SK, Sin DD, Bourbeau J, et al. TNFalpha antagonists for acute exacerbations of COPD: a randomised double-blind controlled trial. *Thorax* 2013;68:142-8.

49 Woodhead M, Blasi F, Ewig S, Garau J, Huchon G, Ieven M, et al. Guidelines for the management of adult lower respiratory tract infections—full version. *Clin Microbiol Infect* 2011;17:E1-59.

50 Nouira S, Marghli S, Belghith M, Besbes L, Elatrous S, Abroug F. Once daily oral ofloxacin in chronic obstructive pulmonary disease exacerbation requiring mechanical ventilation: a randomised placebo-controlled trial. *Lancet* 2001;358:2020-5.

51 Daniels JMA, Snijders D, de Graaff CS, Vlaspolder F, Jansen HM, Boersma WG. Antibiotics in addition to systemic corticosteroids for acute exacerbations of chronic obstructive pulmonary disease. *Am J Respir Crit Care Med* 2010;181:150-7.

52 Ramsay M, Hart N. Current opinions on non-invasive ventilation as a treatment for chronic obstructive pulmonary disease. *Curr Opin Pulm Med* 2013;19:626-30.

53 Chandra D, Stamm JA, Taylor B, Ramos RM, Satterwhite L, Krishnan JA, et al. Outcomes of noninvasive ventilation for acute exacerbations of chronic obstructive pulmonary disease in the United States, 1998-2008. *Am J Respir Crit Care Med* 2012;185:152-9.

54 Woodruff PG, Albert RK, Bailey WC, Casaburi R, Connett JE, Cooper JAD, et al. Randomized trial of zileuton for treatment of COPD exacerbations requiring hospitalization. *COPD* 2011;8:21-9.

55 Osadnik CR, McDonald CF, Miller BR, Hill CJ, Tarrant B, Steward R, et al. The effect of positive expiratory pressure (PEP) therapy on symptoms, quality of life and incidence of re-exacerbation in patients with acute exacerbations of chronic obstructive pulmonary disease: a multicentre, randomised controlled trial. *Thorax* 2014;69:137-43.

56 Greening NJ, Williams JE, Hussain SF, Harvey-Dunstan TC, Bankart MJ, Chaplin EJ, et al. An early rehabilitation intervention to enhance recovery during hospital admission for an exacerbation of chronic respiratory disease: randomised controlled trial. *BMJ* 2014;349:g4315.

57 Han MK, Martinez FJ. Pharmacotherapeutic approaches to preventing acute exacerbations of chronic obstructive pulmonary disease. *Proc Am Thorac Soc* 2011;8:356-62.

58 Poole PJ, Chacko E, Wood-Baker RW, Cates CJ. Influenza vaccine for patients with chronic obstructive pulmonary disease. *Cochrane Database Syst Rev* 2006;1:CD002733.

59 Walters JA, Smith S, Poole P, Granger RH, Wood-Baker R. Injectable vaccines for preventing pneumococcal infection in patients with chronic obstructive pulmonary disease. *Cochrane Database Syst Rev* 2010;11:CD001390.

60 Karner C, Chong J, Poole P. Tiotropium versus placebo for chronic obstructive pulmonary disease. *Cochrane Database Syst Rev* 2012;7:CD009285.

61 Kew K, Mavergames C, Walters J. Long-acting beta2-agonists for chronic obstructive pulmonary disease. *Cochrane Database Syst Rev* 2013;3:CD010177.

62 Nannini L, Lasserson T, Poole P. Combined corticosteroid and long-acting beta-agonist in one inhaler versus long-acting beta-agonists for chronic obstructive pulmonary disease. *Cochrane Database Syst Rev* 2012;9:CD006829.

63 Welte T, Miravitlles M, Hernandez P, Eriksson G, Peterson S, Polanowski T, et al. Efficacy and tolerability of budesonide/formoterol added to tiotropium in patients with chronic obstructive pulmonary disease. *Am J Respir Crit Care Med* 2009;180:741-50.

64 Wedzicha JA, Decramer M, Ficker JH, Niewoehner DE, Sandstrom T, Taylor AF, et al. Analysis of chronic obstructive pulmonary disease exacerbations with the dual bronchodilator QVA149 compared with glycopyrronium and tiotropium (SPARK): a randomised, double-blind, parallel-group study. *Lancet Respir Med* 2013;1:199-209.

65 Fabbri LM, Calverley PM, Izquierdo-Alonso JL, Bundschuh DS, Brose M, Martinez FJ, et al. Roflumilast in moderate-to-severe chronic obstructive pulmonary disease treated with longacting bronchodilators: two randomised clinical trials. *Lancet* 2009;374:695-703.

66 Sethi S, Jones P, Theron M, Miravitlles M, Rubinstein E, Wedzicha J, et al. Pulsed moxifloxacin for the prevention of exacerbations of chronic obstructive pulmonary disease: a randomized controlled trial. *Respir Res* 2010;11:10.

67 Albert RK, Connett J, Bailey WC, Casaburi R, Cooper JA, Criner GJ, et al. Azithromycin for prevention of exacerbations of COPD. *N Engl J Med* 2011;365:689-98.

68 Donath E, Chaudhry A, Hernandez-Aya LF, Lit L. A meta-analysis on the prophylactic use of macrolide antibiotics for the prevention of disease exacerbations in patients with chronic obstructive pulmonary disease. *Respir Med* 2013;107:1385-92.

69 Criner GJ, Connet JE, Aaron SD, Albert RK, Bailey WC. Simvastatin for the prevention of exacerbations in moderate to severe COPD. *N Engl J Med* 2014;370:2201-10.

70 Decramer M, Rutten-van Mölken M, Dekhuijzen PN, Troosters T, van Herwaarden C, Pellegrino R, et al. Effects of N-acetylcysteine on outcomes in chronic obstructive pulmonary disease (Bronchitis Randomized on NAC Cost-Utility Study, BRONCUS): a randomised placebo-controlled trial. *Lancet* 2005;365:1552-60.

71 Tse HN, Raiteri L, Wong KY, Yee KS, Ng LY, Wai KY, et al. High-dose N-acetylcysteine in stable COPD: the 1-year, double-blind, randomized, placebo-controlled hiace study. *Chest J* 2013;144:106-18.

72 Zheng JP, Wen FQ, Bai CX, Wan HY, Kang J, Chen P, et al. Twice daily N-acetylcysteine 600 mg for exacerbations of chronic obstructive pulmonary disease (PANTHEON): a randomised, double-blind placebo-controlled trial. *Lancet Respir Med* 2014;2:187-94.

73 Lehouck A, Mathieu C, Carremans C, Baeke F, Verhaegen J, Van Eldere J, et al. High doses of vitamin D to reduce exacerbations in chronic obstructive pulmonary diseasea randomized trial. *Ann Intern Med* 2012;156:105-14.

74 Niewoehner DE, Rice KL, Cote CG, Paulson D, Cooper JA, Korducki L, et al. Prevention of exacerbations of chronic obstructive pulmonary disease with tiotropium, a once-daily inhaled anticholinergic bronchodilator. A randomized trial. *Ann Intern Med* 2005;143:317-26.

75 Kerwin E, Hebert J, Gallagher N, Martin C, Overend T, Alagappan VKT, et al. Efficacy and safety of NVA237 versus placebo and tiotropium in patients with COPD: the GLOW2 study. *Eur Respir J* 2012;40:1106-14.

76 D'Urzo A, Ferguson GT, van Noord JA, Hirata K, Martin C, Horton R, et al. Efficacy and safety of once-daily NVA237 in patients with moderate-to-severe COPD: the GLOW1 trial. *Respir Res* 2011;12:156.

77 Decramer M, Chapman K, Dahl R, Frith PA, Devouassoux G, Fritscher C, et al. Once-daily indacaterol versus tiotropium for patients with severe chronic obstructive pulmonary disease (INVIGORATE): a randomised, blinded, parallel-group study. *Lancet Respir Med* 2013;1:524-33.

78 Nannini L, Poole P, Milan S, Holmes R, Normansell R. Combined corticosteroid and long-acting beta-agonist in one inhaler versus placebo for chronic obstructive pulmonary disease. *Cochrane Database Syst Rev* 2013;11:CD003794.

79 Agusti A, de Teresa L, De Backer W, Zvarich MT, Locantore N, Barnes N, et al. A comparison of the efficacy and safety of once-daily fluticasone furoate/vilanterol with twice-daily fluticasone propionate/salmeterol in moderate to very severe COPD. *Eur Respir J* 2014;43:763-72.

80 Woodcock A, Bleecker ER, Lötvall J, O'Byrne PM, Bateman ED, Medley H, et al. Efficacy and safety of fluticasone furoate/vilanterol compared with fluticasone propionate/salmeterol combination in adult and adolescent patients with persistent asthma: a randomized trial. *Chest J* 2013;144:1222-9.

81 Suissa S, Patenaude VR, Lapi F, Ernst P. Inhaled corticosteroids in COPD and the risk of serious pneumonia. *Thorax* 2013;68:1029-36.

82 Sin DD, Tashkin D, Zhang X, Radner F, Sjöbring U, Thorén A, et al. Budesonide and the risk of pneumonia: a meta-analysis of individual patient data. *Lancet* 1929;374:712-9.

83 Marzoratti LA, Iannella HA, Waterer GW. Inhaled corticosteroids and the increased risk of pneumonia. *Ther Adv Respir Dis* 2013;7:225-34.

84 Wilson R, Sethi S, Anzueto A, Miravitlles M. Antibiotics for treatment and prevention of exacerbations of chronic obstructive pulmonary disease. *J Infect* 2013;67:497-515.

85 Mosholder AD, Mathew J, Alexander JJ, Smith H, Nambiar S. Cardiovascular risks with azithromycin and other antibacterial drugs. *N Engl J Med* 2013;368:1665-8.

86 Ray WA, Murray KT, Hall K, Arbogast PG, Stein CM. Azithromycin and the risk of cardiovascular death. *N Engl J Med* 2012;366:1881-90.

87 Svanstrom H, Pasternak B, Hviid A. Use of azithromycin and death from cardiovascular causes. *N Engl J Med* 2013;368:1704-12.

88 Wang MT, Lo YW, Tsai CL, Chang LC, Malone DC, Chu CL, et al. Statin use and risk of COPD exacerbation requiring hospitalization. *Am J Med* 2013;126:598-606.

89 Cazzola M, Matera MG. N-acetylcysteine may be beneficial, but for whom? *Lancet Respir Med* 2014;2:166-7.

90 Walters JA, Turnock AC, Walters EH, Wood-Baker R. Action plans with limited patient education only for exacerbations chronic obstructive pulmonary disease. *Cochrane Database Syst Rev* 2010;5:CD005074.

91 Bourbeau J, Julien M, Maltais F, Rouleau M, Beaupre A, Begin R, et al. Reduction of hospital utilization in patients with chronic obstructive pulmonary disease: a disease-specific self-management intervention [see comment]. *Arch Intern Med* 2003;163:585-91.

92 Rice KL, Dewan N, Bloomfield HE, Grill J, Schult TM, Nelson DB, et al. Disease management program for chronic obstructive pulmonary disease. *Am J Respir Crit Care Med* 2010;182:890-6.

93 Fan VGJ, Lew R, Bourbeau J, Adams S, Adams SG, Leatherman S, et al. A comprehensive care management program to prevent chronic obstructive pulmonary disease hospitalizations. *Ann Intern Med* 2012;156:673-83.

94 Compton C, McBryan D, Bucchioni E, Patalano F. The Novartis view on emerging drugs and novel targets for the treatment of chronic obstructive pulmonary disease. *Pulm Pharmacol Therapeut* 2013;26:562-73.

95 Gross NJ. The COPD pipeline XXIV. *COPD* 2013;10:625-7.

96 Calverley P, Martinez F, Fabbri L, Goehring UM, Rabe KF. Does roflumilast decrease exacerbations in severe COPD patients not controlled by inhaled combination therapy? The REACT study protocol. *Int J COPD* 2012;7:375-82.

97 Myou S, Fujimura M, Kamio Y, Ishiura Y, Tachibana H, Hirose T, et al. Bronchodilator effect of inhaled olprinone, a phosphodiesterase 3 inhibitor, in asthmatic patients. *Am J Respir Crit Care Med* 1999;160:817-20.

98 Franciosi LG, Diamant Z, Banner KH, Zuiker R, Morelli N, Kamerling IMC, et al. Efficacy and safety of RPL554, a dual PDE3 and PDE4 inhibitor, in healthy volunteers and in patients with asthma or chronic obstructive pulmonary disease: findings from four clinical trials. *Lancet Respir Med* 2013;1:714-27.

99 Mercer B, D'Armiento J. Emerging role of MAP kinase pathways as therapeutic targets in COPD. *Int J Chron Obstruct Pulm Dis* 2006;1:137-50.

How to investigate a patient with suspected interstitial lung disease

Owen J Dempsey, consultant chest physician[1], Keith M Kerr, professor of pulmonary pathology[2], Hardy Remmen, consultant cardiothoracic surgeon[3], Alan R Denison, clinical senior lecturer and honorary consultant thoracic radiologist[4]

[1]Department of Respiratory Medicine, Aberdeen Royal Infirmary, Foresterhill, Aberdeen AB25 2ZN

[2]Aberdeen University Medical School, Foresterhill, Aberdeen AB25 2ZD

[3]Department of Cardiothoracic Surgery, Aberdeen Royal Infirmary

[4]Aberdeen Biomedical Imaging Centre, Aberdeen Royal Infirmary

Correspondence to: O J Dempsey owen.dempsey@nhs.net

Cite this as: *BMJ* 2010;340:c2843

<DOI> 10.1136/bmj.c2843 http://www.bmj.com/content/340/bmj.c2843

Patients with interstitial lung disease often present with breathlessness, chronic cough, inspiratory crackles on auscultation, and abnormal spirometry.[1 2] Over 200 different types of disease can cause thickening of the pulmonary interstitium, with the common final pathway for many of these being fibrosis (figs 1 and 2) .[3 4] Some forms of interstitial lung disease can be life threatening, such as idiopathic pulmonary fibrosis, approximately 4000 new cases of which are diagnosed in England and Wales each year. Survival rates of 57% at three years and 43% at five years are worse outcomes than those for some cancers.[5] About 3000 new cases of sarcoidosis are diagnosed each year in the UK.[5 6]

Early recognition and treatment of interstitial lung diseases may prevent progression to irreversible pulmonary fibrosis and respiratory failure. This review provides a guide to the initial investigation of patients with suspected interstitial lung disease and provides a summary of further investigations.

Sources and selection criteria

We sought papers that were fully published between 1966 and April 2010 using appropriate index terms (interstitial lung disease, diffuse parenchymal lung disease) the National Library of Medicine's computerised search service (providing access to Medline, PreMedline and other related databases). We also consulted Cochrane database systematic reviews and a personal archive of references.

What are the most common interstitial lung diseases and how are they classified?

Some forms of interstitial lung disease are idiopathic, whereas others are associated with connective tissue diseases, commonly prescribed drugs, smoking, and exposures to environmental factors such as dusts.[7] The histopathological classification of interstitial lung diseases is complex, simplified in figure 3.[3] The key clinical point is to try and identify a known cause if at all possible. The most commonly encountered conditions are:

- Sarcoidosis[6 8]
- Idiopathic pulmonary fibrosis[9] and other less common forms of "idiopathic" interstitial lung diseases[3 4] (fig 4)
- Connective tissue disease associated pulmonary fibrosis—for example, rheumatoid or scleroderma lung[10]
- Hypersensitivity pneumonitis, also known as extrinsic allergic alveolitis (fig 5).[11]

What questions are important to ask when taking a history?

Medication history

Box 1 lists medications that may be associated with adverse effects in the lung. Prescribed and "over the counter" medications, herbal therapies, and illicit drugs have been associated with interstitial lung diseases; www.pneumotox.com provides information about drug induced lung disease.[12 13] Drug induced interstitial lung disease is straightforward to recognise if it develops within days of prescription, but presentation may be subacute (over months) or chronic (years) even with the same drug (for example, nitrofurantoin).[14 15] Similarly, various pathological patterns of interstitial lung disease can occur for the same drug (for example, methotrexate) ranging from a relatively benign interstitial pneumonitis through to life threatening diffuse alveolar damage. If recognised early enough, most forms of drug induced interstitial lung disease are reversible[12 13]

History of a connective tissue disease

Any of the connective tissue diseases may be complicated by interstitial lung disease.[10 16 17] Occasionally patients present with pulmonary symptoms before rheumatological manifestations become obvious. Clinical clues to the possibility of an underlying connective tissue disease are shown in figure 6.

Environmental exposures

Hobbies, occupation, travel, and other possible environmental exposures should be taken into account. Taking a detailed current and previous occupational history can be time consuming;[18] a practical solution is to ask patients in

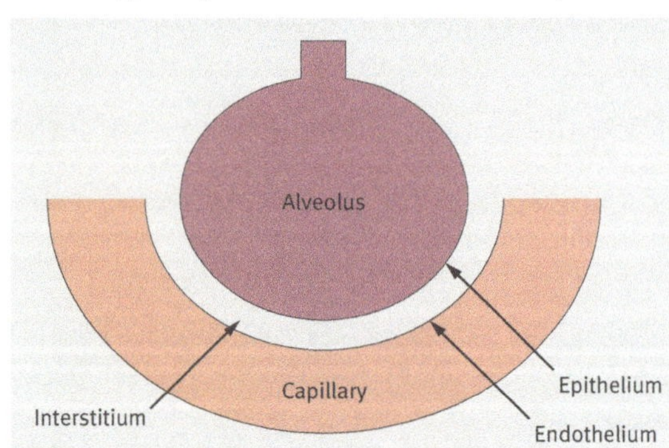

Fig 1 The pulmonary interstitium is the microscopic space between the alveolar epithelium and capillary endothelium and is crucial for gas exchange

SUMMARY POINTS

- Persistent crackles on chest auscultation may be due to interstitial lung disease and should prompt a detailed history and some first line tests including a chest radiograph
- Some commonly prescribed drugs, environmental dusts, smoking, and underlying connective tissue diseases can cause interstitial lung disease
- Detailed pulmonary function tests and high resolution computed tomography are usually done in specialist care and some patients may need a lung biopsy
- Refer to a chest physician with an interest in interstitial lung diseases for diagnosis and management by a multi-disciplinary team, and possible participation in a clinical trial.

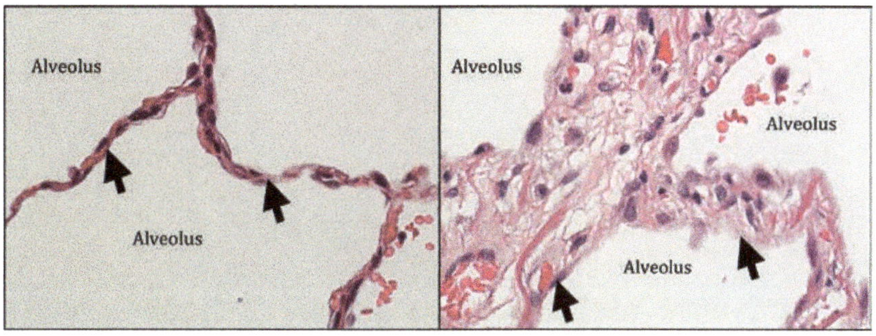

Fig 2 Arrows indicate pulmonary interstitium in (left) healthy lung and (right) pulmonary fibrosis. The grossly thickened interstitium in pulmonary fibrosis impairs gas exchange.

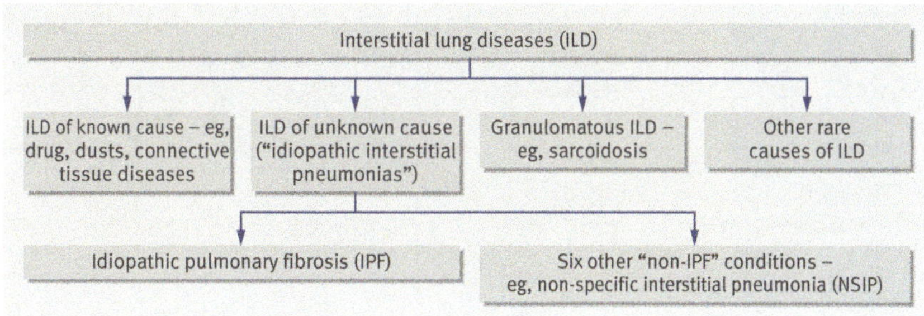

Fig 3 Current classification of interstitial lung disease.[3] Idiopathic interstitial pneumonias refers to a group of seven related interstitial lung diseases, the most common of which is idiopathic pulmonary fibrosis (formerly known as cryptogenic fibrosing alveolitis), which has a particularly poor prognosis

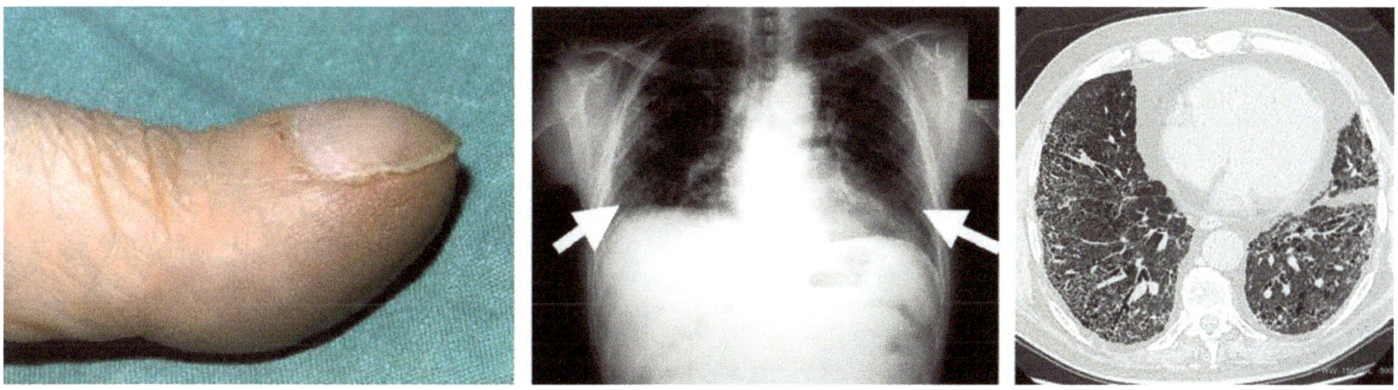

Fig 4 Idiopathic pulmonary fibrosis. (A) Digital clubbing is commonly, but not always, seen. (B) Chest radiograph noting small lungs with bilateral subpleural shadowing with a lower zone predominance (arrows). (C) Computed tomography noting gross abnormalities of both lungs including intralobular and interlobular septal thickening with honeycombing

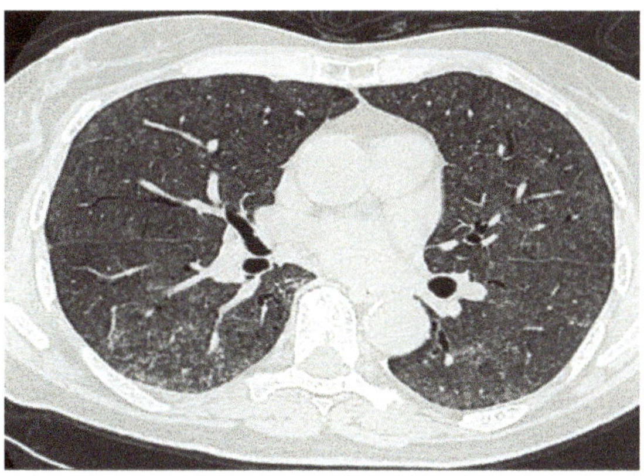

Fig 5 Hypersensitivity pneumonitis resulting from dust exposure. A typical computed tomography image is shown with diffuse centrilobular ground glass nodules.

BOX 1 EXAMPLES OF DRUGS THAT CAN CAUSE INTERSTITIAL LUNG DISEASE[12 13]

- Antibiotics—cephalosporin, minocycline, nitrofurantoin, quinine
- Rheumatology treatments—gold, leflunomide, methotrexate, NSAIDs, penicillamine, sulphasalazine, tumour necrosis factor α blockers (infliximab, etanercept)
- Cardiology treatments—amiodarone, angiotensin converting enzyme inhibitors, aspirin, atenolol, statins
- Oncology treatments—bleomycin, busulfan, chlorambucil, melphalan, methotrexate, mitomycin C, tyrosine kinase inhibitors (dasatnib, imatinib)
- Illicit drugs—cocaine, heroin, intravenous talc, methadone
- Immunomodulators—azathioprine, cyclophosphamide, epidermal growth factor receptor inhibitors (gefitinib, erlotinib), interferons, methotrexate, rapamycin derivatives (sirolimus), tumour necrosis factor α blockers, rituxumab
- Miscellaneous—high flow oxygen, inhalation or aspiration of fat-containing substances (drugs containing mineral oils, certain laxatives, petroleum jelly), paraquat, radiotherapy

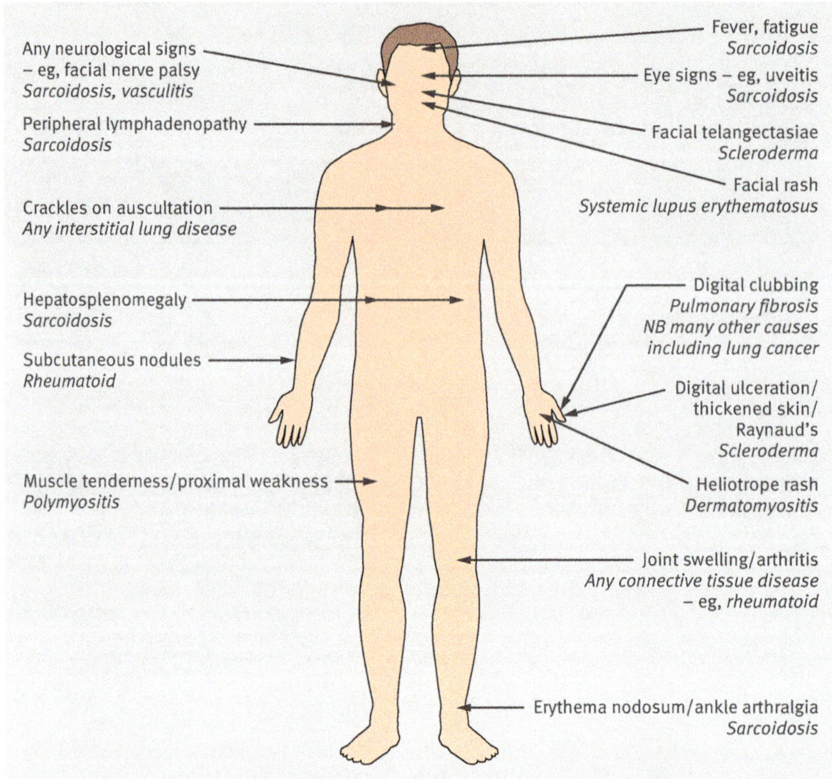

Fig 6 Possible clinical manifestations of interstitial lung disease

advance to prepare a chronological list of jobs and to bring this list to their initial assessment. Inorganic dusts linked with interstitial lung disease include asbestos,[19] coal and silica,[20] and beryllium.[21] New industries have generated new forms of interstitial lung disease, such as flockworker's lung in manufacturers of synthetic microfibres (flock) of nylon,[22] and metalworker's lung in those exposed to metalworking fluid aerosol.[23] Hypersensitivity pneumonitis can be caused by antigens in organic dusts, such as *Saccharopolyspora rectivirgula* in hay, which causes farmer's lung, and proteins in bird droppings and on feathers that cause bird or pigeon fancier's lung.[11] Case reports have associated feathers in duvets with hypersensitivity pneumonitis.[24 25] and more than 20 case reports have linked domestic mould exposure with hypersensitivity pneumonitis.[26 27]

Questions about recreational activities and travel may reveal an important exposure—for example, *Mycobacterium avium* complex causes "hot tub lung" and *Trichoderma koningii* "woodworker's lung."[28] A meta-analysis of six case-control studies conducted in the UK, United States, and Japan reported that smoking (odds ratio 1.58, 95% confidence interval 1.27 to 1.97), agriculture or farming (1.65, 1.20 to 2.26), livestock (2.17, 1.28 to 3.68), wood dust (1.94, 1.34 to 2.81), metal dust (2.44, 1.74 to 3.40), and stone or sand (1.97, 1.09 to 3.55) were associated with an increased risk of idiopathic pulmonary fibrosis.[29]

Smoking

Cigarette smoking is associated with several interstitial lung diseases.[30 31] A recent population based cohort study of 2563 adults in the United States suggested that smoking may cause subclinical parenchymal lung disease that is detectable by spirometry and computed tomography imaging.[32] Curiously, some forms of interstitial lung disease, such as hypersensitivity pneumonitis and sarcoidosis, are less common in smokers.[33 34]

Family history

Although familial clustering is well described for sarcoidosis,[35 36] familial idiopathic pulmonary fibrosis is rare, accounting for only 0.5-2.2% of all cases.[37]

Gastro-oesophageal reflux

The nature of an observed link between chronic recurrent microaspiration of gastric acid and the development of chronic lung disease is not clear.[38] The prevalence of reflux is increased in patients with idiopathic pulmonary fibrosis and scleroderma lung, although whether its development and course can be influenced by anti-reflux treatment is not known.[39 40]

What are the key features on examination?

Clinical examination does not always reveal signs of illness. However, inspiratory crackles may be heard on chest auscultation.[2] Crackles are typically best heard over the lower lobes and axillary regions in patients with idiopathic pulmonary fibrosis. In those with sarcoidosis crackles may be absent, despite radiological abnormality. Mid-inspiratory "squeaks" are suggestive of bronchiolitis. Clubbing of the fingers occurs in about half of patients with idiopathic pulmonary fibrosis and may accompany other interstitial lung diseases. If interstitial lung disease is advanced patients may be cyanosed and show signs of secondary pulmonary arterial hypertension.[41] Examples of extrapulmonary signs that may occur are shown in figure 6.

What first line investigations should be considered before referral?

Figure 7 outlines the initial assessment of patients with suspected interstitial lung disease. Full history and examination may identify known causes of such disease and will help direct subsequent investigations.

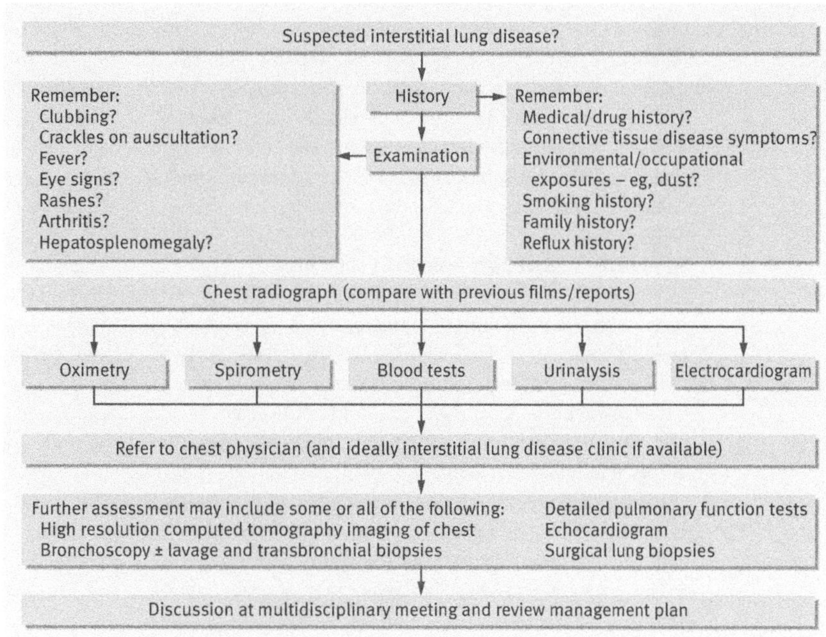

Fig 7 Initial assessment of patients with suspected interstitial lung disease

Chest radiograph

The chest radiograph can be normal in early interstitial lung disease.[42] By the time the disease is clinically apparent chest radiographs will usually be abnormal. Abnormalities include decreased lung volumes, subpleural reticular opacities, peripheral migratory air space shadowing, and mediastinal or hilar lymph node enlargement. For example, bilateral hilar lymphadenopathy with upper lobe pulmonary infiltrates in a young adult suggests sarcoidosis; basal fibrosis with pleural thickening and pleural plaques suggests asbestosis. The chest radiograph may also help to identify lung cancer, infection, or pneumothorax, which may be associated with interstitial disease. Chest radiography has limited sensitivity and lacks specificity for diagnosing subtypes of interstitial lung disease; high resolution computed tomography is more useful in diagnosis and differentiation.[1]

Oximetry

An oxygen saturation of less than 94% at rest is abnormal and should prompt referral for more detailed assessment by a chest physician.

Blood tests

A full blood count, including eosinophils, and a serum biochemistry profile (including renal and liver function tests, calcium, glucose, thyroid function, C reactive protein) are potentially useful baseline investigations in combination with clinical and radiological findings.

Urinalysis

Haematuria or proteinuria may strengthen suspicion of an underling systemic vasculitis.[43] A 24 hour urine collection may identify hypercalcuria in suspected sarcoidosis.[44 45 46]

Electrocardiogram

Since many patients who present with a cough and breathlessness may also have a history of smoking and other cardiovascular risk factors, a baseline electrocardiogram is necessary. It may show signs of right ventricular strain, prompting further investigation of suspected secondary pulmonary vascular disease. Rarely, conduction defects and arrhythmias are found in patients with cardiac sarcoidosis.[47]

What are the second line investigations?

An algorithm for further investigation is presented in figure 7. Some approaches are discussed here.

Other blood tests

An arterial blood gas is needed to confirm respiratory failure in patients with a resting oxygen saturation of less than 94%, in those who are polycythaemic and those with signs suggestive of cor pulmonale. If a connective tissue disease is suspected then an immunology screen (antinuclear antibody, extractable nuclear antigens, rheumatoid factor, and anti-neutrophil cytoplasmic antibody) will be required. If an environmental factor is suspected, specific serum IgG antibody screens can be performed for relevant antigens (such as *Saccharopolyspora rectivirgula, Thermactinomycetes vulgaris, Aspergillus* for mouldy hay).

British Thoracic Society guidelines suggest that measurement of serum angiotensin converting enzyme has a limited role in the diagnosis of suspected sarcoidosis and does not contribute to monitoring patients when added to serial lung function and imaging.[1] Furthermore, assays to detect the enzyme have limited sensitivity and specificity and values are affected by angiotensin converting enzyme gene polymorphisms.[48] Levels of angiotensin converting enzyme are raised in many other conditions including other granulomatous diseases (leprosy, tuberculosis, histoplasmosis), Gaucher's disease, and hyperthyroidism[49] Results are invalidated if a patient is taking an angiotensin converting enzyme inhibitor.

Testing for HIV infection may be helpful, since some forms of interstitial lung disease are associated with immunodeficiency, such as lymphocytic interstitial pneumonia.[50] Brain natriuretic peptide, secreted in response to ventricular stretch by cardiomyocytes, is a marker of right ventricular dysfunction. Although the test is not available in all centres, some studies in patients with interstitial lung disease suggest that elevated levels of the peptide can identify patients with pulmonary hypertension and poorer prognosis.[51 52 53 54] A wide range of serum biomarkers (lung epithelium specific proteins, cytokines, and other biological markers of cellular activity) may also theoretically reflect more severe or widespread interstitial lung disease.[55] However, as yet, no perfect biomarker has been identified, and since the tests are costly and of uncertain clinical usefulness their role is unclear.[56]

What is the role of high resolution computed tomography?

High resolution computed tomography is a specialised imaging test in which thin (<1.5 mm) axial sections of the lungs are acquired with 10 mm or 20 mm gaps between sections. No intravenous contrast is used. Image reconstruction with a high spatial frequency algorithm allows sub-millimetre structures to be visualised. A high resolution computed tomogram is a comparatively low dose test, with a radiation exposure six times less than that of a conventional thoracic computed tomogram, and equivalent to approximately 50 chest radiographs. It is accordingly a sampling examination and should be reserved for patients who have a raised clinical or radiographic suspicion of interstitial lung disease. Interpretation of high resolution computed tomography is best done by radiologists with an interest in thoracic imaging and with ready access to multidisciplinary input.[1] Typical reasons for high resolution computed tomography in interstitial lung disease are:

- To detect interstitial lung disease in patients with normal or equivocal chest radiograph findings
- To focus the differential diagnosis in patients with obvious but non-specific chest radiograph abnormalities
- To guide the type and site of lung biopsy
- To evaluate disease reversibility.

Characteristic features of idiopathic pulmonary fibrosis on high resolution computed tomography (fig 4) include bilateral and symmetrical bibasal pulmonary reticular shadowing with destroyed and fibrotic lung tissue that contains numerous cystic airspaces with thick fibrous walls (honeycombing). The reticular pattern reflects a combination of interlobular septal thickening and intralobular opacities. As the fibrosis progresses, traction bronchiectasis is often present. Ground glass opacity is often present in idiopathic pulmonary fibrosis and in the absence of adjacent fibrosis it is associated with response to treatment and longer survival.[57] Other common features include reactive mediastinal lymphadenopathy and, since many patients are smokers, coexisting emphysema. Most patients with clinical evidence of interstitial lung disease will have abnormal high resolution computed tomography features. High resolution computed tomography has better sensitivity than chest radiography for the detection of interstitial lung disease.[58] However, patients with very early disease may not have imaging abnormalities. Conversely, some patients (in particular older people and smokers) may have parenchymal changes in the absence of clinical or physiological abnormality.[59 60]

The main clinical value of high resolution computed tomography is the identification of interstitial lung disease and the most common variant, idiopathic pulmonary fibrosis. In an appropriate clinical context, the presence of classic features of idiopathic pulmonary fibrosis on high resolution computed tomography allow a confident non-invasive diagnosis without the need for lung biopsy.[61 62] However, diagnostic doubt may often remain because of the considerable overlap between findings in "non-specific interstitial pneumonia" and variants of interstitial lung disease. In a well conducted retrospective study of 92 patients with biopsy proved interstitial lung disease, blinded observers made the correct diagnosis from high resolution computed tomography images in 79% of cases and identified some features that would favour idiopathic pulmonary fibrosis over non-specific interstitial pneumonia,[63] suggesting that a diagnosis of non-specific interstitial pneumonia will usually require a lung biopsy.[64 65] High resolution computed tomography at diagnosis is valuable in determining prognosis. Several recent studies have shown that patients with features of fibrosis at diagnosis (including honeycombing and reticular change) have a worse prognosis and that the extent of lung fibrosis is a predictor of death.[64 66]

What is the role of pulmonary function tests?

Pulmonary function tests offer useful information on the degree of physiological impairment and disease severity, and the results provide a baseline against which disease progression and response to treatment can be measured

Diseases of the lung parenchyma, such as interstitial lung diseases, typically display a "restrictive" pattern on spirometry, as the forced expiratory volume in one second (FEV1) and the forced vital capacity (FVC) are both reduced, which results in a preserved or sometimes increased FEV1:FVC ratio. However, this is not always the case, particularly in smokers who may have coexisting emphysema and have normal, or near normal, lung volumes resulting from the opposing effects of hyperinflation and fibrosis.[67 68 69] Other interstitial lung diseases associated with relative preservation of lung volumes include respiratory bronchiolitis associated interstitial lung disease, Langerhans' cell histiocytosis, and lymphangioleiomyomatosis (either sporadic or in association with tuberous sclerosis). Spirometry is usually done routinely at clinic visits.[70] In patients with idiopathic pulmonary fibrosis, a fall in forced vital capacity of greater than 10% is considered clinically important, and is associated with a 2.4-fold increase in risk of mortality.[1 71]

Transfer factor (also known as diffusing capacity for carbon monoxide) is measured in pulmonary function laboratories, and allows a non-invasive assessment of gas exchange.[72] Transfer factor is typically reduced in patients with interstitial lung disease, secondary to thickening of the alveolar-capillary barrier impairing gas exchange. A spuriously raised transfer factor measurement can occasionally result from minor pulmonary haemorrhage from a systemic vasculitis or, conversely, from anaemia in the context of an interstitial lung disease. In patients with idiopathic pulmonary fibrosis, serial measurement of transfer factor can help to clinicians to estimate prognosis and track progression of disease, and a change may prompt referral for transplant in suitable patients; a change in transfer factor of 15% or greater from baseline is considered clinically important.[1 73] In a UK study of 115 patients with idiopathic pulmonary fibrosis referred to a transplant centre, a transfer factor under 40% (advanced disease) with high resolution computed tomography scoring predicted death within two years with a specificity of 84% and sensitivity of 82%.[74] A disproportionately reduced transfer factor in a patient with relatively normal spirometry may suggest that the underlying disease process is vascular rather than interstitial lung disease and these patients should be screened for pulmonary hypertension.[75]

Exercise tests may help evaluation of disease severity.[76] The six minute walk test records oxygen saturation before, during, and after exercise and measures the total distance walked. Some patients with interstitial lung disease may appear deceptively well at rest, with normal oximetry and spirometry, but become profoundly hypoxic when walking.[76] Exercise associated oxygen desaturation significantly correlates with pulmonary hypertension[75] and patients who have these features merit more detailed assessment for pulmonary artery hypertension including echocardiography.[77] Substantial oxygen desaturation (<88%) during a six minute walk test has been associated with a poor prognosis.[78] For example, in a retrospective study of 105 patients with biopsy proved interstitial lung disease (83 with the "usual interstitial pneumonia" histological pattern, typically associated with idiopathic pulmonary fibrosis), those with a usual interstitial pneumonia pattern who experienced desaturation to less than 88% for a minute or longer during a six minute walk test had significantly reduced survival (hazard ratio 4.47, 95% confidence interval 1.58-12.64).[79] Thus, desaturation during exercise is a useful prognostic marker and identifies patients at high risk who should be screened for pulmonary hypertension and, if appropriate, considered for early transplant referral.

What is the role of echocardiography?

British Thoracic Society guidelines suggest that pulmonary hypertension should be considered in patients with interstitial lung disease who have either breathlessness or lung dysfunction (reduced transfer factor or desaturation on exercise).[1] Pulmonary hypertension is defined as a mean pulmonary artery pressure of greater than 25 mm Hg at rest, or 35 mm Hg or greater during exercise, with normal left atrial pressure.[75] Right heart catheterisation is the gold standard test for measuring pulmonary artery pressure but is invasive, and typically transthoracic echocardiography is performed first.[80 81] Importantly an estimation of systolic pulmonary artery pressure can only be made in patients who have a tricuspid regurgitant jet (70-80%) evident at echocardiography. If so, the systolic pulmonary artery pressure can be estimated and used to calculate the mean pulmonary artery pressure as follows:[82]

$$\text{Mean pulmonary artery pressure} = (0.61\times \textit{systolic pulmonary artery pressure})+2$$

For example, an echocardiography assessed systolic pulmonary artery pressure of 50 mm Hg equates to a mean pulmonary artery pressure of 32 mm Hg.

The prevalence of pulmonary hypertension varies widely according to the disease and severity of lung impairment, but is relatively high (30-40%); higher levels are associated with increased mortality.[77] For example, in a single centre American study of 88 patients with idiopathic pulmonary fibrosis who had a trans-thoracic echocardiograph (allowing estimation of systolic pulmonary artery pressure) within three months of their initial assessment, the median survival for those with a systolic pulmonary artery pressure of ≥0 mm Hg to ≤35 mm Hg was 4.8 years, for those with a systolic pulmonary artery pressure >35 mm Hg to ≤50 mm Hg was 4.1 years, and for those with a systolic pulmonary artery pressure >50 mm Hg was 0.7 years.[83] Patients with systemic sclerosis are particularly at increased risk of pulmonary hypertension (prevalence of 8-12%) and are particularly likely to develop pulmonary hypertension.[84 85 86] British Thoracic Society guidelines advocate annual lung function testing for patients with systemic sclerosis, with echocardiography in patients who have a falling transfer factor or if the transfer factor is less than 50% of the predicted value.[1] Further assessment and management of pulmonary hypertension is a complex topic that is well summarised elsewhere.[87 88 89] Patients with interstitial lung disease who have pulmonary hypertension that is judged to be contributing to symptoms and is disproportionate to the extent of their lung disease, or is severe (systolic pulmonary artery pressure >50 mm Hg) should be considered for referral to the regional specialist pulmonary hypertension centre for assessment and recruitment to high quality trials.

Is lung biopsy necessary?

If key radiological features are present (for example, subpleural, basilar, and reticular abnormalities with traction bronchiectasis and honeycombing in a patient with clinical features consistent with idiopathic pulmonary fibrosis) the diagnostic accuracy of computed tomography approaches 90-100% and most clinicians would not opt for surgical lung biopsy.[90] Such biopsies, which are done under general anaesthetic, are most helpful when clinical and radiological data result in an uncertain diagnosis or when patients are not thought to have idiopathic pulmonary fibrosis.[61]

The site of surgical biopsy is best informed by high resolution computed tomography images of the lung. Video assisted thoracoscopic surgery is now used routinely rather than open thoracotomy. Since a range of interstitial patterns may be seen within the same lung, best practice guidelines encourage sampling from at least two lobes[1 91] and the biopsy with the pathological pattern associated with the poorest prognosis should dictate treatment and estimates of disease prognosis. The risks of video assisted thoracoscopic surgery include persistent air leak (approximately 10-15%), which results in delayed re-expansion of the lung following the procedure, and perioperative bleeding and sepsis. One retrospective cohort study in the United States of 68 patients with interstitial lung disease who had video assisted thoracoscopic surgery reported a mortality rate of 4% (95% confidence interval 1% to 12%) that was associated with the severity of disease, which underlies the importance of careful patient selection for this procedure.[92]

Fibreoptic bronchoscopy, which is typically performed as a day case procedure under local anaesthetic, allows visualisation of proximal airways and sampling of more distal lung using transbronchial biopsy, and bronchoalveolar lavage to exclude infectious causes.[93] It is particularly useful in sarcoidosis, with diagnostic yields of up to 90%.[94] Sampling of lymph nodes adjacent to the airways via endobronchial ultrasound guided aspiration is now also possible.[95 96] Bronchoscopy with lavage and transbronchial biopsies may be diagnostic, or increase diagnostic confidence, in other conditions such as cancer, acute pulmonary eosinophilia, cryptogenic organising pneumonia, subacute hypersensitivity pneumonitis, and some rarer forms of interstitial lung disease such as alveolar proteinosis.[1] However, in most other form of interstitial lung disease bronchoscopy is not particularly helpful since the biopsies obtained are too small to make a confident histopathological diagnosis.

Although lung biopsy will reveal a pathological pattern the final clinical diagnosis still requires integration of clinical, physiological, and radiological data, ideally by a multi-disciplinary team.

ADDITIONAL EDUCATIONAL RESOURCES

Resources for healthcare professionals

- British Thoracic Society (www.brit-thoracic.org.uk)—Recent guidelines on the management of interstitial lung diseases, with useful patient information sheets and management algorithms
- American Thoracic Society (www.thoracic.org/statements/index.php)—Includes consensus statements on classification of idiopathic forms of interstitial lung disease and disease-specific guidelines on sarcoidosis and idiopathic pulmonary fibrosis
- Pneumotox Online (www.pneumotox.com)—Excellent site providing information about drug induced lung diseases
- Ongoing clinical trials (www.clinicaltrials.gov)—Involvement in clinical trials will improve our understanding and management of interstitial lung diseases. This website provides a useful up to date summary of ongoing trials

Resources for patients

- British Lung Foundation (www.lunguk.org)—Useful site with links to patient support groups (Breathe Easy groups)
- Pulmonary Fibrosis UK (www.pulmonaryfibrosis.org.uk)—Excellent site including video about pulmonary fibrosis
- Pulmonary Fibrosis Foundation (www.pulmonaryfibrosis.org)—Support group for patients with pulmonary fibrosis in United States

Who should manage these patients?

Interstitial lung disease clinics that provide multidisciplinary care are now common in the UK and elsewhere. This team approach improves inter-observer agreement, diagnostic confidence,[97 98] and perhaps outcome,[99] and this model of care is advocated in recent guidelines.[1 2] Key individuals in the team typically include chest physicians, pathologists, radiologists, pulmonary physiologists, thoracic surgeons, rheumatologists, palliative care specialists, specialist nurses, and physiotherapists. For example, in an American study of 58 patients with suspected interstitial lung disease, information was provided sequentially to a group of three clinicians, two radiologists, and two pathologists, with each recording their diagnostic impression and diagnostic confidence at each stage.[97] Interobserver agreement improved from beginning to end and after presentation of histopathological information, radiologists changed their diagnostic impressions more than clinicians. Of the 30 patients who had idiopathic pulmonary fibrosis, clinicians identified 75% and radiologists identified 48% before presentation of the histopathological data.[97] Multidisciplinary interaction may prevent unnecessary surgical lung biopsies (when the clinical and radiological impression is consistent with a confident diagnosis of idiopathic pulmonary fibrosis) and identify those in whom a biopsy may be helpful. Links with regional transplant and pulmonary hypertension centres are important and, ideally, patients should have the opportunity to participate in well designed clinical studies where available.[100] Regardless of the model of care available, the patient's general practitioner and local chest physician remain integral to providing continuity and quality of ongoing care.

Contributors: OJD conceived the idea for the article and all authors contributed to the first draft and subsequent revisions. OJD is guarantor.

Funding: No funding was received for this work.

Competing interests: All authors have completed the Unified Competing Interest form at www.icmje.org/coi_disclosure.pdf (available on request from the corresponding author) and declare that they have (1) no support from companies for the submitted work; (2) no relationship with any companies that might have an interest in the submitted work in the previous 3 years; (3) no spouses, partners, or children with financial relationships that may be relevant to the submitted work; and (4) no non-financial interests that may be relevant to the submitted work.

Provenance and peer review: Not commissioned, externally peer reviewed.

1 Bradley B, Branley HM, Egan JJ, Greaves MS, Hansell DM, Harrison NK, et al. Interstitial lung disease guideline: the British Thoracic Society in collaboration with the Thoracic Society of Australia and New Zealand and the Irish Thoracic Society. *Thorax* 2008;63(suppl 5):v1-v58.
2 American Thoracic Society, European Respiratory Society. Idiopathic pulmonary fibrosis: diagnosis and treatment. International consensus statement. *Am J Respir Crit Care Med* 2000;161:646-64.
3 American Thoracic Society, European Respiratory Society. American Thoracic Society/European Respiratory Society international multidisciplinary consensus classification of the idiopathic interstitial pneumonias. *Am J Respir Crit Care Med* 2002;165:277-304.
4 Raghu G, Nicholson AG, Lynch D. The classification, natural history and radiological/histological appearance of idiopathic pulmonary fibrosis and the other idiopathic interstitial pneumonias. *Eur Respir Rev* 2008;17:108-115.
5 Gribbin J, Hubbard RB, Le Jeune I, Smith CJ, West J, Tata LJ. Incidence and mortality of idiopathic pulmonary fibrosis and sarcoidosis in the UK. *Thorax* 2006;61:980-5.
6 Dempsey OJ, Paterson EW, Kerr KM, Denison AR. Sarcoidosis. *BMJ* 2009;339:B3206.
7 Khalil N, Churg A, Muller N, O'Connor R. Environmental, inhaled and ingested causes of pulmonary fibrosis. *Toxicol Pathol* 2007;35:86-96.
8 Iannuzzi MC, Rybicki BA, Teirstein AS. Sarcoidosis. *N Engl J Med* 2007;357:2153-65.
9 Dempsey OJ, Kerr KM, Gomersall L, Remmen H, Currie GP. Idiopathic pulmonary fibrosis: an update. *QJM* 2006;99:643-54.
10 Woodhead F, Wells AU, Desai SR. Pulmonary complications of connective tissue diseases. *Clin Chest Med* 2008;29:149-64.
11 Girard M, Lacasse Y, Cormier Y. Hypersensitivity pneumonitis. *Allergy* 2009;64:322-34.
12 Cottin V, Bonniaud P. Drug-induced infiltrative lung disease. *Eur Respir Mon* 2009;46:287-318.
13 Camus P. Drug-induced and iatrogenic infiltrative lung disease. In: Costabel U, du Bois RM, Egan JJ, eds. Diffuse parenchymal lung disease. Karger, 2007:212-37.
14 Sovijarvi AR, Lemola M, Stenius B, Idanpaan-Heikkila J. Nitrofurantoin-induced acute, subacute and chronic pulmonary reactions. *Scand J Respir Dis* 1977;58:41.
15 Camus P, Kudoh S, Ebina M. Interstitial lung disease associated with drug therapy. *Br J Cancer* 2004;91(suppl 2):S18-S23.
16 Wells AU, Steen V, Valentini G. Pulmonary complications: one of the most challenging complications of systemic sclerosis. *Rheumatology* 2009;48(suppl 3):iii40-4.
17 Nannini C, Ryu JH, Matteson EL. Lung disease in rheumatoid arthritis. *Curr Opin Rheumatol* 2008;20:340-6.
18 Glazer CS, Maier L. Occupational interstitial lung disease. *Eur Respir Mon* 2009;46:265-286.
19 Currie GP, Watt SJ, Maskell NA. An overview of how asbestos exposure affects the lung. *BMJ* 2009;339:b3209.
20 Cohen RA, Patel A, Green FH. Lung disease caused by exposure to coal mine and silica dust. *Semin Respir Crit Care Med* 2008;29:651-61.
21 Santo Tomas LH. Beryllium hypersensitivity and chronic beryllium lung disease. *Curr Opin Pulm Med* 2009;15:165-9.
22 Atis S, Tutluoglu B, Levent E, Ozturk C, Tunaci A, Sahin K, et al. The respiratory effects of occupational polypropylene flock exposure. *Eur Respir J* 2005;25:110-7.
23 Fox J, Anderson H, Moen T, Gruetzmacher G, Hanrahan L, Fink J. Metal working fluid-associated hypersensitivity pneumonitis: an outbreak investigation and case-control study. *Am J Ind Med* 1999;35:58-67.
24 Haitjema T, van Velzen-Blad H, van den Bosch JM. Extrinsic allergic alveolitis caused by goose feathers in a duvet. *Thorax* 1992;47:990-1.
25 Inase N, Ohtani Y, Sumi Y, Umino T, Usui Y, Miyake S, et al. A clinical study of hypersensitivity pneumonitis presumably caused by feather duvets. *Ann Allergy Asthma Immunol* 2006;96:98-104.
26 Diego C, Cullinan P. Extrinsic allergic alveolitis. *Eur Respir Mon* 2009;46:112-25.
27 Enríquez-Matas A, Quirce S, Hernández E, Vereda A, Carnés J, Sastre J. Hypersensitivity pneumonitis caused by domestic exposure to molds. *J Invest Allergol Clin Immunol* 2007;17:126-7.
28 Halpin DM, Graneek BJ, Lacey J, Nieuwenhuijsen MJ, Williamson PA, Venables KM, et al. Respiratory symptoms, immunological responses, and aeroallergen concentrations at a sawmill. *Occup Environ Med* 1994;51:165-172.
29 Taskar VS, Coultas DB. Is idiopathic pulmonary fibrosis and environmental disease? *Proc Am Thorac Soc* 2006;3:293-8.
30 Wells AU, Nicholson AG, Hansell DM. Challenges in pulmonary fibrosis. 4: Smoking-induced diffuse interstitial lung diseases. *Thorax* 2007;62:904-10.
31 Attili AK, Kazerooni EA, Gross BH, Flaherty KR, Myers JL, Martinez FJ. Smoking-related interstitial lung disease: radiologic-clinical-pathologic correlation. *Radiographics* 2008;28:1383-96.
32 Lederer DJ, Enright PL, Kawut SM, Hoffman EA, Hunninghake G, van Beek EJ, et al. Cigarette smoking is associated with subclinical parenchymal lung disease. The multi-ethnic study of atherosclerosis (MESA)-lung study. *Am J Respir Crit Care Med* 2009;180:407-14.
33 Douglas JG, Middleton WG, Gaddie J, Petrie GR, Choo-Kang YF, Prescott RJ, et al. Sarcoidosis: a disorder commoner in non-smokers? *Thorax* 1986;41:787-91.

34 Warren CP. Extrinsic allergic alveolitis: a disease commoner in non-smokers. *Thorax* 1977;32:567-9.
35 Rybicki BA, Iannuzzi MC, Frederick MM, Thompson BW, Rossman MD, Bresnitz EA, et al. Familial aggregation of sarcoidosis. A case-control etiologic study of sarcoidosis. *Am J Respir Crit Care Med* 2001;164:2085-91.
36 McGrath DS, Daniil Z, Foley P, du Bois JL, Lympany PA, Cullinan P, et al. Epidemiology of familial sarcoidosis in the UK. *Thorax* 2000;55:751-4.
37 Marshall RP, Puddicombe A, Cookson WO, Laurent GJ. Adult familial cryptogenic fibrosing alveolitis in the United Kingdom. *Thorax* 2000;55:143-6.
38 Sweet MP, Patti MG, Hoopes C, Hays SR, Golden JA. Gastro-oesophageal reflux and aspiration in patients with advanced lung disease. *Thorax* 2009;64:167-73.
39 Tobin RW, Pope CE 2nd, Pellegrini CA, Emond MJ, Sillery J, Raghu G. Increased prevalence of gastroesophageal reflux in patients with idiopathic pulmonary fibrosis. *Am J Respir Crit Care Med* 1998;158:1804-8.
40 Savarino E, Bazzica M, Zentilin P, Pohl D, Parodi A, Cittadini G, et al. Gastroesophageal reflux and pulmonary fibrosis in scleroderma: a study using pH-impedance monitoring. *Am J Respir Crit Care Med* 2009;179:408-13.
41 Patel NM, Lederer DJ, Borczuk AC, Kawut SM. Pulmonary hypertension in idiopathic pulmonary fibrosis. *Chest* 2007;132:998-1006.
42 Epler GR, McLoud TC, Gaensler EA, Mikus JP, Carrington CB. Normal chest roentgenograms in chronic diffuse infiltrative lung disease. *N Engl J Med* 1978;298:934-9.
43 Specks U. Pulmonary vasculitis: update on the management of ANCA-associated vasculitis. *Eur Respir Mon* 2009;46:251-64.
44 Lebacq E, Desmet V, Verhaegen H. Renal involvement in sarcoidosis. *Postgrad Med J* 1970;46:526-9.
45 Sharma OP, Trowell J, Cohen N, et al. Abnormal calcium metabolism in sarcoidosis. In: Turiaf J, Chabot J, eds. La sarcoidose: rapports de la IV conference internationale. (proceedings of the IV international conference on sarcoidosis). Masson and Cie, 1967:627-31.
46 Sharma OP. Renal sarcoidosis and hypercalcaemia. *Eur Respir Mon* 2005;32:220-32.
47 Kim JS, Judson MA, Donnino R, Gold M, Cooper LT Jr, Prystowsky EN, et al. Cardiac sarcoidosis. *Am Heart J* 2009;157:9-21.
48 Marshall BG, Shaw RJ. Association between angiotensin II receptor gene polymorphism and serum angiotensin converting enzyme (SACE) activity in patients with sarcoidosis. *Thorax* 1998;53:439-40.
49 Baughman RP, Lower EE. Sarcoidosis. In: Warrell DA, Cox TM, Firth DM, eds. Oxford textbook of medicine, 4th ed. Oxford University Press, 2003:1464-71.
50 Nicholson AG. Lymphocytic interstitial pneumonia and other lymphoproliferative disorders in the lung. *Semin Respir Crit Care Med* 2001;22:409-22.
51 Leuchte HH, Neurohr C, Baumgartner R, Holzapfel M, Giehrl W, Vogeser M, et al. Brain natriuretic peptide and exercise capacity in lung fibrosis and pulmonary hypertension. *Am J Respir Crit Care Med* 2004;170:360-5.
52 Song JW, Song JK, Kim DS. Echocardiography and brain natriuretic peptide as prognostic indicators in idiopathic pulmonary fibrosis. *Respir Med* 2009;103:180-6.
53 Corte TJ, Wort SJ, Gatzoulis M, Engel R, Giannakoulas G, Macdonald PM, et al. Elevated brain natriuretic peptide predicts mortality in interstitial lung disease. *Eur Respir J* 2010; published online 11 March.
54 Leuchte HH, Baumgartner RA, Nounou ME, Vogeser M, Neurohr C, Trautnitz M, et al. Brain natriuretic peptide is a prognostic parameter in chronic lung diseases. *Am J Respir Crit Care Med* 2006;173:744-50.
55 Nukiwa T. The role of biomarkers in management of interstitial lung disease: implications of biomarkers derived from type II pneumocytes. *Eur Respir Mon* 2009;46:47-66.
56 Tzouvelekis A, Kouliatsis G, Anevlavis S, Bouros D. Serum biomarkers in interstitial lung diseases. *Respir Res* 2005;6:78.
57 Wells AU, Rubens MB, du Bois RM, Hansell DM. Serial CT in fibrosing alveolitis: prognostic significance of the initial pattern. *Am J Roentgenol* 1993;161:1159-65.
58 Padley SP, Adler B, Muller NL. High-Resolution computed tomography of the chest: current indications. *J Thoracic Imaging* 1993;8:189-99.
59 Copley SJ, Wells AU, Hawtin KE, Gibson DJ, Hodson JM, Jacques AE, et al. Lung morphology in the elderly: comparative CT study of subjects over 75 years old versus those under 55 years old. *Radiology* 2009;251:566-73.
60 Remy-Jardin M, Edme JL, Boulenguez C, Remy J, Mastora I, Sobaszek A. Longitudinal follow-up study of smoker's lung with thin-section CT in correlation with pulmonary function tests. *Radiology* 2002;222:261-70.
61 Hunninghake GW, Zimmerman MB, Schwartz DA, King TE Jr, Lynch J, Hegele R, et al. Utility of a lung biopsy for the diagnosis of idiopathic pulmonary fibrosis. *Am J Respir Crit Care Med* 2001;164:193-6.
62 Lynch JP 3rd, Saggar R, Weigt SS, Zisman DA, White ES. Usual interstitial pneumonia. *Semin Respir Crit Care Med* 2006;27:634-51.
63 Sumikawa H, Johkoh T, Ichikado K, Taniguchi H, Kondoh Y, Fujimoto K, et al. Usual interstitial pneumonia and chronic idiopathic interstitial pneumonia: analysis of CT appearances in 92 patients. *Radiology* 2006;241:258-66.
64 Silva CI, Muller NL. Idiopathic interstitial pneumonias. *J Thorac Imaging* 2009;24:260-73.
65 Silva CI, Müller NL, Hansell DM, Lee KS, Nicholson AG, Wells AU. Non-specific interstitial pneumonia and idiopathic pulmonary fibrosis: change in pattern and distribution of disease over time. *Radiology* 2008;247:251-59.
66 Gay SE, Kazerooni EA, Toews GB, Lynch JP 3rd, Gross BH, Cascade PN, et al. Idiopathic pulmonary fibrosis: predicting response to therapy and survival. *Am J Respir Crit Care Med* 1998;157:1063-72.
67 Wiggins J, Strickland B, Turner-Warwick M. Combined cryptogenic fibrosing alveolitis and emphysema; the value of high resolution computed tomography in assessment. *Respir Med* 1990;84:365-9.
68 Doherty MJ, Pearson MG, O'Grady EA, Pellegrini V, Calverley PM. Cryptogenic fibrosing alveolitis with preserved lung volumes. *Thorax* 1997;52:998-1002.
69 Munson JC. Combined pulmonary fibrosis and emphysema: a high-pressure situation. *Eur Respir J* 2010;35:9-11.
70 Miller MR, Hankinson J, Brusasco V, Burgos F, Casaburi R, Coates A, et al. Standardisation of spirometry. *Eur Respir J* 2005;26:319-38.
71 King TE Jr, Safrin S, Starko KM, Brown KK, Noble PW, Raghu G, et al. Analyses of efficacy end points in a controlled trial of interferon-gamma 1b for idiopathic pulmonary fibrosis. *Chest* 2005;127:171-7.
72 Macintyre N, Crapo RO, Viegi G, Johnson DC, van der Grinten CP, Brusasco V, et al. Standardisation of the single-breath determination of carbon monoxide uptake in the lung. *Eur Respir J* 2005;26:720-35.
73 Latsi PI, du Bois RM, Nicholson AG, Colby TV, Bisirtzoglou D, Nikolakopoulou A, et al. Fibrotic idiopathic interstitial pneumonia: the prognostic value of longnitudinal functional trends. *Am J Respir Crit Care Med* 2003;168:531-7.
74 Mogulkoc N, Brutsche MH, Bishop PW, Greaves SM, Horrocks AW, Egan JJ, et al. Pulmonary function in idiopathic pulmonary fibrosis and referral for lung transplantation. *Am J Respir Crit Care Med* 2001;164:103-8.
75 Task Force for Diagnosis and Treatment of Pulmonary Hypertension of European Society of Cardiology, European Respiratory Society, International Society of Heart and Lung Transplantation, Galiè N, Hoeper MM, Humbert M, et al. Guidelines for the diagnosis and treatment of pulmonary hypertension. *Eur Respir J* 2009;34:1219-63.
76 Han MK, Martinez FJ. Exercise testing in interstitial lung disease diagnosis and management. *Eur Respir Mon* 2009;46:7-23.
77 Behr J, Ryu JH. Pulmonary hypertension in interstitial lung disease. *Eur Respir J* 2008;31:1357-67.
78 Flaherty KR, Andrei AC, Murray S, Fraley C, Colby TV, Travis WD, et al. Idiopathic pulmonary fibrosis: prognostic value of changes in physiology and six-minute walk test. *Am J Respir Crit Care Med* 2006;174:803-9.
79 Lama VN, Flaherty KR, Toews GB, Colby TV, Travis WD, Long Q, et al. Prognostic value of desaturation during a 6-minute walk test in idiopathic interstitial pneumonia. *Am J Respir Crit Care Med* 2003;168:1084-90.
80 Arcasoy SM, Christie JD, Ferrari VA, Sutton MS, Zisman DA, Blumenthal NP, et al. Echocardiographic assessment of pulmonary hypertension in patients with advanced lung disease. *Am J Respir Crit Care Med* 2003;167:735-40.
81 Denton CP, Cailes JB, Phillips GD, Wells AU, Black CM, Bois RM. Comparison of Doppler echocardiography and right heart catheterization to assess pulmonary hypertension in systemic sclerosis. *Br J Rheumatol* 1997;36:239-43.
82 Chemla D, Castelain V, Humbert M, Hébert JL, Simonneau G, Lecarpentier Y, et al. New formula for predicting mean pulmonary artery pressure using systolic artery pressure. *Chest* 2004;126:1313-7.
83 Nadrous HF, Pellikka PA, Krowka MJ, Swanson KL, Chaowalit N, Decker PA, et al. The impact of pulmonary hypertension on survival in patients with idiopathic pulmonary fibrosis. *Chest* 2005;128:616S-7S.
84 Mukerjee D, St George D, Coleiro B, Knight C, Denton CP, Davar J, et al. Prevalence and outcome in systemic sclerosis associated pulmonary arterial hypertension: application of a registry approach. *Ann Rheum Dis* 2003;62:1088-93.
85 McLaughlin V, Humbert M, Coghlan G, Nash P, Steen V. Pulmonary arterial hypertension: the most devastating vascular complication of systemic sclerosis. *Rheumatology* 2009;48(Suppl 3):iii25-31.
86 Hachulla E, Gressin V, Guillevin L, Carpentier P, Diot E, Sibilia J, et al. Early detection of pulmonary arterial hypertension in systemic sclerosis: a French nationwide prospective multicenter study. *Arthritis Rheum* 2005;52:3792-800.
87 National Pulmonary Hypertension Centres of the UK and Ireland. Consensus statement on the management of pulmonary hypertension in clinical practice in the UK and Ireland. *Thorax* 2008;63(suppl 2):ii1-ii41.
88 Corte TJ, Wort SJ, Wells AU. Pulmonary hypertension in idiopathic pulmonary fibrosis: a review. *Sarcoidosis Vasc Diffuse Lung Dis* 2009;26:7-19.
89 Patel NM, Lederer DJ, Borczuk AC, Kawut SM. Pulmonary hypertension in idiopathic pulmonary fibrosis. *Chest* 2007;132:998-1006.
90 Huang SK, Myers JL, Flaherty KR. Diagnosing idiopathic interstitial pneumonias: utility of surgical lung biopsy. *Eur Respir Mon* 2009;46:24-45.
91 Flaherty KR, Travis WD, Colby TV, Toews GB, Kazerooni EA, Gross BH, et al. Histopathologic variability in usual and nonspecific interstitial pneumonias. *Am J Respir Crit Care Med* 2001;164:1722-7.
92 Kreider ME, Hansen-Flaschen J, Ahmad NN, Rossman MD, Kaiser LR, Kucharczuk JC, et al. Complications of video-assisted thoracoscopic lung biopsy in patients with interstitial lung disease. *Ann Thorac Surg* 2007;83:1140-4.

93 British Thoracic Society Bronchoscopy Guidelines Committee. British Thoracic Society guidelines on diagnostic flexible bronchoscopy. *Thorax* 2001;56(suppl 1):i1-21.

94 Shorr AF, Torrington KG, Hnatiuk OW. Endobronchial involvement and airway hyperreactivity in patients with sarcoidosis. *Chest* 2001;120:881-6.

95 Cameron SE, Andrade RS, Pambuccian SE. Endobronchial ultrasound-guided transbronchial needle aspiration cytology: a state of the art review. *Cytopathology* 2010;21:6-26.

96 Medford AR, Agrawal S, Bennett JA. Sarcoidosis. Technique to enable diagnosis. *BMJ* 2009;339:b3962.

97 Flaherty KR, King TE Jr, Raghu G, Lynch JP 3rd, Colby TV, Travis WD, et al. Idiopathic interstitial pneumonia: what is the effect of a multidisciplinary approach to diagnosis? *Am J Respir Crit Care Med* 2004;170:904-10.

98 Flaherty KR, Andrei AC, King TE Jr, Flaherty KR, Andrei AC, King TE Jr, et al. Idiopathic interstitial pneumonia: do community and academic physicians agree on diagnosis? *Am J Respir Crit Care Med* 2007;175:1054-60.

99 Lok SS. Interstitial lung disease clinics for the management of idiopathic pulmonary fibrosis: a potential advantage to patients. Greater Manchester Lung Fibrosis Consortium. *J Heart Lung Transplant* 1999;18:884-90.

100 Behr J, Noble PW. Clinical trials in interstitial lung disease. *Eur Respir Mon* 2009;46:67-84.

BMJ
BPP UNIVERSITY SCHOOL OF HEALTH

Paediatric obstructive sleep apnoea

Steven Powell, specialist registrar, otolaryngology[1], Haytham Kubba, consultant paediatric otolaryngologist[2], Chris O'Brien, consultant paediatrician[3], Mike Tremlett, consultant anaesthetist[4]

[1]Department of Otolaryngology, James Cook University Hospital, Middlesbrough TS4 3BW

[2]Department of Paediatric Otolaryngology, Royal Hospital for Sick Children, Glasgow G3 8SJ

[3]Department of Paediatric Respiratory Medicine, Royal Victoria Infirmary, Newcastle upon Tyne NE1 4LP

[4]Department of Anaesthesia, James Cook University Hospital, Middlesbrough TS4 3BW

Correspondence to: S Powell steven_m_powell@hotmail.com

Cite this as: *BMJ* 2010;340:c1918

‹DOI› 10.1136/bmj.c1918
http://www.bmj.com/content/340/bmj.c1918

Habitual snoring occurs in 12% of children in the United Kingdom.[1] Two large cross sectional studies from the UK and Italy found that the prevalence of obstructive sleep apnoea in children was 0.7% to 1.8%.[1 2] A recent, well designed cross sectional study of 700 children in the United States found that the prevalence of primary snoring was 15.5% and of sleep apnoea 1.2%.[3] Delayed diagnosis of obstructive sleep apnoea can lead to neurobehavioural consequences and even serious cardiorespiratory morbidity.[4] History and examination alone are insufficient to distinguish reliably those with sleep apnoea from those who simply snore.[5] Paediatric obstructive sleep apnoea has completely different clinical features and requires different management strategies from adult obstructive sleep apnoea. In this review we provide an overview of the diagnosis and management of children with obstructive sleep apnoea, from primary to specialist care. The review is based on the best available evidence, which for much of obstructive sleep apnoea comprises longitudinal or cohort studies.

How do snoring and obstructive sleep apnoea differ?

Sleep disordered breathing refers to the whole spectrum of breathing disturbance during sleep, from primary snoring through to obstructive apnoea. Obstructive sleep apnoea is defined as a disorder of breathing during sleep that is characterised by prolonged partial upper airway obstruction and/or intermittent complete obstruction that adversely affects ventilation during sleep and disrupts normal sleep patterns.[6] Snoring is noisy breathing caused by turbulent airflow through the upper airway without the sequelae of obstructive apnoea, frequent arousals from sleep, or disordered gas exchange.[6]

The normal sleep pattern has several phases. Muscle relaxation usually occurs during rapid eye movement sleep, possibly as a protective mechanism to prevent sleep movements during dreaming. A child's soft pharyngeal upper airway is held open only by active pharyngeal muscle tone. Relaxation of the pharyngeal constrictor muscles narrows the airway at the pharynx. Obstructive sleep apnoea may be caused by anatomical obstruction in the pharyngeal airway or a reduction of pharyngeal muscle tone, or a combination of both.[7] Negative pharyngeal pressure is generated by the diaphragm to compensate for the upper airway resistance, which contributes to airway obstruction.

Are diagnoses of obstructive sleep apnoea in children increasing?

Obstructive sleep apnoea in children has existed for a long time without being widely recognised as a clinical syndrome. In 1889 Hill published an article in the *BMJ* on "some causes of backwardness and stupidity in children."[8] Several startling revelations appear in this work—for example, Hill identified the symptoms of obstructive sleep apnoea: ". . . children, the victims of nasal and pharyngeal obstructions, often suffer from headaches especially when engaged in study, and frequently evince marked inability to fix their attention on their lessons or work for any length of time . . ."[8]

In the 1960s and '70s tonsillectomy was almost routine in children for a range of perceived clinical reasons, including blocked noses and frequent upper respiratory infections. Many children may have had unrecognised sleep disordered breathing. The first case series describing obstructive sleep apnoea in children was not published until 1976.[9] The increasing interest in the condition has led to more diagnoses, and a position paper published by ENT-UK (the British Association of Otorhinolaryngology—Head and Neck Surgery) has estimated that about a quarter of the 27 400 paediatric tonsillectomies in 2008-9 in the UK were carried out for obstructive conditions.[10] In many countries the adenotonsillectomy rate has fallen, and the Australasian College of Physicians and the Australian Society of Otolaryngology Head and Neck surgery conclude in their position paper that too few adenotonsillectomies are performed in Australia and New Zealand for obstructive sleep apnoea.[11]

Who gets obstructive sleep apnoea?

Children with no underlying medical diagnosis can get physical obstruction of the nasal airway by enlarged adenoids and of the oropharyngeal airway by enlarged tonsils, resulting in increased airway resistance. The peak incidence of obstructive sleep apnoea in this group occurs in those aged 3 to 6 years, coinciding with the time when the adenoids and tonsils undergo hypertrophy.[7] The situation is more complex than simple obstruction by adenoid and tonsil hypertrophy as not all children with large lymphoid tissue have obstructive sleep apnoea; this reflects variation between individuals in pharyngeal muscle tone and anatomical differences.[7]

The increasing prevalence of obesity in children has led to the emergence of a second group in whom obstructive sleep apnoea can occur.[12] The pathogenesis is multifactorial,

SOURCES AND SELECTION CRITERIA

We conducted a Medline search using the key words "sleep apnoea", "sleep disordered breathing", "upper airways resistance", and "snoring". We limited our search to the English language and to children (age 0-18). We searched the Cochrane database. We hand searched reference lists to check that we had considered all relevant articles. We selected articles for this review if they were the best evidence available on a particular point or the best summary of the evidence. We included some articles to place the review in historical context.

SUMMARY POINTS

- Obstructive sleep apnoea has a prevalence of 0.7% to 1.8% in the paediatric population
- The condition can be difficult to diagnose clinically
- Even mild to moderate obstructive sleep apnoea can result in adverse neurobehavioural consequences and negatively affect quality of life
- Adenotonsillectomy is an effective treatment in most uncomplicated cases
- More complex cases need management by paediatric and ear, nose, and throat teams in hospitals with appropriate support facilities

with pharyngeal adipose tissue and decreased respiratory capacity contributing, but the exact mechanism is unclear.[12]

In a third group of children (those with congenital abnormalities such as achondroplasia or craniofacial abnormalities) the cause of obstructive sleep apnoea is complex. Children with such congenital abnormalities have narrow pharyngeal airways, which will predispose them to obstruction. Children with Down's syndrome have both an abnormally narrow upper airway and reduced pharyngeal muscle tone. Two thirds of children with Down's syndrome have some form of sleep disordered breathing, and regular screening for obstructive sleep apnoea is advised.[13] Box 1 lists conditions associated with an increased risk of obstructive sleep apnoea.

What symptoms and signs might the child have?

Children with obstructive sleep apnoea are different from adults with the syndrome. In adults, daytime sleepiness and snoring are the predominant features of obstructive sleep apnoea.[14] In children, tiredness is not a prominent symptom. The symptoms may be divided into daytime and night time symptoms.

During the night the universal symptoms of obstructive sleep apnoea are habitual snoring, restless sleep, and possibly witnessed apnoeas. The symptoms may be exacerbated when the child has an upper respiratory tract infection. The parents may report the child sleeping in a position with the head extended in an effort to open his or her airway. Reports of apnoea differ, but a well designed prospective cohort study showed that even a history of apnoea episodes could not predict obstructive sleep apnoea reliably.[5] Parents may often be anxious about their child's breathing during sleep. Parents may report secondary enuresis, which is thought to result from decreased appropriate arousals during sleep.[15] Evidence also exists of an association of primary enuresis with habitual snoring from a population based study.[16]

A systematic review of observational studies has concluded that a suggestive history is an unreliable predictor of a diagnosis of obstructive sleep apnoea.[17] This review was somewhat limited as nearly a half of the studies were retrospective, although others were well designed cohort studies. A meta-analysis of the raw data showed history and examination to have poor positive predictive value for obstructive sleep apnoea.

During the daytime, neurobehavioural symptoms such as irritability, behavioural problems, and poor concentration predominate. These result not only from hypoxia but also from sleep fragmentation.[18] In experimental models hypoxia has resulted in neuronal cell loss, which has detrimental effects on memory and cognition.[15] A review identified 22 studies that compared children with obstructive sleep apnoea with controls using tools such as the child behaviour checklist, Conners' rating scale, and the child health questionnaire.[19] Although the studies provided a low standard of evidence, they showed almost universally poorer concentration, attention, behaviour, and quality of life in the group with obstructive sleep apnoea.

In the most severe cases the child may fail to thrive.[20] Pulmonary complications arise from complex mechanisms that increase pulmonary vessel resistance. When this becomes persistent pulmonary hypertension and cor pulmonale can occur.[15] Serious complications leading to death are rare.[6]

What is the differential diagnosis?

A child who snores may simply have primary snoring or may have obstructive sleep apnoea. Apnoeas without respiratory effort can occur with central apnoea as a result of a lack of neural drive. Describing other sleep problems is beyond the scope of this article, but these are discussed in a recent excellent review.[21]

What history can be taken in primary care?

We recommend taking a sleep history for all children presenting with symptoms of blocked nose, recurrent nasal or throat infections, and recurrent ear infections, and for children whose parents are concerned about snoring. Snoring sounds (stertor) are different from the higher pitched sounds (stridor) that arise from a narrowed larynx

BOX 1 CONDITIONS THAT CARRY AN INCREASED RISK OF OBSTRUCTIVE SLEEP APNOEA[13]

- Down's syndrome
- Neuromuscular disease
- Craniofacial abnormalities
- Achondroplasia
- Mucopolysaccharidoses
- Prader-Willi syndrome

BOX 2 TAKING A SLEEP HISTORY

Ask about night time symptoms

- Do they snore?
- Do they get a good night's sleep or are they restless?
- Do they wake through the night?
- Do they struggle with their breathing or stop breathing?
- Do they sleep in an unusual position (such as with extended head)?
- Do they sweat excessively?
- Do they wet the bed?

Ask about daytime symptoms

- Do they have any behavioural or concentration problems?
- Do they breathe through their mouth?
- Are they growing normally?

BOX 3 GRADING OF TONSIL SIZE BY HOW MUCH OF THE OROPHARYNGEAL AIRWAY IS OCCUPIED[22]

- Grade 0: Within tonsillar fossa
- Grade 1: 0-25% of oropharyngeal airway
- Grade 2: 26-50%
- Grade 3: 51-75%
- Grade 4: >75%

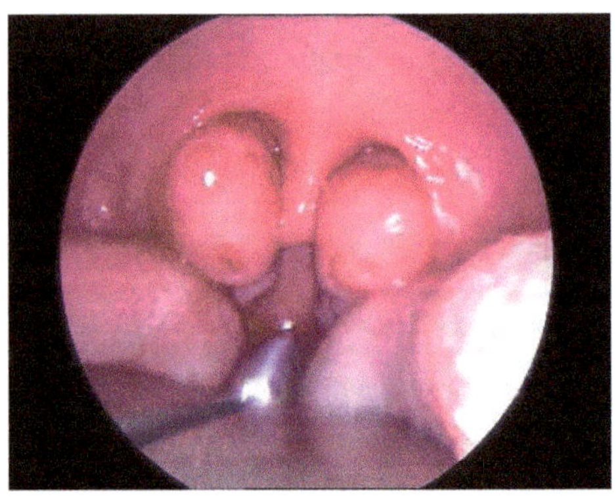

Fig 1 Enlarged tonsils in patient with obstructive sleep apnoea under general anaesthetic for adenotonsillectomy (endotracheal tube and tonsillar gag are visible)

or trachea. In our experience children with sleep apnoea may have several seemingly unrelated symptoms, such as failure to thrive and poor concentration, and nocturnal symptoms are not volunteered unless a sleep history is routinely taken. Box 2 lists questions that might be used to elicit daytime and night time symptoms associated with disordered breathing.

What examinations can be performed in primary care?

An assessment of nasal airflow can be performed by holding a cold spatula or tongue depressor under the nose. Misting of the cold metal indicates airflow. A lack of airflow may indicate nasopharyngeal obstruction resulting from enlarged adenoids or nasal obstruction, usually caused by rhinitis. The nasal cavity may be examined using a headlight or an otoscope for the presence of rhinitis or obstructive polyps.

Assessing the mouth and pharynx elicits information on tonsillar size and any abnormality of the palate. Tonsils can be graded by size (box 3). Examine the neck for any lymphadenopathy and the ears for glue ear, which may coexist with adenoid hypertrophy.

BOX 4 INDICATIONS FOR PAEDIATRIC RESPIRATORY INVESTIGATIONS[25]

- Unclear or inconsistent diagnosis of obstructive sleep apnoea
- Age <2 years
- Weight <15 kg
- Down's syndrome
- Cerebral palsy
- Hypotonia or neuromuscular disorders
- Craniofacial anomalies
- Mucopolysaccharidoses
- Obesity (body mass index >95th centile for age and sex)
- Important comorbidity such as congenital heart disease, chronic lung disease
- Residual symptoms after adenotonsillectomy

BOX 5 CHILDREN WHO SHOULD BE REFERRED FOR TREATMENT IN A SPECIALIST CENTRE (NOT A DISTRICT GENERAL HOSPITAL)[25]

- Age <2 years
- Weight <15 kg
- Failure to thrive (weight <5th centile for age)
- Obesity (body mass index >95th centile for age and sex)
- Severe cerebral palsy
- Hypotonia or neuromuscular disorders (moderately severely or severely affected)
- Serious craniofacial anomalies
- Mucopolysaccharidoses and syndromes associated with difficult airway
- Serious comorbidity (such as congenital heart disease; chronic lung disease; ASA 3 or above—that is, grade 3 in the American Society of Anesthesiologists' physical status classification system)
- Electrocardiographic or echocardiographic abnormalities
- Severe obstructive sleep apnoea (described by polysomnographic indices including an obstructive index >10, a respiratory disturbance index >40, and an oxygen saturation nadir <80%)

Who should be referred and where should they be sent?

Children with clinical evidence of adenotonsillar hypertrophy (fig 1) and symptoms of persistent snoring plus any of the daytime or night time features of obstructive sleep apnoea require referral, in the first instance to an ear, nose, and throat surgeon with an interest in paediatrics.

Children with underlying diagnoses, such as those listed in box 1, and any of the clinical features of obstructive sleep apnoea need to be investigated. If the child is already in the care of a paediatric team, then liaising with that team, which can refer the child to the paediatric respiratory/sleep team, is the most appropriate route.

Children with obesity and features suggestive of obstructive sleep apnoea can be referred, usually to a paediatrician in the first instance.

How are children with sleep disordered breathing investigated and managed in secondary care?

An ear, nose, and throat surgeon will take a sleep history with reference to presenting symptoms and may ask about symptoms of hearing loss. A full ear, nose, and throat examination will be done, with a hearing assessment if indicated. The clinician will then decide if investigations are indicated. There are two common investigations for this condition: overnight pulse oximetry and polysomnography.

Overnight pulse oximetry provides information, on heart rate and oxygen saturation, which may be valuable if more detailed tests of sleep disordered breathing are not available. This does not always require an overnight hospital admission as the family can go home with portable pulse oximetry equipment. Periods of apnoea are indicated by occasions when the oxygen saturation drops; these episodes are usually accompanied by a rise in heart rate (fig 2). A group of Canadian researchers devised an oximetry scoring system, which they tested in a prospective cohort study, and found that higher scores were associated with increasing severity of obstructive sleep apnoea.[23] Oximetry has a high positive predictive value (97%) for diagnosis of obstructive sleep apnoea, but because not all apnoeas result in a drop in saturations the negative predictive value is low (53%).[24]

Polysomnography (a sleep study) is currently the optimal investigation. The minimum elements of investigation should comprise measurements of oxygen saturation, airflow, and respiratory effort; electrocardiography; and videotaping with sound.[13] Polysomnography can measure apnoeas (cessation in airflow) or hypopnoeas (reduction in airflow). These two measures are often combined as the apnoea-hypopnoea index, which is the total number of apnoeas and hypopnoeas per hour of sleep. Other additional measurements can be included in a sleep study, such as results from electroencephalography, electro-oculography, or electromyography.

In the United States the American Academy of Pediatrics' management guideline recommends polysomnography

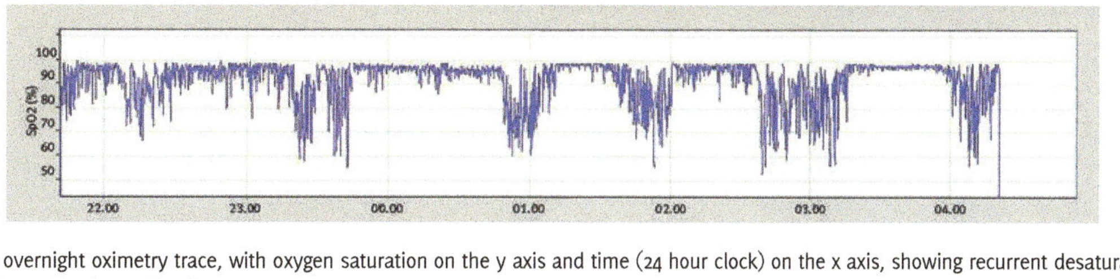

Fig 2 An overnight oximetry trace, with oxygen saturation on the y axis and time (24 hour clock) on the x axis, showing recurrent desaturations in a patient with obstructive sleep apnoea

as the optimal investigation and oximetry or abbreviated studies if this is not available.[6]

The UK Royal College of Paediatrics and Child Health's working group concluded in its management guideline that oximetry is a useful screening tool but that to discriminate reliably primary snoring from obstructive sleep apnoea polysomnography would be required.[13]

A UK working party consensus statement endorsed by the British Association of Paediatric Otolaryngology, ENT-UK, the Association of Paediatric Anaesthetists, the Royal College of Anaesthetists, and the Royal College of Paediatrics and Child Health was published in 2009.[25] The statement recognised that in the UK the decision to operate on children with sleep disordered breathing is a clinical one, based on symptom severity.

If the symptoms are inconsistent and the child is very young or at the extremes of the weight centiles then investigations are indicated. In patients with a suspected underlying syndrome or serious illness then investigations are essential before further management. Box 4 lists indications for considering investigation before treatment in a child suspected of having obstructive sleep apnoea.

As a history and examination alone cannot reliably differentiate between obstructive sleep apnoea and primary snoring, if a strategy of surgery without respiratory investigations is adopted, some children with primary snoring may have adenotonsillectomy.[17] However, it is not logistically possible for all snoring children to have polysomnography. A pragmatic approach is taken, and the decision to treat is based on the severity of the daytime and nocturnal symptoms reported and on the occurrence of early complications associated with obstructive sleep apnoea. These children are diagnosed with sleep disordered breathing with a suspicion of obstructive sleep apnoea.

What are the possible treatments?

For the child with no underlying medical condition and with clinical evidence of adenotonsillar hypertrophy an adenotonsillectomy would be the most appropriate treatment. As discussed above, adenotonsillectomy is appropriate in some children without further investigations if they have clinical features suggestive of obstructive sleep apnoea.[25] The symptoms and signs need to be considered along with other indications for tonsillectomy and adenoidectomy, such as recurrent tonsillitis or glue ear. Children with fewer symptoms of sleep disorder may still require adenoidectomy or tonsillectomy for other indications. A Cochrane review of treatment of obstructive apnoea by adenotonsillectomy found only one paper meeting the Cochrane criteria,[26] and this was primarily concerned with surgical technique.[27] The patients were randomised either to radiofrequency tonsil reduction and adenoidectomy or to conventional adenotonsillectomy. The outcome measures did not differ.

The main physiological outcome is the apnoea-hypopnoea index, calculated from polysomnography results as described above. Several studies show a reduction in the apnoea-hypopnoea index after adenotonsillectomy, and these have been summarised in a recent meta-analysis.[28] The inclusion criteria for the meta-analysis included paediatric patients with no underlying syndrome or diagnosis who had adenotonsillectomy with preoperative and postoperative polysomnography. The meta-analysis pooled data on 355 children from 14 series. The data are limited by the fact that they come from case series and no control groups were included. An improvement in the polysomnography results to normal occurred in 83%, and a reduction in the apnoea-hypopnoea index of 14 events an hour was found.

Measuring outcomes other than the physiological sleep outcomes—such as neurocognitive outcomes and quality of life by proxy—is of increasing interest. The only UK study to have measured quality of life improvement was by Georgalas and colleagues.[29] In a cohort of patients, adenotonsillectomy improved all domains of the child health questionnaire. In North America disease-specific quality of life measures such as the OSA-18 are widely used.[30] A review article found 11 publications measuring changes in behaviour, neurocognition, and quality of life after adenotonsillectomy.[19] The authors of the review over-rate the quality of evidence as these studies are generally prospective, single sample, observational studies, although five of the 11 do include a control group. Universal improvement in quality of life is reported in these studies. Behaviour and neurocognitive measures also show improvement. Longer term studies show that the quality of life improvement can be sustained over a couple of years but may be less pronounced than initially.[31]

Adenotonsillectomy can still be done if an underlying condition or syndrome is present, but the surgery needs to be evaluated carefully as the obstructive sleep apnoea in this group is likely to be multifactorial. Continuous positive airway pressure may need to be considered if adenotonsillectomy is contraindicated or unlikely to help. A randomised control trial of continuous versus bilevel positive airway pressure in children with obstructive sleep apnoea who were unsuitable for adenotonsillectomy found no difference between the methods.[32]

Nasal steroids can be used to treat rhinitis if nasal obstruction is thought to be making a substantial contribution. A well produced, double blind, randomised control trial of nasal steroids (six weeks of fluticasone) showed a reduction in the apnoea-hypopnoea index.[33] The only long term data relate to a non-randomised longitudinal study, which found that symptom scores in mild obstructive sleep apnoea decreased after four weeks of a nasal steroid and remained at this level nine months later.[34]

In specific circumstances such as craniofacial abnormality, specific surgery or dental appliances such as advancement splints may be required.

Can complications of treatment occur?

The main risk of adenotonsillectomy is of postoperative haemorrhage, which has a rate of 3.5%.[35] Clinicians are concerned that children who have obstructive sleep apnoea may be at increased risk of perioperative respiratory complications. They may be more sensitive to opiates and inhalational anaesthetic agents. Postoperative desaturations can occur in up to 10% of children.[4] Rarely, children can develop pulmonary oedema. This happens as a result of the loss of the positive end expiratory pressure they experienced secondary to the airway obstruction. With relief of the obstruction a transudate and pulmonary oedema can develop.[4] In children who have been identified as high risk (box 5), surgery should be performed in a hospital with paediatric intensive care facilities. Careful preoperative investigation is essential.[25]

We thank Mr D Bosman for the clinical photograph.

Contributors: SP did the literature review and wrote the first draft. All authors redrafted the article and produced the final draft.

Funding: No special funding.

A PARENT'S PERSPECTIVE

A parent of a child with obstructive sleep apnoea treated by adenotonsillectomy: "Before the operation, my son had noisy breathing, and even with the television on you could hear his breathing when he slept. He had loud snoring, and I could tell something was not right. During the day he seemed to have a cold all the time. He had an operation to remove his tonsils and adenoids. He came through this well and didn't have too many problems with pain. He ate and drank well. The results from this were fantastic. His symptoms vanished after the operation. He now makes no noise when he sleeps and seems to have a better night's sleep. His speech is clearer—before, he always seemed to talk with a blocked nose. During the day he seems happier and more settled than he was before the operation."

UNANSWERED QUESTIONS

- Can a clinical assessment be designed to detect sleep apnoea accurately?
- What should be the consensus definition for paediatric obstructive sleep apnoea based on polysomnographic criteria?
- What is the natural course of mild obstructive sleep apnoea?
- At what level of mild obstructive sleep apnoea should surgical intervention take place, and who could be treated conservatively?
- How does paediatric obstructive sleep apnoea affect the long term risk of developing adult obstructive sleep apnoea?
- What is the significance of the metabolic changes that occur in obstructive sleep apnoea?[36]

TIPS FOR NON-SPECIALISTS

- Take a full sleep history in children presenting with symptoms of upper respiratory infection and ear infection
- Consider referral of patients with habitual snoring and other daytime or nocturnal symptoms of obstructive sleep apnoea
- Uncomplicated cases with symptoms suggestive of obstructive sleep apnoea and evidence of adenotonsillar hypertrophy can be referred to an ear, nose, and throat specialist
- Patients with congenital abnormalities, syndromes, comorbidity, or obesity can be referred to the paediatric team in the first instance

ADDITIONAL EDUCATIONAL RESOURCES

For professionals

- Royal College of Paediatric and Child Health Working Party on Sleep Physiology and Respiratory Control Disorders in Childhood. *Standards for services for children with disorders of sleep physiology*. 2009. www.rcpch.ac.uk/Research/ce/Guidelines-frontpage/Guideline-Appraisals-by-Organisation/RCPCH-Working-Party. (This is a comprehensive review of children's sleep disorders, including obstructive sleep apnoea)
- Lim J, McKean MC. Adenotonsillectomy for obstructive sleep apnoea in children. *Cochrane Database Syst Rev* 2009;(2):CD003136.
- Hill W. On some causes of backwardness and stupidity in children. *BMJ* 1889;2:771-2. (Available from *BMJ* archive, www.bmj.com/cgi/reprint/2/1500/711.)

For parents

- ENT-UK (www.entuk.org/patient_info/throat/tonsil_html)—A guide to tonsil surgery
- ENT-UK (www.entuk.org/patient_info/throat/adenoid)—A guide to adenoid surgery
- American Academy of Otolaryngology-Head and Neck Surgery (www.entnet.org/HealthInformation/Could-Child-Have-Sleep-Apnea.cfm)— Fact sheet: *Could My Child Have Sleep Apnea?*

Competing interests: None declared.

Provenance and peer review: Not commissioned; externally peer reviewed.

Patient consent obtained.

1 Ali NJ, Pitson DJ, Stradling JR. Snoring, sleep disturbance, and behaviour in 4-5 year olds. *Arch Dis Child* 1993;68:360-6.
2 Brunetti L, Rana S, Lospalluti ML, Pietrafesa A, Francavilla R, Fanelli M, et al. Prevalence of obstructive sleep apnea syndrome in a cohort of 1,207 children of southern Italy. *Chest* 2001;120:1930-5.
3 Bixler EO, Vgontzas AN, Lin H-M, Liao D, Calhoun S, Vela-Bueno A, et al. Sleep disordered breathing in children in a general population sample: prevalence and risk factors. *Sleep* 2009;32:731-6.
4 Blum RH, McGowan FX Jr. Chronic upper airway obstruction and cardiac dysfunction: anatomy, pathophysiology and anesthetic implications. *Paediatr Anaesth* 2004;14(1):75-83.
5 Carroll JL, McColley SA, Marcus CL, Curtis S, Loughlin GM. Inability of clinical history to distinguish primary snoring from obstructive sleep apnea syndrome in children. *Chest* 1995;108:610-8.
6 Section on Pediatric Pulmonology and Subcommittee on Obstructive Sleep Apnea Syndrome. Clinical practice guideline: diagnosis and management of childhood obstructive sleep apnea syndrome. *Pediatrics* 2002;109:704-12.
7 Marcus CL. Pathophysiology of childhood obstructive sleep apnea: current concepts. *Respir Physiol* 2000;119(2-3):143-54.
8 Hill W. On some causes of backwardness and stupidity in children. *BMJ* 1889;2:771-2.
9 Guilleminault C, Eldridge FL, Simmons FB, Dement WC. Sleep apnea in eight children. *Pediatrics* 1976;58(1):23-30.
10 ENT UK. Indications for tonsillectomy: position paper. 2009. www.entuk.org/position_papers/documents/tonsillectomy
11 Royal Australasian College of Physicians and the Australian Society of Otolaryngology Head and Neck Surgery. Indications for tonsillectomy and adenotonsillectomy in children. A joint position paper. 2008. www.racp.edu.au/page/policy-and-advocacy/paediatrics-and-child-health
12 Shine NP, Coates HL, Lannigan FJ. Obstructive sleep apnea, morbid obesity, and adenotonsillar surgery: a review of the literature. *Int J Pediatr Otorhinolaryngol* 2005;69:1475-82.
13 Royal College of Paediatric and Child Health Working Party on Sleep Physiology and Respiratory Control Disorders in Childhood. Standards for services for children with disorders of sleep physiology. 2009. www.rcpch.ac.uk/Research/ce/Guidelines-frontpage/Guideline-Appraisals-by-Organisation/RCPCH-Working-Party.
14 Johns MW. A new method for measuring daytime sleepiness: the Epworth sleepiness scale. *Sleep* 1991;14:540-5.
15 Gozal D, O'Brien LM. Snoring and obstructive sleep apnoea in children: why should we treat? *Paediatr Respir Rev* 2004;5(suppl A):S371-6.
16 Alexopoulos EI, Kostadima E, Pagonari I, Zintzaras E, Gourgoulianis K, Kaditis AG. Association between primary nocturnal enuresis and habitual snoring in children. *Urology* 2006;68:406-9.
17 Brietzke SE, Katz ES, Roberson DW. Can history and physical examination reliably diagnose pediatric obstructive sleep apnea/hypopnea syndrome? A systematic review of the literature. *Otolaryngol Head Neck Surg* 2004;131:827-32.
18 Hill CM, Hogan AM, Karmiloff-Smith A. To sleep, perchance to enrich learning? *Arch Dis Child* 2007;92:637-43.
19 Mitchell RB, Kelly J. Behavior, neurocognition and quality-of-life in children with sleep-disordered breathing. *Int J Pediatr Otorhinolaryngol* 2006;70:395-406.
20 Freezer NJ, Bucens IK, Robertson CF. Obstructive sleep apnoea presenting as failure to thrive in infancy. *J Paediatr Child H* 1995;31:172-5.
21 Kotagal S, Pianosi P. Sleep disorders in children and adolescents. *BMJ* 2006;332:828-32.
22 Brodsky L. Modern assessment of tonsils and adenoids. *Pediatr Clin North Am* 1989;36:1551-69.
23 Nixon GM, Kermack AS, Davis GM, Manoukian JJ, Brown KA, Brouillette RT. Planning adenotonsillectomy in children with obstructive sleep apnea: the role of overnight oximetry. *Pediatrics* 2004;113(1, part 1):e19-25.
24 Brouillette RT, Morielli A, Leimanis A, Waters KA, Luciano R, Ducharme FM. Nocturnal pulse oximetry as an abbreviated testing modality for pediatric obstructive sleep apnea. *Pediatrics* 2000;105:405-12.
25 Robb P, Bew S, Kubba H, Murphy N, Primhak R, Rollin A-M, et al. Tonsillectomy and adenoidectomy in children with sleep related breathing disorders: consensus statement of a UK multidisciplinary working party. *Clin Otolaryngol* 2009;34:61-3.
26 Lim J, McKean MC. Adenotonsillectomy for obstructive sleep apnoea in children. *Cochrane Database Syst Rev* 2009;(2):CD003136.
27 Coticchia JM, Yun RD, Nelson L, Koempel J. Temperature-controlled radiofrequency treatment of tonsillar hypertrophy for reduction of upper airway obstruction in pediatric patients. *Arch Otolaryngol Head Neck Surg* 2006;132:425-30.
28 Brietzke SE, Gallagher D. The effectiveness of tonsillectomy and adenoidectomy in the treatment of pediatric obstructive sleep apnea/hypopnea syndrome: a meta-analysis. *Otolaryngol Head Neck Surg* 2006;134:979-84.
29 Georgalas C, Babar-Craig H, Arora A, Narula A. Health outcome measurements in children with sleep disordered breathing. *Clin Otolaryngol* 2007;32:268-74.
30 Sohn H, Rosenfeld RM. Evaluation of sleep-disordered breathing in children. *Otolaryngol Head Neck Surg* 2003;128:344-52.
31 Mitchell RB, Kelly J, Call E, Yao N. Long-term changes in quality of life after surgery for pediatric obstructive sleep apnea. *Arch Otolaryngol Head Neck Surg* 2004;130:409-12.
32 Marcus CL, Rosen G, Ward SLD, Halbower AC, Sterni L, Lutz J, et al. Adherence to and effectiveness of positive airway pressure therapy in children with obstructive sleep apnea *Pediatrics* 2006;117(3):e442-51.
33 Brouillette RT, Manoukian JJ, Ducharme FM, Oudjhane K, Earle LG, Ladan S, et al. Efficacy of fluticasone nasal spray for pediatric obstructive sleep apnea. *J Pediatr* 2001;138:838-44.
34 Alexopoulos EI, Kaditis AG, Kalampouka E, Kostadima E, Angelopoulos NV, Mikraki V, et al. Nasal corticosteroids for children with snoring. *Pediatr Pulmonol* 2004;38:161-7.
35 Lowe D, van der Meulen J, Cromwell D, Lewsey J, Copley L, Browne J, et al. Key messages from the National Prospective Tonsillectomy Audit. *Laryngoscope* 2007;117:717-24.
36 Gozal D, Capdevila OS, Kheirandish-Gozal L. Metabolic alterations and systemic inflammation in obstructive sleep apnea among

nonobese and obese prepubertal children. *Am J Respir Crit Care Med* 2008;177:1142-9.

BMJ

An overview of how asbestos exposure affects the lung

Graeme P Currie, consultant chest physician[1], Stephen J Watt, consultant chest physician[1], Nick A Maskell, consultant chest physician[2]

[1]Chest Clinic C, Aberdeen Royal Infirmary, Aberdeen AB25 2ZN

[2]North Bristol Lung Centre, Southmead Hospital, University of Bristol, Bristol BS10 5NB

Correspondence to: G P Currie graeme.currie@nhs.net

Cite this as: *BMJ* 2009;339:b3209

<DOI> 10.1136/bmj.b3209
http://www.bmj.com/content/339/bmj.b3209

People exposed to asbestos often develop lung disease in later life; manifestations include benign, malignant, or diffuse interstitial lung disease. This evidence based review covers who is considered to be at risk, different ways that exposure to asbestos affect the lung, and matters relating to compensation. Because many doctors in primary and secondary care encounter patients who have been exposed to asbestos, they need to be aware of how different people can be affected.

Who is at risk of asbestos related lung disease?

All people who have worked with asbestos are at potential risk of asbestos related lung disease through inhalation of fibres. Asbestos is a mineral silicate that occurs naturally in various forms. It is resistant to heat and other means of destruction, which explains its extensive use during the 19th and 20th centuries. The fibrous nature of asbestos allows it to be woven into cloth or incorporated into cement materials, ceiling tiles, brake and clutch linings, pipe and boiler insulation, flooring, resins, polymers, and filter papers.

Historically, people with the highest exposures worked in asbestos mining, milling, and production of asbestos textiles. Countries that currently produce large amounts of asbestos include Russia, Kazakhstan, China, and Canada. In the 1920s to 1940s asbestosis developed in textile workers with a latency of only a few years and progressed rapidly to death, because exposure was high.[1 w1 w2] The risk to people using asbestos products was recognised in shipyard workers in the 1950s, and an association with mesothelioma was determined in the 1960s through a case-control study in South African miners.[2] However, one of the first suggestions that exposure to asbestos can cause lung disease was in 1899 in an industrial diseases board of enquiry.[3] Today, most people with asbestos related lung disease have a clear history of exposure, such as mixing asbestos cement or fitting insulation (builders), working with asbestos insulation materials (plumbers and electricians), or cutting asbestos cement sheet materials, although some may have been exposed without their knowledge (for example, shipyard workers or ship engineering workers). The lifetime risk of developing mesothelioma was highlighted in a recent study in which joiners, plumbers, electricians, painters, and construction workers had a greater likelihood of being diagnosed within the general population.[4] The occurrence of asbestos related lung disease in spouses who laundered the clothing of workers exposed to asbestos is also well established.[5] A detailed occupational history—to determine the occupation, what it involved, dates of employment, and length of asbestos exposure—is therefore important in all patients presenting with respiratory symptoms.[w3] Because of the unregulated use of asbestos in developing countries, the incidence of asbestos related lung disease worldwide is likely to rise significantly in the years ahead.

SOURCES AND SELECTION CRITERIA

We comprehensively searched articles published up to February 2009 using PubMed and Medline. Key words and phrases used were "asbestos", "malignant mesothelioma", "pleural plaques", "pleural thickening", "asbestosis", "lung cancer", "cigarette smoking", "pleural effusions", "compensation", "occupation", "chemotherapy", "radiotherapy", "surgery", "treatment", and "survival"

SUMMARY POINTS

- The risk of asbestos related lung disease is dose related and depends on fibre type
- Joiners, plumbers, electricians, painters, shipyard workers, builders, engineers, and asbestos miners are at greatest risk
- Asbestos exposure can cause benign disease (pleural plaques, pleural thickening, benign pleural effusions), malignant disease (mesothelioma, lung cancer), and interstitial lung disease (asbestosis)
- Mesothelioma will peak in incidence between 2011 and 2015; it should be considered in all patients with a pleural effusion, chest pain, and history of asbestos exposure
- Treatment options in asbestosis are limited
- Some patients are entitled to compensation and should seek advice from the Department of Work and Pensions or dedicated charity organisations

How does asbestos affect the lung?

The shape of asbestos fibres results in their retention within the lung. Clearance from the lung occurs by the mucociliary ladder and phagocytic ingestion by macrophages or endocytosis by pneumocytes, but migration to the pleural surface can occur via the lymphatic system.[6] The common forms of asbestos exist as serpentine curved fibres (chrysotile (white)) or amphibole straight fibres (crocidolite (blue), amosite (brown), and anthophyllite). Curved fibres carry a slightly lower risk of lung disease than straight fibres,[w4] although no safe threshold of exposure to asbestos of any type exists.

What sort of lung disease can asbestos cause?

Benign pleural disease

Pleural plaques

Pleural plaques consist of layers of hyalinised collagen fibres usually found on the parietal pleura, and they occur in 20-60% of people who have been exposed to asbestos.[7 w5] They most commonly appear as calcified areas adjacent to the sixth to ninth ribs and along the surface of the diaphragm, but they tend not to be evident at the lung apices or costophrenic angles. Pleural plaques can usually be identified on a chest radiograph (fig 1), although computed tomography is more sensitive and distinguishes them from solid tumours if the diagnosis is uncertain. They do not undergo malignant change or generally cause symptoms, although pleural plaques have been associated with anginal pain.[8]

Diffuse pleural thickening

Diffuse thickening of the pleura is less specific to asbestos exposure than pleural plaques. It may occur after exposure to asbestos, but other causes include previous haemothorax,

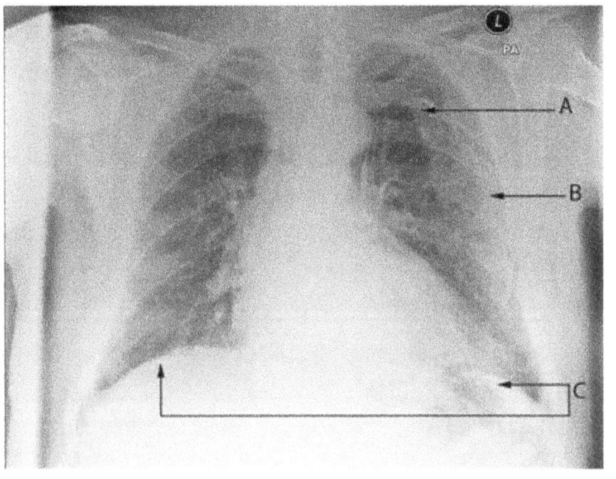

Fig 1 Chest radiograph showing pleural plaques (A), pleural thickening (B), and calcification of the diaphragm (C)

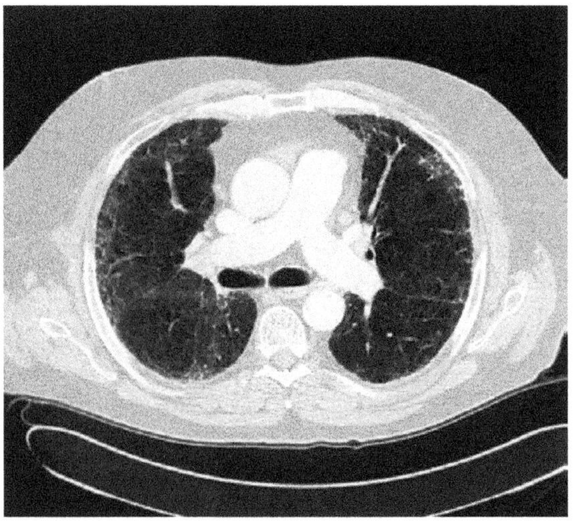

Fig 2 Computed tomograph showing typical features of asbestosis; note the peripheral interstial change

tuberculosis, chest surgery, radiation, infection, and exposure to drugs such as methysergide. Diffuse pleural thickening on a chest radiograph is characterised by a smooth continuous pleural density affecting at least 25% of the lateral chest wall, with or without blunting of the costophrenic angle.[w6] It has also been defined on computed tomography as a continuous sheet of pleural thickening (>5 cm wide, >8 cm in craniocaudal extent, and >3 mm thick).[9] In extensive diffuse pleural thickening, patients may become breathless and have a restrictive ventilatory defect on lung function tests. In diffuse thickening (which is usually bilateral), the pleura will appear smooth, and the mediastinal border will be unaffected, whereas in mesothelioma, the pleura is likely to be unilaterally irregularly thickened and the mediastinal border affected. If the diagnosis is uncertain, computed tomography and biopsy are warranted.

Benign asbestos related pleural effusion

Benign exudative pleural effusions are often preceded by episodes of "asbestos pleurisy." They can occur within 15 years of asbestos exposure[10] but may also appear much later.[w7] Because of confusion with a malignant effusion, a pleural biopsy is usually needed, and this shows non-specific inflammation. Benign effusions may resolve spontaneously (often leaving an area of pleural thickening) or require drainage if large enough to cause symptoms.

Interstitial lung disease

Asbestosis

Asbestosis is caused by inhalation of asbestos fibres and is a typical pneumoconiosis (interstitial lung disease caused by inhaled inorganic dusts). The condition is directly related to the magnitude and duration of exposure to asbestos.[11] After a latent period of 20-30 years, patients with developing asbestosis experience an insidious onset of breathlessness and reduced exercise tolerance; cough, sputum production, and wheezing are less common. As the condition progresses, fine bilateral inspiratory crackles, finger clubbing, and cor pulmonale may occur. Data from the Health and Safety Executive indicated that 111 deaths in the United Kingdom in 2006 were caused by asbestosis, and that 393 death certificates mentioned asbestosis (www.hse.gov.uk/statistics/causdis/asbestosis/index.htm).

Pulmonary function tests show reduced gas transfer, reduced lung volumes, a restrictive ventilatory defect, and exercise related hypoxaemia. Chest radiography may be normal,[12] but usually shows bilateral lower zone interstitial changes, often with pleural plaques and thickening. High resolution computed tomography is a more sensitive tool (fig 2), and characteristic features include coarse parenchymal bands, subpleural linear densities, interstitial fibrotic change, and honeycombing in advanced disease.[13] In contrast to idiopathic pulmonary fibrosis, confluent ground glass changes are rare in asbestosis, whereas thick band-like opacities are more common[w8]; the most discriminatory feature is concomitant pleural disease in asbestosis. Histological evidence is not necessary for the diagnosis to be made: typical clinical features along with previous asbestos exposure, consistent pulmonary function abnormalities, interstitial fibrosis (with no alternative explanation), plus other radiographic changes seen after exposure to asbestos are usually adequate. No specific treatment is available other than that for chronic obstructive pulmonary disease and cor pulmonale if present, smoking cessation, and prevention of further exposure to asbestos. The prognosis of asbestosis is highly variable and depends on the extent of lung involvement and severity of coexisting chronic obstructive pulmonary disease and presence of other comorbidities.

Malignant disease

Lung cancer

Exposure to asbestos causes lung cancer independently of cigarette smoking.[14 w9] In an analysis of 23 epidemiological studies, asbestos exposure increased the risk of lung cancer by a similar factor in non-smokers and smokers, with a synergistic (multiplicative) interaction seen between asbestos exposure and cigarette smoking.[14] Even in the absence of asbestosis, very heavy asbestos exposure may cause lung cancer.[w10] Lung cancer should be considered in patients with asbestosis who have haemoptysis, worsening cough, chest pain and breathlessness, weight loss, and anorexia. Diagnostic and management strategies are the same as those for lung cancer in general (www.sign.ac.uk; www.nice.org.uk).

Mesothelioma

Malignant mesothelioma is an aggressive pleural tumour with increasing incidence.[15 16] Data from the UK mesothelioma register indicated that the annual number of deaths from mesothelioma had risen from 153 in 1968 to 1848 in 2001, and it is predicted to peak at 1950-2450 cases annually between 2011 and 2015.[17] In 2006, the UK Health and Safety Executive gave the number of deaths from mesothelioma on death certificates as 2056 (85% male; www.hse.gov.uk/statistics/causdis/mesothelioma/). However, official mortality data may underestimate the extent by 10%.[w11]

In one well conducted study of 622 patients with mesothelioma (512 men), disease was caused by occupational or domestic asbestos exposure in 86% of men and 38% of women. Around half of the men were construction workers, and only four had worked for more than five years in the manufacture of asbestos products.[4] The lag period between initial exposure and death varies, but one retrospective analysis (1105 patients with definite mesothelioma) found a median latency of 32 years, with 96% of cases occurring after at least 20 years.[w12]

Focus on mesothelioma

The diagnosis of malignant mesothelioma is based on a combination of clinical, radiological, and histological features. However, a clear histological diagnosis removes any uncertainty and makes compensation claims more straightforward.

Clinical presentation

British Thoracic Society guidelines suggest that malignant mesothelioma should be considered in any patient with a pleural effusion or pleural thickening, especially if a history of asbestos exposure and chest pain is present.[15] Characteristically, the pain is dull, diffuse, progressive, and occasionally pleuritic. Breathlessness may be caused by a pleural effusion or circumferential pleural thickening. Patients may also present with a palpable chest wall mass, finger clubbing (usually caused by underlying asbestosis), and features of a pericardial effusion caused by local extension in progressive disease. Ascites caused by peritoneal mesothelioma and secondary hydropneumothorax are uncommon but recognised presentations.

Investigations

Chest radiography and computed tomography may show a pleural effusion, lobulated or nodular pleural changes, a pleural mass, rib destruction, chest wall involvement, or a small hemithorax as a result of lung entrapment (fig 3); other features of exposure to asbestos may also be present.

Pleural fluid in patients with mesothelioma is straw coloured or blood stained. Cytological analysis of pleural fluid occasionally leads to the diagnosis, although a pleural biopsy is usually needed. Percutaneous pleural biopsy has historically been performed using an Abram's needle,[18 19] although this procedure is no longer recommended because of the availability and superiority of ultrasound or computed tomography guided percutaneous biopsy.[15] For example, in one study, 50 patients with a cytologically negative (although suspected malignant) pleural effusion were randomised to either Abram's pleural biopsy or computed tomography guided biopsy.[20] The first method correctly diagnosed malignancy in eight of 17 patients (sensitivity 47%, specificity 100%), whereas computed tomography guided biopsy diagnosed malignancy in 13 of 15 (sensitivity 87%, specificity 100%; difference in sensitivity between procedures 40%, 95% confidence interval 10% to 69%, P=0.02). An alternative surgical diagnostic procedure consists of a video assisted thoracoscopic approach that allows multiple biopsies to be taken under direct visualisation; this technique also allows talc pleurodesis to be performed at the same time if malignancy is highly likely. Thoracoscopy under local anaesthetic (enabling drainage of pleural fluid, biopsy, and pleurodesis) is becoming increasingly available across the UK and may be carried out by appropriately trained physicians.

Treatment

Patients with mesothelioma should be discussed at a lung multidisciplinary team meeting (comprising chest physicians, surgeons, radiologists, pathologists, oncologists, and specialist nurses; see box).[15 w13] Although the benefits are uncertain, prophylactic radiotherapy to the pleural puncture site is often considered in patients who have had large chest wall incisions (during thoracoscopy or insertion of a large bore chest tube) to reduce the chance of tumour cells seeding along the track to the skin surface.[21]

Palliative chemotherapy is offered to fit patients, despite a paucity of data showing any survival advantage. In one study, 448 patients were randomised to receive pemetrexed plus cisplatin or cisplatin alone. Median survival with permetrexed and cisplatin was 12 months versus nine months with cisplatin alone (P=0.002).[22] In another study of 250 patients,[23] raltitrexed and cisplatin significantly improved overall survival compared with cisplatin alone, although no differences in quality of life were seen, and the study had no placebo arm. The role of surgery is controversial,[24] but recent data suggest that extrapleural pneumonectomy is not useful in the management of mesothelioma[25]; however, the results of other trials are awaited (MesoVATS and MARS2). Lung sparing debulking procedures are now gaining popularity and should be considered for patients within the context of randomised trials.

The prognosis of malignant mesothelioma—especially in older men who are unfit and have peritoneal mesothelioma and sarcomatoid histology—is poor. The median survival in a variety of studies is between eight and 14 months from diagnosis.[15]

Who is entitled to compensation?

Patients with asbestos related lung disease may be eligible for compensation through Industrial Injuries Disablement Benefit (IIDB) from the Department of Social Security or a civil law claim for damages from the employer under whose auspices exposure occurred (table). Under the UK Limitation Act 1980, patients have only three years in which

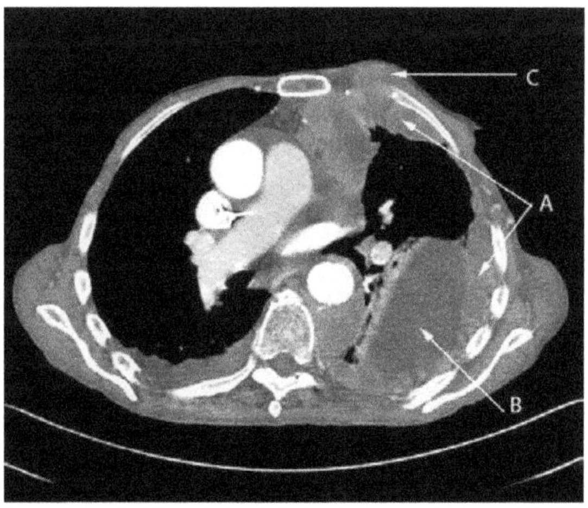

Fig 3 Computed tomography showing typical features of mesothelioma (A, pleural based masses; B, pleural fluid; C, palpable chest wall mass; note the reduction in size of the left hemithorax)

Compensation options according to type of lung disease

Condition	Type of compensation possible	Notes
Pleural plaques	None	Existing legislation currently being reviewed*
Diffuse pleural thickening	IIDB and lump sum under PWCA; civil claim	For a civil claim, patients must have loss of respiratory reserve plus evidence of diffuse bilateral pleural thickening on computed tomography
Asbestos related lung cancer	IIDB and lump sum under PWCA; civil claim	For a civil claim, patients need to have asbestosis plus lung cancer, or a high enough degree of asbestos exposure to have doubled the risk of lung cancer
Asbestosis	IIDB and lump sum under PWCA; civil claim	For a civil claim, patients must have loss of respiratory reserve plus evidence of asbestosis on computed tomography
Mesothelioma with occupational asbestos exposure	IIDB payable weekly and lump sum under PWCA; civil claim	
Mesothelioma with non-occupational asbestos exposure	Lump sum under the Mesothelioma Lump Sum Payments Regulation; no IIDB; possible civil claim	Mesothelioma Lump Sum Payments Regulations (available from October 2008); civil claim may be possible with secondary asbestos history (for example, spouse washing husband's overalls)

**Currently, legislation in Scotland differs from that in the rest of the United Kingdom.*

IIDB = Industrial Injuries Disablement Benefit; PWCA = Pneumoconiosis Workers' Compensation Act 1979.

MANAGEMENT STRATEGIES IN MESOTHELIOMA

- Discuss at a multidisciplinary team meeting
- Skilful and empathetic communication of the diagnosis is needed, with provision of written patient centred information
- Provide the patient with access to specialist nurses
- Liaise closely with primary care and arrange secondary care follow-up
- Discuss compensation with the patient
- Drain pleural effusions then carry out pleurodesis (talc is most effective)
- Consider an indwelling pleural catheter if pleurodesis is unsuccessful or a trapped lung is present
- Consider prophylactic or palliative radiotherapy to large biopsy or drainage sites
- Consider chemotherapy
- Consider surgery
- Consider entry into a clinical trial
- Provide the patient with access to palliative care professionals and pain clinics

ADDITIONAL EDUCATIONAL RESOURCES

Additional resources for healthcare professionals

- British Thoracic Society (www.brit-thoracic.org.uk)—The main UK respiratory society for clinicians
- Mesothelioma Framework (www.dh.gov.uk/prod_consum_dh/groups/dh_digitalassets/documents/digitalasset/dh_072347.pdf)—Department of Health website that provides advice on how to organise services for patients with mesothelioma

Resources for patients

- National Asbestos Helpline (www.nationalasbestos.co.uk)—Provides help on legal matters for patients with asbestos related lung disease
- Macmillan Cancer Support (www.macmillan.org.uk)—UK charity that aims to improve the lives of people affected by cancer
- Mesothelioma UK (www.mesothelioma.uk.com/)—Provides impartial up to date information for patients diagnosed with mesothelioma and their carers
- Cancer research UK (www.cancerresearchuk.org/)—UK charity dedicated to cancer research
- British Lung Foundation (www.lunguk.org)—A leading UK charity helping those with respiratory disorders

TIPS FOR NON-SPECIALISTS

- Take a detailed occupational history in all patients with symptoms and signs of lung disease
- Ask specifically about previous asbestos exposure in patients with chest wall pain, haemoptysis, and breathlessness
- Find out about any previous asbestos exposure in patients with a pleural effusion, features of interstitial lung disease, a lung mass, or diagnosed lung cancer
- Make sure compensation has been discussed with patients with an asbestos related lung disease
- Emphasise the importance of smoking cessation in people who have been exposed to asbestos; explain that continuing to smoke increases the risk of lung cancer
- Refer patients with a suspected asbestos related lung disease to a chest physician

to make a civil claim from the date they became aware of a serious injury caused by an act or omission of the proposed defendant. Patients should be advised to consult their local Department of Work and Pensions benefit agency for advice on benefits that may be claimed (which may include attendance allowance and disability living allowance). Various charities can also provide help and support on compensation. Some compensation requests involve lengthy periods of negotiation (especially civil claims), and patients should be made aware of this to help minimise psychological distress. Former Ministry of Defence personnel who develop asbestos related diseases are unable to sue the crown for an industrial injury that occurred before 1987 because of "crown immunity," although they may be eligible to receive a war pension.

Thanks to Peter Montgomery for reviewing the section on compensation.

Contributors: GPC had the original idea for the manuscript and wrote it along with SJW and NAM. GPC is guarantor.

Competing interests: None declared.

Provenance and peer review: Commissioned based on an idea from the author; externally peer reviewed.

1 Wood WB, Gloyne SR. Pulmonary asbestosis. *Lancet* 1930;i:445.
2 Wagner JC, Sleggs CA, Marchand P. Diffuse pleural mesothelioma and asbestos exposure in the North Western Cape Province. *Br J Ind Med* 1960;17:260-71.
3 Tweedale G, Hansen P. Protecting the workers: the medical board and the asbestos industry, 1930s-1960s. *Med Hist* 1998;42:439-57.
4 Rake C, Gilham C, Hatch J, Darnton A, Hodgson J, Peto J. Occupational, domestic and environmental mesothelioma risks in the British population: a case-control study. *Br J Cancer* 2009;100:1175-83.
5 Ferrante D, Bertolotti M, Todesco A, Mirabelli D, Terracini B, Magnani C. Cancer mortality and incidence of mesothelioma in a cohort of wives of asbestos workers in Casale Monferrato, Italy. *Environ Health Perspect* 2007;115:1401-5.
6 Brody AR, Hill LH, Adkins B Jr, O'Connor RW. Chrysotile asbestos inhalation in rats: deposition pattern and reaction of alveolar epithelium and pulmonary macrophages. *Am Rev Respir Dis* 1981;123:670-9.
7 Merchant JA. Human epidemiology: a review of fiber type and characteristics in the development of malignant and nonmalignant disease. *Environ Health Perspect* 1990;88:287-93.
8 Mukherjee S, de Klerk N, Palmer LJ, Olsen NJ, Pang SC, Musk AW. Chest pain in asbestos-exposed individuals with benign pleural and parenchymal disease. *Am J Respir Crit Care Med* 2000;162:1807-11.
9 Lynch DA, Gamsu G, Aberle DR. Conventional and high resolution computed tomography in the diagnosis of asbestos-related diseases. *Radiographics* 1989;9:523-51.
10 Wagner GR. Asbestosis and silicosis. *Lancet* 1997;349:1311-5.
11 Wagner GR. The fallout from asbestos. *Lancet* 2007;369:973-4.
12 Kipen HM, Lilis R, Suzuki Y, Valciukas JA, Selikoff IJ. Pulmonary fibrosis in asbestos insulation workers with lung cancer: a radiological and histopathological evaluation. *Br J Ind Med* 1987;44:96-100.
13 Fletcher DE, Edge JR. The early radiological changes in pulmonary and pleural asbestosis. *Clin Radiol* 1970;21:355-65.
14 Lee PN. Relation between exposure to asbestos and smoking jointly and the risk of lung cancer. *Occup Environ Med* 2001;58:145-53.
15 British Thoracic Society. BTS statement on malignant mesothelioma in the UK, 2007. *Thorax* 2007;62(suppl 2):ii1-19.

16 Mak V, Davies E, Putcha V, Choodari-Oskooei B, Moller H. The epidemiology and treatment of mesothelioma in South East England 1985-2002. *Thorax* 2008;63:160-6.
17 Hodgson JT, McElvenny DM, Darnton AJ, Price MJ, Peto J. The expected burden of mesothelioma mortality in Great Britain from 2002 to 2050. *Br J Cancer* 2005;92:587-93.
18 Walshe AD, Douglas JG, Kerr KM, McKean ME, Godden DJ. An audit of the clinical investigation of pleural effusion. *Thorax* 1992;47:734-7.
19 McLaughlin KM, Kerr KM, Currie GP. Closed pleural biopsy to diagnose mesothelioma: Dead or alive? *Lung Cancer* 2009;65:388-98.
20 Maskell NA, Gleeson FV, Davies RJ. Standard pleural biopsy versus CT-guided cutting-needle biopsy for diagnosis of malignant disease in pleural effusions: a randomised controlled trial. *Lancet* 2003;361:1326-30.
21 Davies HE, Musk AW, Lee YC. Prophylactic radiotherapy for pleural puncture sites in mesothelioma: the controversy continues. *Curr Opin Pulm Med* 2008;14:326-30.
22 Vogelzang NJ, Rusthoven JJ, Symanowski J, Denham C, Kaukel E, Ruffie P, et al. Phase III study of pemetrexed in combination with cisplatin versus cisplatin alone in patients with malignant pleural mesothelioma. *J Clin Oncol* 2003;21:2636-44.
23 Van Meerbeeck JP, Gaafar R, Manegold C, Van Klaveren RJ, Van Marck EA, Vincent M, et al. Randomized phase III study of cisplatin with or without raltitrexed in patients with malignant pleural mesothelioma: an intergroup study of the European Organisation for Research and Treatment of Cancer Lung Cancer Group and the National Cancer Institute of Canada. *J Clin Oncol* 2005;23:6881-9.
24 Treasure T, Utley M. Ten traps for the unwary in surgical series: a case study in mesothelioma reports. *J Thorac Cardiovasc Surg* 2007;133:1414-8.
25 Flores RM, Pass HI, Seshan VE, Dycoco J, Zakowski M, Carbone M, et al. Extrapleural pneumonectomy versus pleurectomy/decortication in the surgical management of malignant pleural mesothelioma: results in 663 patients. *J Thorac Cardiovasc Surg* 2008;135:620-6.

BMJ BPP UNIVERSITY SCHOOL OF HEALTH

The changing epidemiology of lung cancer with a focus on screening

Gerard A Silvestri, professor of medicine[1], Anthony J Alberg, associate professor of epidemiology [2], James Ravenel, associate professor of radiology[3]

[1]Division of Pulmonary and Critical Care Medicine, Medical University of South Carolina, Charleston, SC 29425, USA

[2]Hollings Cancer Center and Department of Biostatistics, Bioinformatics, and Epidemiology, Medical University of South Carolina

[3]Department of Radiology, Medical University of South Carolina

Correspondence to: G A Silvestri silvestri@musc.edu

Cite this as: *BMJ* 2009;339:b3053

‹DOI› 10.1136/bmj.b3053 http://www.bmj.com/content/339/bmj.b3053

Lung cancer is a global public health problem of epidemic proportions, and the number of people affected is expected to grow in the near future. Worldwide, in 2002 more than 1.3 million people were newly diagnosed with lung cancer.[1] It is the leading global cause of death from cancer, and it accounts for 18% of all deaths from cancer and more than one million deaths a year since as far back as 1993.[2] [3] Lung cancer is the 10th leading overall cause of death, and it is expected to move to fifth place as its incidence rises in developing countries. Lung cancer is a disease that seems to fit the profile for a successful screening programme. However, developing an efficacious screening test that meets the established criteria for screening has proved elusive, despite evidence from many screening trials, and screening remains controversial. This review aims to shed light on the questions surrounding screening for lung cancer.

What are the established causes of lung cancer?

Active cigarette smoking is the main cause—it accounts for 85-90% of all lung cancers.[2] [w1-w5] In addition, exposure to secondhand cigarette smoke; pipe and cigar smoking; occupational exposure to agents such as asbestos, nickel, chromium, and arsenic; exposure to radiation, including radon gas in homes; and exposure to air pollution are all established risk factors for lung cancer.[2] There has been longstanding interest in genetic susceptibility to lung cancer, and results of recent genome-wide association studies consistently point to the long arm of chromosome 15 as being linked to increased risk.[4] [5] [w6-w8]

What is the emerging global picture of lung cancer?

Whereas in the mid-1900s the lung cancer epidemic was largely confined to developed nations, by 2002 the absolute numbers of newly diagnosed lung cancers occurring in developed and developing countries were nearly equal.[1] [6]

Considerable geographical variation exists, with a greater than 20-fold variation in occurrence across countries (figure).[2] [7] As of 2002, the age adjusted annual incidence ranges from a high of 65.7 per 100 000 in Central and Eastern Europe to less than 25 per 100 000 in Africa, with most of that continent at less than five per 100 000 (figure).[1] [7] The occurrence of lung cancer is so strongly determined by cigarette smoking that historical and current smoking prevalence data can help reliably forecast the future patterns of occurrence.

Countries where the lung cancer epidemic is in its infancy, or it is in full force without signs of coming under control, are of greatest public health concern. The hallmark characteristics of a country in transition from lower to higher rates of lung cancer are a low current incidence of lung cancer but a high current prevalence of cigarette smoking. The high prevalence of smoking in these countries foretells a future epidemic of lung cancer. Countries in the middle of an uncontrolled epidemic of lung cancer are those with high current mortality from lung cancer coupled with a high current prevalence of cigarette smoking. The populations of such countries are at the highest risk at present and for the foreseeable future. Korea, the Russian Federation, Kazakhstan, Poland, and Hungary fall into this last category as far as men are concerned, whereas in Venezuela, Germany, Norway, the United States, and Denmark women are at the greatest current and future risk.[8]

Populations may avoid the lung cancer epidemic entirely if cigarette smoking never becomes prevalent, as has historically been the case in many African countries. Unfortunately, several African countries have recently experienced a surge in cigarette smoking.[9] Conversely, the high burden of lung cancer currently seen in some countries will decrease because public health efforts have reduced the prevalence of smoking. Risks are now lower for men in Singapore, Canada, Germany, the United Kingdom, the US, the Netherlands, and Belgium, and for women in Malaysia, Korea, Bahrain, the Philippines, Canada, and Belgium.

Chinese men will strongly influence the global burden of lung cancer in the 21st century because they have a high prevalence of cigarette smoking and they form a large proportion of the world's population. Per capita cigarette consumption among Chinese men has risen from one cigarette per day in 1952, to four in 1972, to 10 in 1992.[10] The rate of smoking among Chinese men today is equivalent to the highest rates ever seen in developed countries. The incidence of lung cancer has already risen, with more substantial increases yet to come.[11] Socioeconomic status is inversely associated with the incidence of lung cancer and mortality. A recent study of nearly 400 000 Europeans found a higher risk of lung cancer in the least well educated populations (a proxy for socioeconomic status). Adjustment for smoking reduced the risk of lung cancer by 50% in men and women in all regions and for all histological types.[12]

With a sustained global burden of lung cancer projected for the coming decades, a method of early detection that could effectively reduce mortality from lung cancer would potentially have an enormous public health benefit.

SUMMARY POINTS

- Lung cancer is the most common cancer worldwide
- Incidence varies greatly between countries because of the varying prevalence of cigarette smoking
- The epidemic of lung cancer has just begun in developing countries, although a decrease is being seen in some developed countries
- Screening for lung cancer using low dose computed tomography has not been proved to be efficacious
- Several large randomised controlled trials to assess the efficacy of screening for lung cancer are under way
- Screening for lung cancer cannot be recommended outside a well designed clinical trial

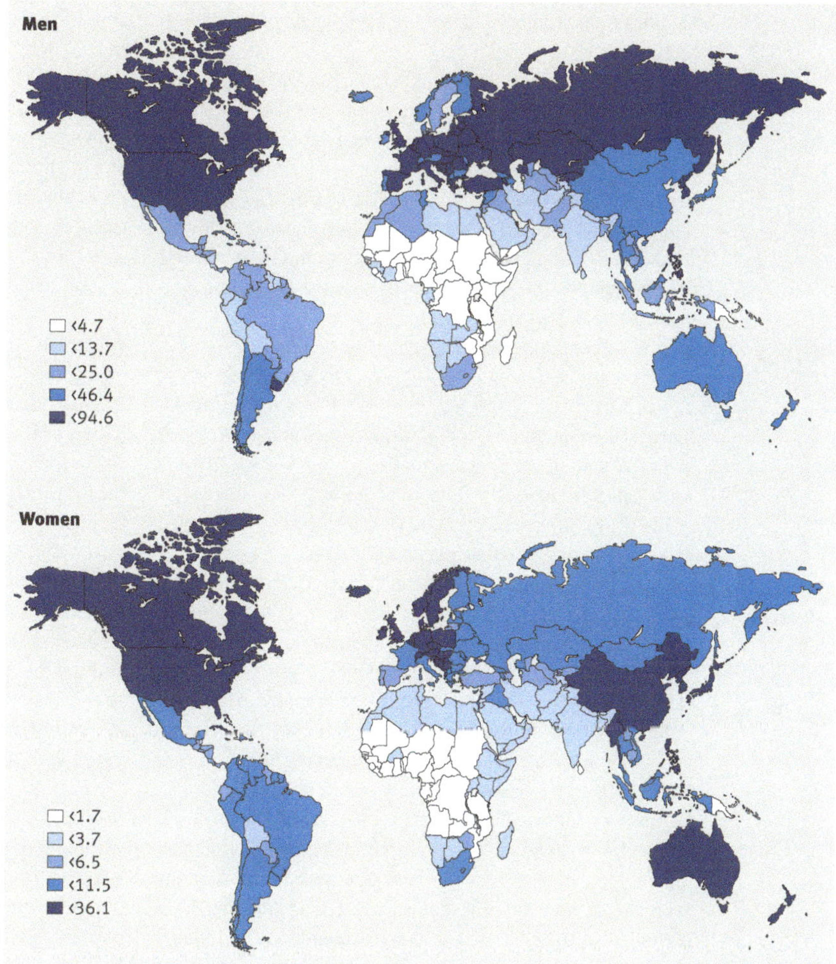

Global annual incidence (per 100 000) of lung cancer in men and women. Adapted, with permission, from GLOBOCAN 2002[7]

Why consider screening for lung cancer?

Three quarters of patients with lung cancer present with symptoms of advanced incurable disease.[13] Despite advances in treatment, the five year survival rate for all stages combined is around 16%.[14] Outcomes are significantly better in patients diagnosed at earlier stages, with a five year survival for stage I disease of 60-75%.[15 w9-w11] An efficacious screening test that could result in early detection and reduced mortality would thus represent a major advance in combating mortality from lung cancer.

TEN CRITERIA FOR EFFECTIVE SCREENING

- The disease has serious consequences
- The screening population has a high prevalence of detectable preclinical disease
- The screening test detects little pseudodisease (overdiagnosis)
- The screening test has high accuracy for detecting preclinical disease
- The screening test detects disease before the critical point
- The screening test causes little morbidity
- The screening test is affordable and available
- Treatment exists
- Treatment is more effective when applied before symptomatic detection
- Treatment is not too risky or toxic

Does screening lead to reduced mortality from lung cancer?

Principles of a screening test

Screening is the process of detecting disease before it becomes symptomatic. For a screening test to be effective, certain criteria must be met regarding the disease, the proposed screening test, and treatment (box).[16] The disease must have serious consequences and be readily detectable in the preclinical phase. The test should have a high accuracy, detect the disease before a critical point, cause little morbidity, be available and affordable, and result in little overdiagnosis. Finally, treatment for the disease must exist, and it must be effective before symptoms occur, with little risk or morbidity. Both chest radiography and computed tomography have been evaluated as screening tests for lung cancer.

Findings from studies evaluating chest radiography

Several randomised trials in the 1960-1980s screened for lung cancer using chest radiography and found no difference in mortality between the screened and unscreened groups, even though more early stage cancers were identified in the screening group.[17] Late stage cancers were not reduced, and deaths from lung cancer were higher in the screened group after 20 years of follow-up, probably because of overdiagnosis.[18 w12-w17]

Findings from studies of screening using chest computed tomography

Low radiation dose computed tomography uses lower doses of radiation than standard techniques to generate an image. Nodules as small as 2-3 mm can be detected, which means that this method detects at least three times as many small lung nodules as a standard chest radiograph.[19] The only evidence on screening for lung cancer using this method is from observational cohort studies that provide information on the distribution of disease stage and survival of the screened population but do not measure efficacy of screening in reducing mortality.

Cohort studies conducted in Japan which included 15 050 at risk participants detected 72 lung cancers during prevalence screening (0.5%), 57 of which were stage IA.[20 21 22] In 21 762 annual incidence screens, 60 (0.3%) new cancers were detected, of which 50 were stage IA.

The Early Lung Cancer Action Project (ELCAP) screened 1000 asymptomatic volunteers with at least a 10 pack year (number of cigarettes smoked each day times number of years smoked) history of smoking with chest radiography and low radiation dose computed tomography.[23] Non-calcified lung nodules were detected in 23% using computed tomography and 7% using chest radiography. Malignant nodules were detected in 2.7% by computed tomography compared with 0.7% by chest radiography. Twenty seven lung cancers were identified and 23 were stage I.

This was followed by a prospective study at the Mayo Clinic of low radiation dose computed tomography screening in 1520 high risk subjects.[19] One year after baseline scanning, a total of 2244 non-calcified lung nodules were identified in 1000 of the 1520 participants (66%). Twenty five cases of lung cancer were diagnosed (22 prevalent cases and three incident cases), and 22 patients underwent surgical resection. Twelve of the 21 non-small cell cancers detected were stage IA at diagnosis. After five years of annual computed tomography scanning,[24] a total of 3356 non-calcified nodules were found in 73.5% of the cohort; about 95% of the nodules were found to be benign with clinical follow-up or surgical biopsy. Sixty eight primary lung tumours were documented in 66 participants, 34 on annual (incidence) studies and three interval lung cancers not detected through annual screening. Of the incident cancers, 21 were stage I and 11 presented at stage III or IV. The large proportion of non-calcified nodules found (5-51%) is problematic because most will turn out to be benign but will require further evaluation, including serial computed tomography scans, biopsy, or in some cases surgical resection, which can carry serious morbidity and a low but real risk of death.

A large multicentre multinational non-randomised trial, the International ELCAP (I-ELCAP) was recently reported.[25] This trial screened 31 567 subjects using low radiation dose computed tomography. Lung cancer was detected in 484 patients (1.3%), 412 of whom had stage I disease. Estimated 10 year survival was 80% for all patients regardless of stage and treatment, and 88% for stage I cancer. This study confirmed earlier observations that lung cancers detected by computed tomography screening are at an early stage and are highly treatable.

This study provides a basis for optimism, but it cannot confirm the efficacy of screening for lung cancer with low radiation dose computed tomography because, although survival was higher in people diagnosed with early stage lung cancer, the study was not designed to assess whether screening reduces overall mortality in patients with lung cancer. A comment on the study gave four reasons why the findings did not make a persuasive case for screening.[26] Firstly, the lack of a control group precluded the study from investigating what would happen to a similar group of patients in the absence of screening. Secondly, lack of an unbiased outcome measure meant that the confounding features of lead time, length time, and overdiagnosis bias were not controlled for. Thirdly, the study did not take into account what is already known about lung cancer screening, particularly the evidence for overdiagnosis bias arising in single arm studies from Japan.[22] Finally, although the study emphasised the positive aspects of screening, it did not discuss potential harms, especially the unnecessary investigation or treatment of benign disease.

The positive findings of the I-ELCAP trial contrast with those from a longitudinal study that examined three populations of current or former smokers, one in Italy and two in the US. The study screened 3246 people annually with computed tomography and had a median follow-up of 3.9 years.[27] The numbers of observed new cases of lung cancer, resections for lung cancer, cases of advanced lung cancer, and deaths from lung cancer were compared with the numbers predicted using two validated models. One hundred and forty four people were diagnosed with lung cancer compared with 44.5 expected cases (relative risk 3.2, 95% confidence interval 2.7 to 3.8; P<0.001). The rate of lung cancer resection was 10 times higher than expected—109 compared with the 10.9 predicted for that cohort (10.0, 8.2 to 11.9; P<0.001). There were 42 cases of advanced lung cancer compared with 33.4 expected cases and 38 deaths, which is the number predicted for that cohort (1.0, 0.7 to 1.3; P=0.90). This study showed that screening with low radiation dose computed tomography increased the detection of lung cancers and the numbers of tumours resected, but it did not reduce the risk of advanced lung cancer or of overall mortality from lung cancer. The survival of patients with stage I tumours that were resected was similar to that seen by the I-ELCAP investigators.

What can we conclude?

Results from observational computed tomography studies show that low radiation dose computed tomography can detect early lung cancer in asymptomatic people. However, we still do not know whether early detection reduces mortality from lung cancer or is cost effective.[28] For this reason, the National Cancer Institute has instituted the National Lung Screening Trial (NLST; www.cancer.gov/nlst). The NLST is a randomised controlled trial that by 2004 recruited nearly 50 000 current or former smokers and randomised them to screening with chest radiography (the control group) or helical computed tomography. Subjects were screened for three years and are now being followed up. The NLST is powered to detect a 20% reduction in mortality from lung cancer by screening with spiral computed tomography compared with chest radiography.

The NELSON trial is a European computed tomography based screening trial being conducted in the Netherlands and Denmark.[29] Almost 20 000 at risk participants have been randomised to computed tomography screening versus no screening. It is designed to have 80% power to show at least a 25% reduction in mortality from lung cancer 10 years after randomisation.

Evidence based reviews have concluded that current evidence does not support computed tomography screen-

ONGOING RESEARCH AND UNANSWERED QUESTIONS

- Two large randomised controlled trials of more than 70 000 people assessing the efficacy of screening with low radiation dose computed tomography for lung cancer are under way
- If lung cancer screening is found to be efficacious how would the health system implement mass screening?
- Would it be better to use scarce healthcare resources to prevent people starting to smoke or to provide better tools for smoking cessation?

TIPS FOR NON-SPECIALISTS

- Counselling patients about smoking cessation is the most effective way to reduce the risk of lung cancer
- Screening for lung cancer using chest radiography or low dose computed tomography of the chest is not currently recommended
- At risk patients who are interested in screening should be counselled about the potential harms of screening, including further unnecessary testing and complications associated with the evaluation of screen detected findings

ADDITIONAL EDUCATIONAL RESOURCES

Resources for healthcare professionals

- Manser R, Irving LB, Stone C, Byrnes G, Abramson MJ, Campbell D. Screening for lung cancer. *Cochrane Database Syst Rev* 2004;(1):CD001991.
- Bach BP, Silvestri GA, Hanger M, Jett JR. Screening for lung cancer: ACCP evidence-based clinical practice guidelines (2nd ed). *Chest* 2007;132 (supp):69S-77S.
- These two references provide an evidenced based review of screening for lung cancer

Resources for patients

- Welch HG. Should I be tested for cancer? Maybe not and here's why. Berkeley: University of California Press, 2004

ing for lung cancer outside the auspices of a well designed clinical trial.[30 31 w18] The upsurge in smoking in developing countries has thwarted the tremendous strides in tobacco control that have been made in many developed countries. The net result is that global mortality from lung cancer will rise in the short term.

Even if screening is found to be efficacious and new treatments are developed, global reductions in smoking initiation combined with effective smoking cessation strategies in those who currently smoke will have the biggest effect on mortality from lung cancer.

Contributors: All authors helped equally in researching and writing this article. GAS edited the final manuscript and responses to the critique and is guarantor.

Competing interests: None declared.

Provenance and peer review: Commissioned; externally peer reviewed.

1 Parkin DM, Bray F, Ferlay J, Pisani P. Global cancer statistics, 2002. *CA: Cancer J Clin* 2005;55:74-108.
2 Alberg AJ, Ford JG, Samet JM. Epidemiology of lung cancer: ACCP evidence-based clinical practice guidelines (2nd edition). *Chest* 2007;132:29S-55S.
3 Rosen G. *A history of public health. Expanded ed.* Baltimore, MD: Johns Hopkins University Press, 1993.
4 Amos CI, Wu X, Broderick P, Gorlov IP, Gu J, Eisen T, et al. Genome-wide association scan of tag SNPs identifies a susceptibility locus for lung cancer at 15q25.1. *Nat Genet* 2008;40:616-22.
5 Hung RJ, McKay JD, Gaborieau V, Boffetta P, Hashibe M, Zaridze D, et al. A susceptibility locus for lung cancer maps to nicotinic acetylcholine receptor subunit genes on 15q25. *Nature* 2008;452:633-7.
6 Ezzati M, Lopez AD. Estimates of global mortality attributable to smoking in 2000. *Lancet* 2003;362:847-52.
7 Ferlay J, Bray F, Pisani P, Parkin DM. *GLOBOCAN 2002: cancer incidence, mortality and prevalence worldwide.* IARC Cancer base no 5. version 2.0. IARC Press, 2004. www-dep.iarc.fr/.
8 Alberg AJ, Nonemaker J. Who is at high risk for lung cancer? Population-level and individual-level perspectives. *Semin Respir Crit Care Med* 2008;29:223-32.
9 Lam WK, White NW, Chan-Yeung MM. Lung cancer epidemiology and risk factors in Asia and Africa. *Int J Tuberc Lung Dis* 2004;8:1045-57.
10 Yang L, Parkin D, Ferlay J. Estimates of cancer incidence in China for 2000 and projections for 2005. *Cancer Epidemiol Biomarkers Prev* 2005;14:243-50.
11 Liu BQ, Peto R, Chen ZM, Boreham J, Wu YP, Li JY, et al. Emerging tobacco hazards in China: 1. Retrospective proportional mortality study of one million deaths. *BMJ* 1998;317:1411-22.
12 Menvielle G, Boshuizen H, Kunst AE, Dalton SO, Vineis P, Bergmann MM, et al. The role of smoking and diet in explaining educational inequalities in lung cancer incidence. *J Natl Cancer Inst* 2009;101:321-30.
13 Molina JR, Adjei AA, Jett JR. Advances in chemotherapy of non-small cell lung cancer. *Chest* 2006;130:1211-9.
14 American Cancer Society. *Cancer facts and figures 2007* . ACS, 2007.
15 Scott WJ, Howington J, Feigenberg S, Movsas B, Pisters K; American College of Chest Physicians. Treatment of non-small cell lung cancer stage I and stage II. *Chest* 2007;132:234S-42S.
16 Obuchowski NA, Graham RJ, Baker ME, Powell KA. Ten criteria for effective screening: their application to multislice CT screening for pulmonary and colorectal cancers. *AJR Am J Roentgenol* 2001;176:1357-62.
17 Bach PB, Niewoehner DE, Black WC. Screening for lung cancer: the guidelines. *Chest* 2003;123:83-8.
18 Marcus PM, Bergstralh EJ, Fagerstrom RM, Williams DE, Fontana R, Taylor WF, et al. Lung cancer mortality in the Mayo lung project: impact of extended follow-up. *J Natl Cancer Inst* 2000;92:1308-16.
19 Swensen SJ, Jett JR, Sloan JA, Midthun DE, Hartman TE, Sykes AM, et al. Screening for lung cancer with low-dose spiral computed tomography. *Am J Respir Crit Care Med* 2002;165:508-13.
20 Nawa T, Nakagawa T, Kusano S, Kawasaki Y, Sugawara Y, Nakata H. Lung cancer screening using low-dose spiral CT: results of baseline and 1-year follow-up studies. *Chest* 2002;122:15-20.
21 Sobue T, Moriyama N, Kaneko M. Screening for lung cancer with low-dose helical computed tomography: anti-lung cancer association project. *J Clin Oncol* 2002;20:911-20.
22 Sone S, Li F, Yang Z, Honda T, Maruyama Y, Takashima S, et al. Results of three-year mass screening programme for lung cancer using mobile low-dose spiral computed tomography scanner. *Br J Cancer* 2001;84:25-32.
23 Henschke CI, McCauley DI, Yankelevitz DF, Naidich DP, McGuinness G, Miettinen OS, et al. Early Lung Cancer Action Project: overall design and findings from baseline screening. *Lancet* 1999;354:99-105.
24 Swensen SJ, Jett JR, Hartman TE, Midthun DE, Mandrekar SJ, Hillman SL, et al. CT screening for lung cancer: five-year prospective experience. *Radiology* 2005;235:259-65.
25 Henschke CI, Yankelevitz DF, Libby DM, Pasmantier MW, Smith JP, Miettinen OS. Survival of patients with stage I lung cancer detected on CT screening. *N Engl J Med* 2006;355:1763-71.
26 Welch HG, Woloshin S, Schwartz LM, Gordis L, Gotzsche PC, Harris R, et al. Overstating the evidence for lung cancer screening: the International Early Lung Cancer Action Program (I-ELCAP) study. *Arch Int Med* 2007;167:2289-95.
27 Bach PB, Jett JR, Pastorino U, Tockman MS, Swensen SJ, Begg CB. Computed tomography screening and lung cancer outcomes. *JAMA* 2007;297:953-61.
28 Mahadevia PJ, Fleisher LA, Frick KD, Eng J, Goodman SN, Powe NR. Lung cancer screening with helical computed tomography in older adult smokers: a decision and cost-effectiveness analysis. *JAMA* 2003;289:313-22.
29 Van Iersel CA, de Koning HJ, Draisma G, Mali WP, Scholten ET, Nackaerts K, et al. Risk-based selection from the general population in a screening trial: selection criteria, recruitment and power for the Dutch-Belgian randomised lung cancer multi-slice CT screening trial (NELSON). *Int J Cancer* 2007;120:868-74.
30 Bach PB, Silvestri GA, Hanger M, Jett JR. Screening for lung cancer: ACCP evidence-based clinical practice guidelines (2nd edition). *Chest* 2007;132:69S-77S.
31 Manser R, Irving LB, Stone C, Byrnes G, Abramson MJ, Campbell D. Screening for lung cancer. *Cochrane Database Syst Rev* 2004;(1):CD001991.

BMJ BPP UNIVERSITY SCHOOL OF HEALTH

Sarcoidosis

Owen J Dempsey, consultant chest physician[1], Edward W Paterson, specialist registrar in respiratory medicine[1], Keith M Kerr, professor of pulmonary pathology[2], Alan R Denison, clinical senior lecturer[3]

[1]Department of Respiratory Medicine, Aberdeen Royal Infirmary, Foresterhill, Aberdeen AB25 2ZN

[2]Aberdeen University Medical School, Foresterhill, Aberdeen AB25 2ZD

[3]Aberdeen Biomedical Imaging Centre, University of Aberdeen Royal Infirmary, Foresterhill, Aberdeen AB25 2ZD

Correspondence to: O J Dempsey owen.dempsey@nhs.net

Cite this as: *BMJ* 2009;339:b3206

<DOI> 10.1136/bmj.b3206
http://www.bmj.com/content/339/bmj.b3206

Around 3000 new cases of sarcoidosis are diagnosed each year in the United Kingdom.[1] General practitioners play a key role in the early recognition of the most common clinical presentations of this multifaceted disease, and they usually direct initial assessment and specialist referral. Although prognosis is excellent for most patients, a minority will develop life threatening complications and may need potentially toxic treatments. Most patients are young and understandably alarmed at having sarcoidosis, which can be difficult to explain and understand. This review provides a summary of the management of sarcoidosis and includes updates from the recently revised British Thoracic Society (BTS) guidelines.[2]

What is sarcoidosis and who gets it?

Sarcoidosis is a multisystem granulomatous disease of unknown cause, first described in 1877.[3] Although sarcoidosis may occur at any age, it is usually seen in adults under the age of 50. It is slightly more common in women and certain racial groups, such as African-Americans and Scandinavians. Estimates of incidence and prevalence vary widely. In a well conducted five year study from a health maintenance organisation in the United States, annual age adjusted incidence was 10.9 per 100 000 for white Americans and 35.5 per 100 000 for African-Americans. The lifetime risk of sarcoidosis was estimated at 0.85% for white Americans and 2.4% for African-Americans.[4] In a UK general practice with 10 000 patients, one to two patients will develop sarcoidosis each year.

How does it present?

Sarcoidosis is remarkable in that it can affect any organ. Some common patterns of presentation are discussed below, with an estimate of how frequently they are seen; these estimates are based on data from US and European studies.[5,6] Up to half of patients have asymptomatic disease, which is sometimes identified when chest radiography is performed for other reasons.[w1]

SOURCES AND SELECTION CRITERIA

We searched for papers published between 1966 and March 2009 using appropriate index terms and the National Library of Medicine's computerised search service (providing access to Medline, PreMedline, and other related databases). We also consulted Cochrane database systematic reviews and used our personal archive of references.

SUMMARY POINTS

- Sarcoidosis is a multisystem granulomatous disease of unknown cause, typically affecting young and middle aged adults
- Three thousand new cases are diagnosed each year in the United Kingdom
- Any organ can be affected—mostly lungs, skin, and eyes—and patients often feel tired and generally unwell
- Most patients do not need systemic treatment, and disease often regresses spontaneously, especially in those presenting with erythema nodosum
- A minority have potentially life threatening progressive organ dysfunction; these patients need active management including oral corticosteroids

Lungs (>90%)—Non-productive cough, breathlessness, and sometimes wheeze (if endobronchial involvement is present) are common. Chest examination may be normal, despite an abnormal chest radiograph (fig 1). In more advanced disease fine interstitial crackles may be audible, particularly anteriorly, because the disease has a predilection for the upper lobes. Finger clubbing is rare, and when present alternative diagnoses should be considered—for example, malignancy; other forms of chronic lung disease, such as bronchiectasis or idiopathic pulmonary fibrosis; or infection, such as tuberculosis. The pleura can be affected, but this is unusual. Patients who develop pulmonary fibrosis can develop secondary complications including infection (aspergilloma, mycobacterial), pneumothorax, respiratory failure, and cor pulmonale (fig 1).

Fatigue (66%)—Profound fatigue is under-recognised by health professionals. It is present in two thirds of patients and has a negative effect on quality of life.[6,7] It may be associated with fever, weight loss, general malaise, depression, and raised C reactive protein.

Skin (24%)—Erythema nodosum is one of the most recognisable manifestations of sarcoidosis (fig 2). Lofgren's syndrome (erythema nodosum, arthralgia, systemic malaise, and bilateral hilar lymphadenopathy on chest radiography) is associated with an excellent prognosis, and patients usually recover spontaneously.[w2,w3] A wide variety of other skin abnormalities may be seen, including maculopapular lesions, lupus pernio (often associated with more chronic disease), nodules, and hyperpigmentation or hypopigmentation. Ask the patient about scars, such as appendicectomy scars or tattoos, because these are often infiltrated by granulomas and are easy to biopsy (fig 3).[w4]

Lymphadenopathy (15%)—Extrathoracic lymphadenopathy is common and may cause alarm, given the possibility of diagnoses such as lymphoma and tuberculosis. Fine needle aspiration, or ideally excision biopsy, can lead to rapid diagnosis.

Ocular (12%)—Sight threatening uveitis is a complication of sarcoidosis, and patients may not always be symptomatic—for example, if they have posterior uveitis—so a slit lamp examination of the eyes is mandatory in all patients. Uveoparotid fever (Heerfordt's syndrome) includes a combination of uveitis, parotid gland enlargement, and facial nerve palsy.[w5] Many other ocular problems can occur including conjunctival nodules, lacrimal gland enlargement, cataracts, glaucoma, retinal ischaemia, optic neuropathy, and papillo-oedema.[w6]

Hepatic or gastrointestinal (18%)—Typically this is asymptomatic, with liver enzymes being slightly raised. Hepatosplenomegaly, intrahepatic cholestasis, and portal hypertension are rare.[w7]

Renal (5%)—Extrarenal production of calcitriol by macrophages can result in renal calculi, nephrocalcinosis, interstitial nephritis, and renal failure.[w8]

Neurological (5%)—This is a rare yet potentially devastating complication of sarcoidosis, especially if the

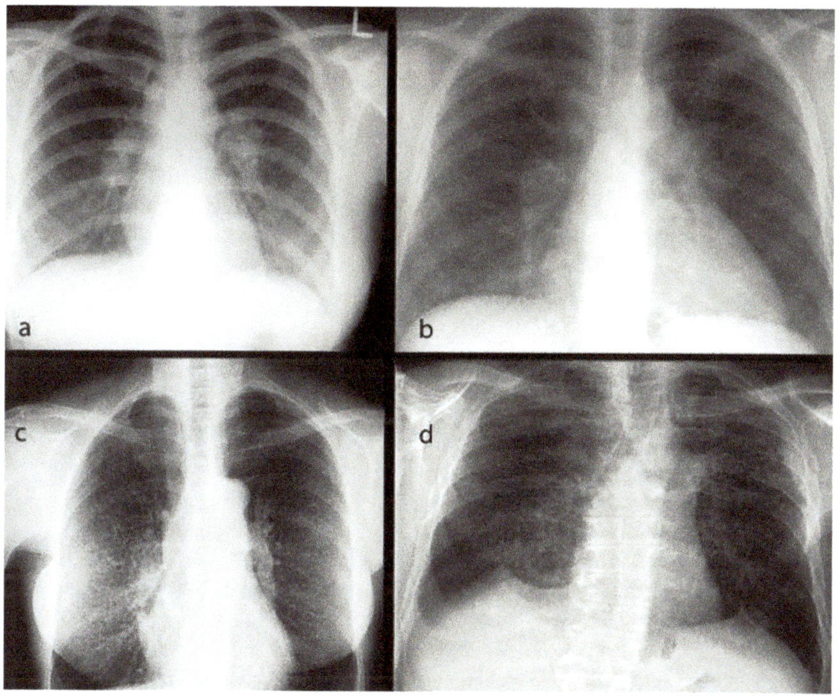

Fig 1 Patients with sarcoidosis may present at any radiographic stage. Panel (a): stage 1—bilateral hilar lymphadenopathy only (likelihood of spontaneous remission 55-90%); panel (b): stage 2—bilateral hilar lymphadenopathy plus pulmonary infiltrates (40-70%); panel (c): stage 3—pulmonary infiltrates only (10-20%); panel (d): stage 4—pulmonary fibrosis (0%)

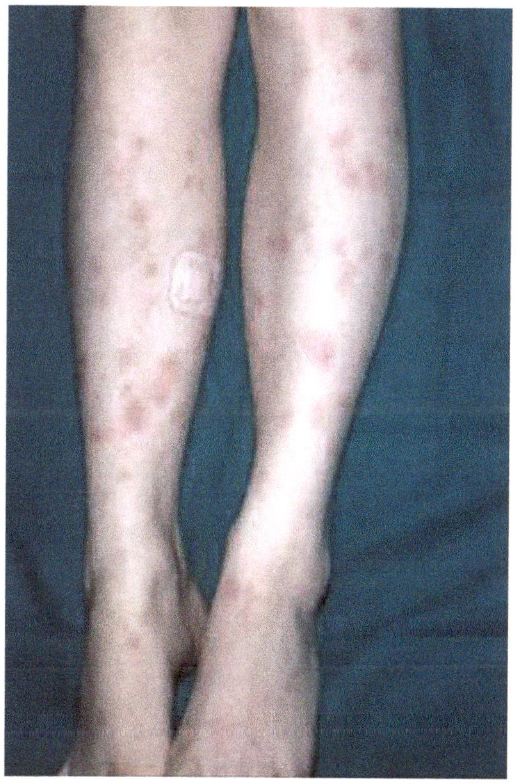

Fig 2 Erythema nodosum in a patient with sarcoidosis

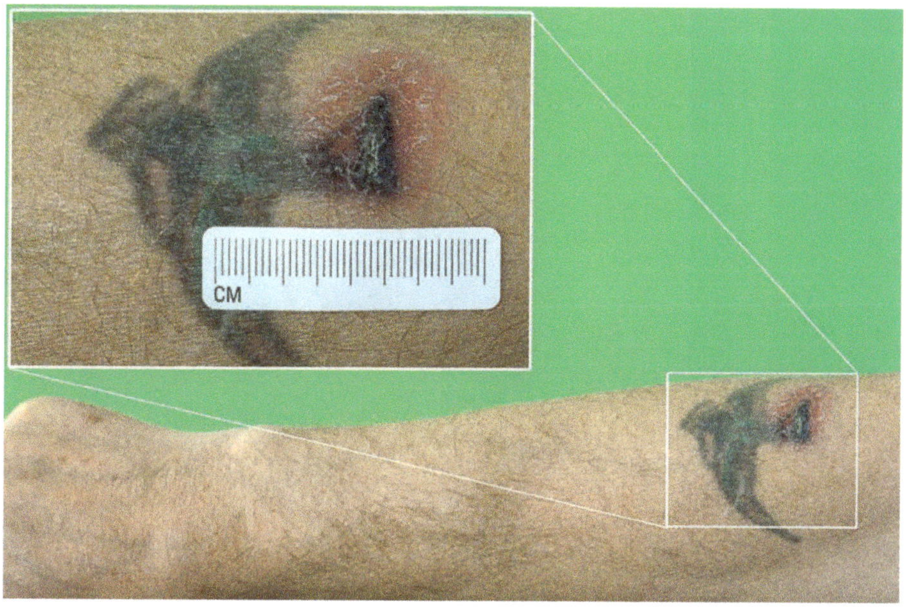

Fig 3 Forearm of a patient with cutaneous sarcoidosis affecting the tail of his swallow tattoo, confirmed on biopsy (arrow). The inflammation resolved with treatment

central nervous system is affected. It includes meningeal inflammation or infiltration, hypothalamic-pituitary effects (for example, diabetes insipidus), encephalopathy, vasculopathy, seizures, aseptic meningitis, hydrocephalus, and mass lesions. Effects on the peripheral nervous system include cranial nerve palsy, most commonly facial, and peripheral or small fibre neuropathy.[w9]

Cardiac (2%)—Although rare, this can cause sudden death so all patients with cardiac symptoms, such as palpitations or abnormalities on electrocardiography, should be referred for specialist cardiology assessment, typically including a Holter monitor, echocardiography, and cardiac magnetic resonance imaging or positron emission tomography. Electrophysiological studies may also be helpful.[w10]

Bone, joint, or muscle (0.9%)—Arthralgia is the most common locomotor symptom. Rarely, bone cysts can occur and muscles can be affected (nodules, myositis, or chronic myopathy).[w11]

Mode of presentation and severity of disease are influenced by ethnicity and sex. African-Americans are more likely than Europeans to develop skin, liver, lymph node, and ocular disease, often with greater severity. Erythema nodosum, commonly seen in white Europeans, is rare in black and Japanese people. In a large US study of patients with recently diagnosed sarcoidosis, women were more likely to have eye and neurological involvement, erythema nodosum, and to be aged 40 years or more, whereas men were more likely to have hypercalcaemia.[5]

How should suspected sarcoidosis be investigated before hospital referral?

History—A detailed history is needed, remembering that sarcoidosis may have extrapulmonary symptoms often relating to skin, eyes, and joints. Consider the possibility of alternative diagnoses that can mimic sarcoidosis. For example, tuberculosis and lymphoma can also cause bilateral hilar lymphadenopathy on chest radiography. A detailed history of occupational and environmental dust exposure may suggest diagnoses such as hypersensitivity pneumonitis. Some patients will have a family history of sarcoidosis.[8]

Examination—Symptoms will help direct clinical examination and may identify potential biopsy sites, such as lymphadenopathy, skin lesions, old scars, and tattoos (fig 3).

Blood tests—A full blood count, liver function tests, and measurement of serum electrolytes, calcium, and immunoglobulins should be performed. Immunoglobulin measurements can help exclude common variable immunodeficiency, which can present in a similar way but is associated with reduced IgG and IgA (and sometimes IgM) rather than the polyclonal gammopathy usually seen in sarcoidosis.[w12] Many clinicians check serum angiotensin converting enzyme (ACE) concentrations, although BTS guidelines suggest it has a limited role in diagnosis and does not contribute to monitoring patients when added to serial lung function and imaging. Furthermore it has limited sensitivity and specificity,[w13] and because values are influenced by *ACE* gene polymorphisms.[w14]

Chest radiography—Chest radiography allows the disease to be staged, which is of prognostic value (fig 1). Comparison with previous chest radiographs (or reports) can be helpful.

Urine dipstick—This is a standard test in any patient with suspected interstitial lung disease, principally to exclude vasculitis and nephritis.

Spirometry—Spirometry is mandatory in patients with respiratory symptoms.

Electrocardiography—Look for evidence of arrhythmia or conduction delay, which can identify latent cardiac sarcoidosis.[w10]

What tests are used in hospital?

Tissue diagnosis

This will be necessary in most patients, but a clinical diagnosis may suffice (fig 2) in those with a classic presentation, such as Lofgren's syndrome. Common biopsy sites include skin, peripheral nodes, lacrimal glands, and conjunctiva. If the lungs are affected, bronchoscopy with biopsy of central (endobronchial) and peripheral (transbronchial) airways is helpful. Patients with mediastinal lymphadenopathy may need a mediastinoscopy.

Importantly, non-caseating granulomas (fig 4) are a non-specific finding and not diagnostic of sarcoidosis.[9] Granulomatous conditions that can mimic sarcoidosis include lymphoma, mycobacterial infections (notably tuberculosis), and fungal infections. Less commonly, sarcoid-like granulomas can form in response to malignancy, foreign bodies, occupational exposure to beryllium, and

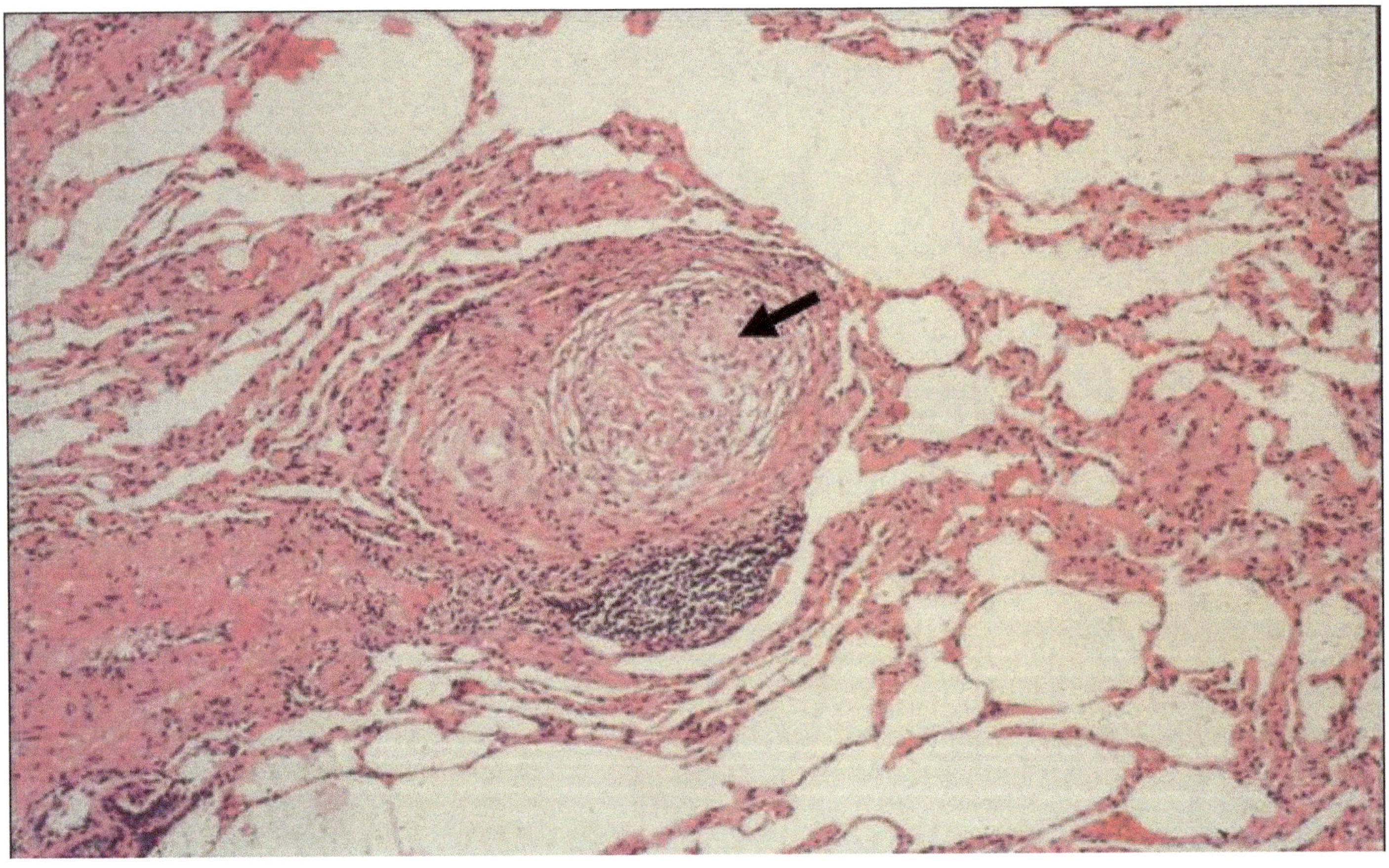

Fig 4 Sarcoid granuloma (arrow)—the histological hallmark of the disease—seen in the interstitium of the lungs, but found potentially in any organ (magnification ×100, haematoxylin and eosin stain)

in common variable immunodeficiency.[w12] Some medical treatments—for example, interferon alfa for hepatitis[w15] or highly active antiretroviral therapy for HIV infection,[w16] can promote granulomatous reactions. Pathologists routinely stain tissue samples to exclude mycobacterial and fungal disease, although false negative stains do occur, and ideally tissue should also be sent (in saline rather than formalin) to microbiology for prolonged culture.

Tuberculin skin test (Mantoux)

This test is classically negative in patients with sarcoidosis because activated T cells are sequestered in the lung, leading to peripheral depletion. If the test is positive, this raises the possibility of tuberculosis, which must be actively excluded.

Further imaging

A high resolution computed tomography scan of the chest is a standard investigation; it assesses pulmonary involvement, strengthens diagnostic confidence, and identifies abnormal nodes for biopsy. In more advanced disease it can detect complications such as fibrobullous disease, aspergilloma, and bronchiectasis. Gadolinium enhanced magnetic resonance imaging should be considered in patients with suspected myocardial sarcoidosis or neurosarcoidosis. Radionuclide imaging techniques can provide functional imaging of pulmonary and extrapulmonary lesions.[w17 w18] Gallium-67 uptake correlates well with alveolar inflammation because the agent localises to alveolar macrophages, but this technique has limited spatial resolution. Integrated fluorodeoxyglucose-positron emission tomography-computed tomography imaging has better diagnostic performance and can identify areas of sarcoidosis not detected by ^{67}Ga imaging (fig 5). It is also useful for monitoring response to treatment in patients with multisystem and complex forms of disease.[w17 w18]

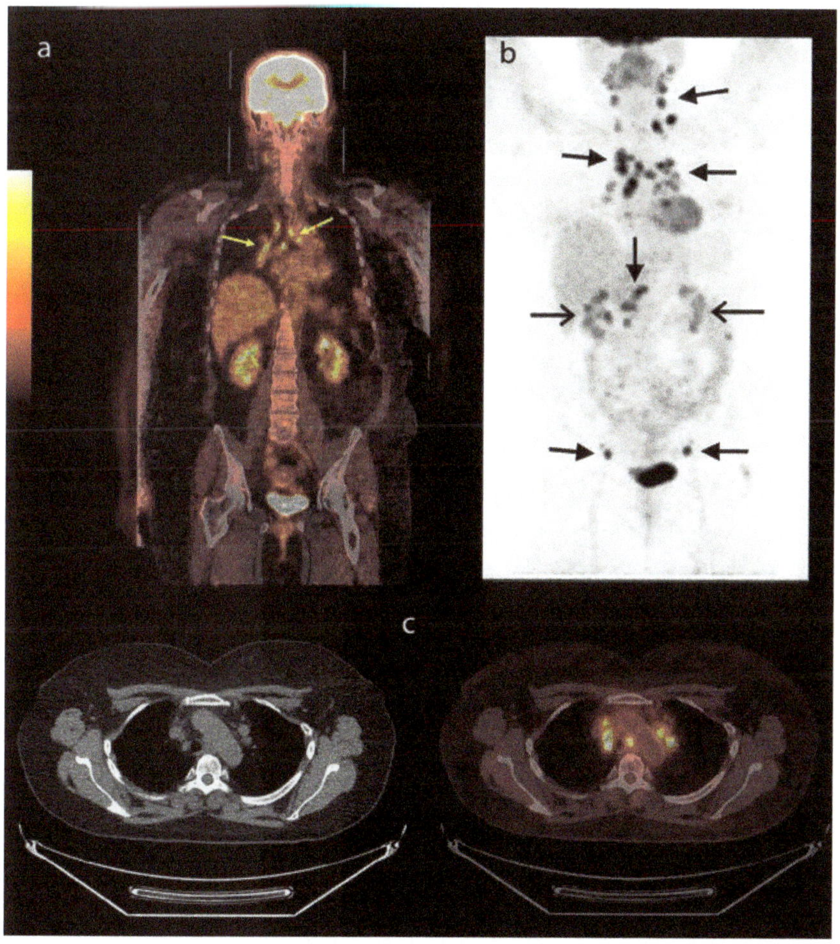

Fig 5 Integrated fluorodeoxyglucose positron emission tomography-computerised tomography can identify biopsy sites and extrapulmonary disease. In this patient with sarcoidosis, the technique identified active disease, the extent of which was not apparent on computed tomography imaging alone. Panel (a) is a fusion image showing increased uptake in mediastinal nodes (arrows); panel (b) is a maximum intensity projection image showing increased uptake in neck, mediastinal, coeliac, and inguinal nodes (closed arrows) and physiological uptake in kidneys (open arrows); panel (c) is an axial computed tomography and fused image at the level of the aortic arch showing increased fluorodeoxyglucose uptake in prevascular, left paratracheal, and right paratracheal nodes, none of which are enlarged by conventional size criteria

Detailed pulmonary function tests

The severity of lung disease, disease progression, and response to treatment are assessed by spirometry, gas transfer, and an exercise test. They may be normal in milder disease, but spirometry typically becomes restrictive in pulmonary fibrosis (although it can be obstructive if there is endobronchial involvement). As the disease progresses, gas transfer may be impaired and exercise associated desaturation may occur.

Ophthalmology review

Guidelines recommend that all patients should have a slit lamp examination to identify symptomatic and potentially sight threatening uveitis that needs treatment.[9 w6]

What causes sarcoidosis?

The cause of sarcoidosis remains elusive.[10] The current hypothesis is that it occurs in genetically susceptible people exposed to specific but unknown environmental agents.[11] Evidence for genetic susceptibility comes from multiple family and case-control studies, recently comprehensively reviewed.[12] A major association has been suggested between sarcoidosis and the class II major histocompatibility complex region (MHC) of chromosome 6. Particular phenotypes of sarcoidosis such as Lofgren's syndrome seem to be associated with particular MHC haplotypes—for example, erythema nodosum or Lofgren's syndrome is strongly associated with *HLA* DQB1*0201 in British and Dutch patients.[w19] A mutation of another MHC gene, *BTNL-2*, is associated with sarcoidosis and other inflammatory disorders; the product of the non-mutated gene inhibits the proliferation of T cells.[w20]

Epidemiological studies have reported clustering of cases within families, geographically and seasonally.[w21] Geographical clusters suggest person to person transmission or shared exposure to an environmental agent. Case clustering in winter and early spring is reported. Suggested infective triggers, such as mycobacteria and *Propionibacterium acnes*, are unconfirmed.[13] Studies exploring occupational risk factors have also been inconclusive, despite detailed occupational and environmental questionnaires, although exposures associated with increased risk include insecticides, agricultural employment, and microbial bioaerosols.[14] A negative association with smoking has often been seen.[w22]

Does it run in families?

Familial clustering of sarcoidosis is well described.[15] In a large multicentre US based case-control study, first degree and second degree relatives of patients with sarcoidosis had a significantly increased risk of sarcoidosis compared with relatives of matched controls. Siblings had the highest relative risk (odds ratio 5.8, confidence interval 2.1 to 15.9).[15] In the UK, a questionnaire based study of 268 patients with sarcoidosis reported that 5.9% had at least one other relative (first, second, or third degree) with biopsy confirmed disease.[8] A recently published Danish-Finnish study found that, compared with the general population, co-twins of affected monozygotic brothers or sisters had an 80-fold increased risk of developing sarcoidosis. The increased risk in dizygotic twins was only sevenfold, suggesting that genetic factors play an important role in susceptibility to the disease.[16]

Immunology of sarcoidosis

This is a complex topic, comprehensively reviewed elsewhere.[w23] Interaction between an unknown antigen and antigen presenting cells is thought to result in a T helper 1 biased CD4 positive response. Affected organs are infiltrated by CD4 positive T cells, and in the lungs a striking T cell alveolitis is seen. A complex inflammatory cascade ensues with other inflammatory cells, notably alveolar macrophages, playing a part. Various chemokines and cytokines are released, ultimately resulting in formation of non-specific inflammatory granulomas (fig 4). In most patients this process regresses spontaneously, but in some patients fibroblasts are recruited and production of matrix proteins increases, ultimately resulting in irreversible fibrosis.

Some investigators have highlighted the "immune paradox" of sarcoidosis—affected organs such as the lungs show an intense immune response, yet relative anergy exists elsewhere (such as the negative response to the Mantoux test).[17] A disequilibrium between effector and regulatory T cells has been hypothesised. For example, patients with sarcoidosis have recently been shown to have reduced numbers of regulatory T cells called CD1d restricted natural killer T cells.[w24] These cells may function as an immunological "brake" and have been shown to protect against disorders with increased CD4 positive T helper 1 responses in animals. Loss of immunoregulation by these natural killer cells could explain the amplified and persistent T cell activity that characterises sarcoidosis and other autoimmune diseases, such as diabetes mellitus and multiple sclerosis.[w24] Patients with Lofgren's syndrome have normal numbers of natural killer cells, which may explain why their prognosis is so good. The role of these and other regulatory T cells in sarcoidosis has been reviewed.[w25]

What is the prognosis?

Sarcoidosis generally has a good prognosis.[18 w26] Many patients are asymptomatic, and spontaneous resolution occurs in as many as 60% of these patients. Nonetheless, some patients do have chronic progressive disease, and mortality has been reported to be 1-6%. The disease can wax and wane, either spontaneously or in response to treatment. Patients with lupus pernio, chronic uveitis, chronic hypercalcaemia, nephrocalcinosis, progressive pulmonary sarcoidosis, nasal mucosal involvement, cystic bone lesions, neurosarcoidosis, and myocardial involvement have a less favourable prognosis, as do black people and those aged 40 or more at onset.[18 w2]

Who needs treatment?

US guidelines and recently updated BTS guidelines (in collaboration with colleagues from Australia, New Zealand, and Ireland) are excellent and discuss treatment options in detail.[2 9] Treatment decisions should balance the risks of using corticosteroids, the most common treatment, against the potential benefits. A general rule is to consider starting treatment when organ function is threatened. The main conclusions reached are[2]:

- Many patients do not need treatment and the disease may spontaneously regress.
- Erythema nodosum can be painful, and short term use of regular paracetamol and a non-steroidal anti-inflammatory drug can be helpful.
- Treatment is not indicated for asymptomatic stage 1 disease or patients with asymptomatic stable stage 2 or 3 disease who have only mildly abnormal lung function.
- Oral steroids may be of benefit for patients with stage 2 or 3 disease who have moderate to severe or progressive symptoms or changes on chest radiography.
- Absolute indications for oral steroids include hypercalcaemia, neurological involvement, cardiac involvement, or ocular involvement (the last one if topical treatment has failed).
- Inhaled corticosteroids are not beneficial as initial treatment or maintenance treatment, although they are sometimes tried in patients with intractable cough.

What should I do if a patient needs oral corticosteroids?

UK guidelines advocate initial treatment with prednisolone, 0.5 mg/kg/day for four weeks.[2] The dose is then gradually reduced over the next six months, ideally to a maintenance dose of around 10 mg or less a day. To prevent corticosteroid induced bone loss, patients are usually started (empirically) on an oral bisphosphonate, and baseline bone densitometry is performed. Duration of treatment varies but is often six to 24 months at least.

What happens if steroids cannot be reduced or stopped?

Some patients will need more than 10 mg/day of prednisolone to control their sarcoidosis. In these circumstances a "steroid sparing" agent can be added, with the aim of subsequently reducing the prednisolone dose to 10 mg/day or less. Unfortunately, no high quality evidence is available to support the use of treatments commonly cited including hydroxychloroquine, methotrexate, azathioprine, and cyclophosphamide.[19] These drugs can be highly toxic and should be given under expert supervision only. For patients who have failed a trial of these agents, treatment with a tumour necrosis factor inhibitor can be considered. The most commonly used is infliximab, although other agents include etanercept and adalimumab. The use of these inhibitors has recently been expertly reviewed.[20] Factors associated with a good response to these agents include more severe pulmonary disease, chronic extrapulmonary disease, longer disease duration, and impaired quality of life.

How effective are corticosteroids in sarcoidosis?

We do not know which dose or duration of corticosteroids is most effective, or whether treatment alters the course of the disease. For patients in whom crucial organs are affected, corticosteroids can be life saving. For patients with milder pulmonary disease the evidence is weak. A systematic review of eight randomised placebo controlled trials of oral or inhaled corticosteroids in patients with pulmonary disease concluded that oral steroids improved appearances on chest radiography and a global score of such appearances, symptoms, and spirometry over three to 24 months. However, it found little evidence of improvement

ADDITIONAL EDUCATIONAL RESOURCES

Resources for healthcare professionals

- British Thoracic Society (www.brit-thoracic.org.uk)—Recently published guidelines on the initial assessment, investigations, and management of sarcoidosis and other forms of interstitial lung disease are available here
- American Thoracic Society (www.thoracic.org/sections/publications/statements/index.html)—Although published nine years ago, these guidelines cover all aspects of the disease
- Ongoing clinical trials (www.clinicaltrials.gov)—Involvement in clinical trials will improve our understanding and management of sarcoidosis and other lung diseases. This website provides a useful up to date summary of ongoing trials

Resources for patients

- British Lung Foundation (www.lunguk.org/sarcoidosis.asp)—Useful site with links to patient support groups (breathe easy groups)
- Sarcoidosis and Interstitial Lung Association (www.sila.org.uk)—UK support group
- National Heart Lung and Blood Institute (www.nhlbi.nih.gov/health/dci/Diseases/sarc/sarc_all.html)—Provides comprehensive information for patients
- Sarcoid Networking Association (www.sarcoidosisnetwork.org)—US based site with multiple links to resources for patients with sarcoidosis

TIPS FOR NON-SPECIALISTS

- Always consider alternative diagnoses, such as lymphoma or tuberculosis. Confirmation with tissue biopsy is needed unless clinical confidence is high
- Remember that granulomatous inflammation is consistent with, but not specific for, sarcoidosis and can occur with other illnesses
- A diagnosis of sarcoidosis is often frightening for patients, and vetted patient information leaflets and website links can be helpful
- Ask about cardiac symptoms, such as palpitations and syncope. Although cardiac sarcoidosis is rare, it can cause sudden death, and early identification may allow lifesaving treatment

in lung function, and only limited data to indicate that oral steroids affect long term disease progression.[21]

Who should manage these patients?

Patients with sarcoidosis should be offered regular hospital clinic review by the appropriate specialist(s). The lungs are affected in most patients, so chest physicians are usually involved, and BTS guidelines recommend multidisciplinary care at interstitial lung disease clinics.[2] Clinic review is typically every three to six months initially, and more often if drugs have been started. Patients with clinically stable disease are seen less often. Patients with stage 2-4 disease are often followed up indefinitely, but stable patients with milder (stage 0-1 disease) can often be discharged by two years. At hospital visits patients should be assessed clinically (symptoms, signs), radiologically (usually chest radiography), and physiologically (pulmonary function tests). They may need blood tests, especially if they previously had hypercalcaemia, impaired renal or hepatic function, or raised serum angiotensin converting enzyme concentrations. Rarely, patients with progressive pulmonary sarcoidosis, who are otherwise medically fit, are considered for lung transplantation.

Contributors: OD conceived the idea for the article, and all authors helped in the first draft and subsequent revisions. OD is guarantor.

Funding: No special funding received.

Competing interests: None declared.

Provenance and peer review: Not commissioned; externally peer reviewed.

Patient consent obtained.

1 Gribbin J, Hubbard RB, Le Jeune I, Smith CJ, West J, Tata LJ. Incidence and mortality of idiopathic pulmonary fibrosis and sarcoidosis in the UK. *Thorax* 2006;61:980-5.

2 Bradley B, Branley HM, Egan JJ, Greaves MS, Hansell DM, Harrison NK, et al. Interstitial lung disease guideline: the British Thoracic Society in collaboration with the Thoracic Society of Australia and New Zealand and the Irish Thoracic Society. *Thorax* 2008;63(suppl 5):v1-58.

3 Hutchinson J. Anomalous diseases of skin and fingers: case of livid papillary psoriasis? In: *Illustrations of clinical surgery* . London: J and A Churchill, 1877:42-3.

4 Rybicki BA, Major M, Popovich J, Maliank MJ, Iannuzzi. Racial differences in sarcoidosis incidence: a 5-year study in a health maintenance organization. *Am J Epidemiol* 1997;145:234-41.

5 Baughman RP, Teirstein AS, Judson MA, Rossman MD, Yeager H Jr, Bresnitz EA, et al. Clinical characteristics of patients in a case control study of sarcoidosis. *Am J Respir Crit Care Med* 2001;164:1885-9.

6 Drent M, Wirnsberger RM, de Vries J, van Dieijen-Visser MP, Wouters EFM, Schols AMWJ. Association of fatigue with an acute phase response in sarcoidosis. *Eur Respir J* 1999;13:718-22.

7 Cox CE, Donohue JF, Brown CD, Kataria YP, Judson MA. Health-related quality of life of persons with sarcoidosis. *Chest* 2004;125:997-1004.

8 McGrath DS, Daniil Z, Foley P, du Bois JL, Lympany PA, Cullinan P, et al. Epidemiology of familial sarcoidosis in the UK. *Thorax* 2000;55:751-4.

9 American Thoracic Society. Statement on sarcoidosis. *Am J Resp Crit Care Med* 1999;160:736-55.

10 Taylor AN, Cullinan P. Sarcoidosis: in search of the cause. *Am J Respir Crit Care Med* 2004;170:1268-9.

11 Newman LS. Aetiologies of sarcoidosis. *Eur Respir Mon* 2005;32:23-48.

12 Du Bois RM, Beirne PA, Anevlavis SE. Genetics. *Eur Respir Mon* 2005;32:64-81.

13 Gupta D, Agarwal R, Aggarwal AN, Jindal SK. Molecular evidence for the role of mycobacteria in sarcoidosis: a meta-analysis. *Eur Respir J* 2007;30:508-16.

14 Newman LS, Rose CS, Bresnitz EA, Rossman MD, Barnard J, Frederick M, et al. A case control etiologic study of sarcoidosis: environmental and occupational risk factors. *Am J Respir Crit Care Med* 2004;170:1324-30.

15 Rybicki BA, Iannuzzi MC, Frederick MM, Thompson BW, Rossman MD, Bresnitz EA, et al. Familial aggregation of sarcoidosis. A case-control etiologic study of sarcoidosis. *Am J Respir Crit Care Med* 2001;164:2085-91.

16 Sverrild A, Backer V, Kyvik KO, Kaprio J, Milman N, Svendsen CB, et al. Heredity in sarcoidosis: a registry-based twin study. *Thorax* 2008;63:894-6.

17 Miyara M, Amoura Z, Parizot C, Badoual C, Dorgham K, Trad S, et al. The immune paradox of sarcoidosis and regulatory T cells. *J Exp Med* 2006;203:359-70.

18 MacFarlane JT. Prognosis in sarcoidosis. *BMJ* 1984;288:1557-8.

19 Paramothayan S, Lasserson TJ, Walters EH. Immunosuppressive and cytotoxic therapy for pulmonary sarcoidosis. *Cochrane Database Syst Rev* 2003;(3):CD003536.

20 Baughman RP, Lower EE, Drent M. Inhibitors of tumor necrosis factor (TNF) in sarcoidosis: who, what, and how to use them. *Sarcoidosis Vasc Diffuse Lung Dis* 2008;25:76-89.

21 Paramothayan NS, Lasserson TJ, Jones PW. Corticosteroids for pulmonary sarcoidosis. *Cochrane Database Syst Rev* 2000;(1):CD001114.

More titles in The BMJ Clinical Review Series

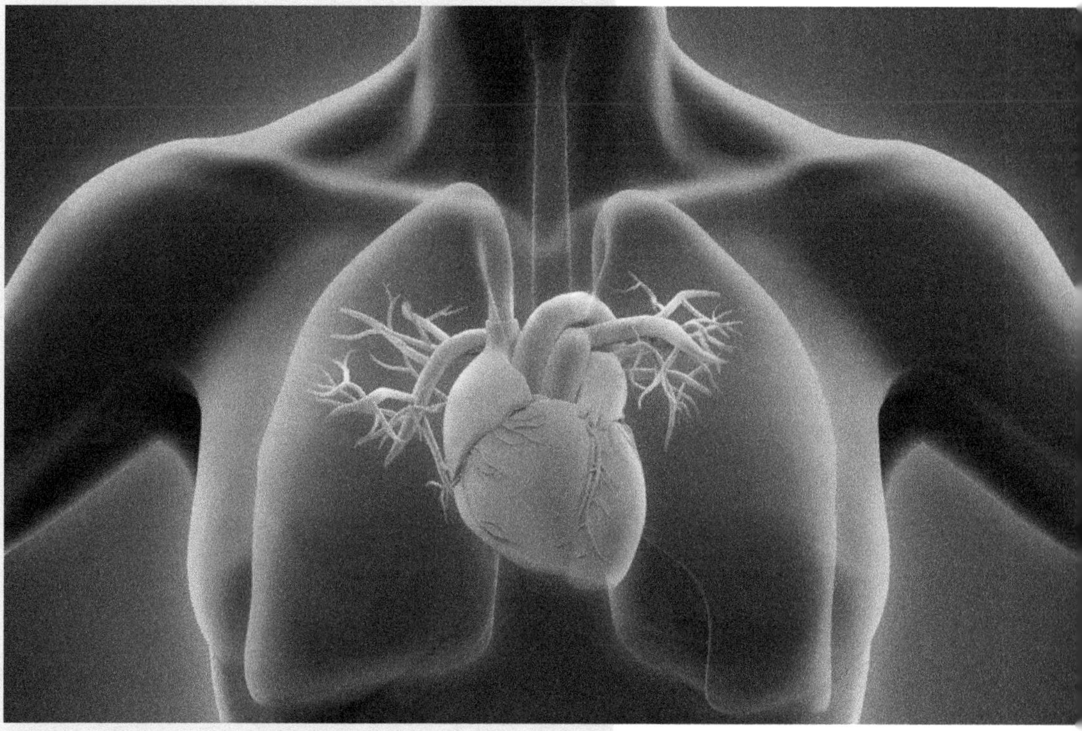

BMJ

BPP UNIVERSITY SCHOOL OF HEALTH

More titles in The Progressing your Medical Career Series

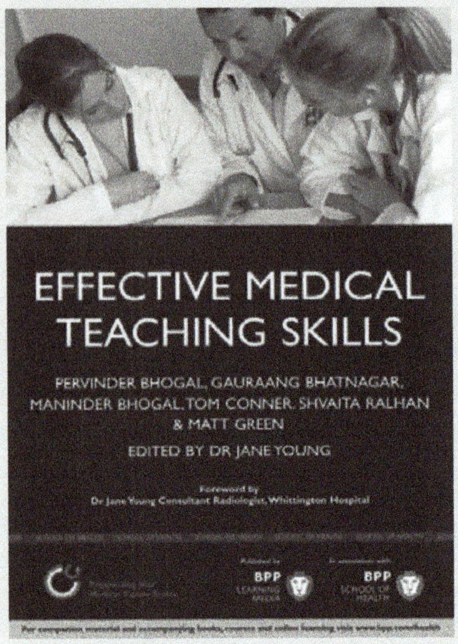

£19.99

September 2011

Paperback

978-1-445379-56-2

We can all remember a teacher that inspired us, encouraged us and helped us to excel. But what is it that makes a good teacher and are these skills that can be learned and improved?

As doctors and healthcare professionals we are all expected to teach, to a greater or lesser degree, and this carries a great deal of responsibility. We are helping to develop the next generation and it is essential to pass on the knowledge that we have gained during our experience to date.

This book aims to cover the fundamentals of medical education. It has been designed to be a guide for the budding teacher with practical advice, hints, tips and essential points of reflection designed to encourage the reader to think about what they are doing at each step.

By taking the time to read through this book and completing the exercises contained within it you should:

- Understand the needs of the learner
- Understand the skills required to be an effective teacher
- Understanding the various different teaching scenarios, from lectures to problem based teaching, and how to use them effectively
- Understand the importance and sources of feedback
- Be aware of assessment techniques, appraisal and revalidation

This book aims to provide you with a foundation in medical education upon which you can build the skills and attributes to become a competent and skilled teacher.

BPP UNIVERSITY SCHOOL OF HEALTH

www.bpp.com/medical-series

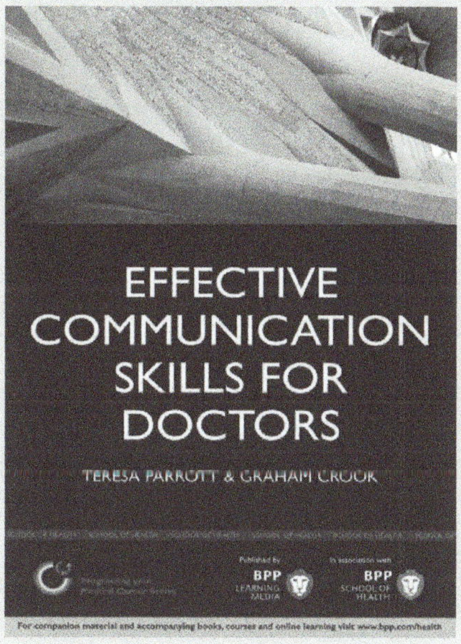
EFFECTIVE COMMUNICATION SKILLS FOR DOCTORS
TERESA PARROTT & GRAHAM CROOK
BPP LEARNING MEDIA
BPP SCHOOL OF HEALTH

BMJ BPP UNIVERSITY SCHOOL OF HEALTH

More titles in The Progressing your Medical Career Series

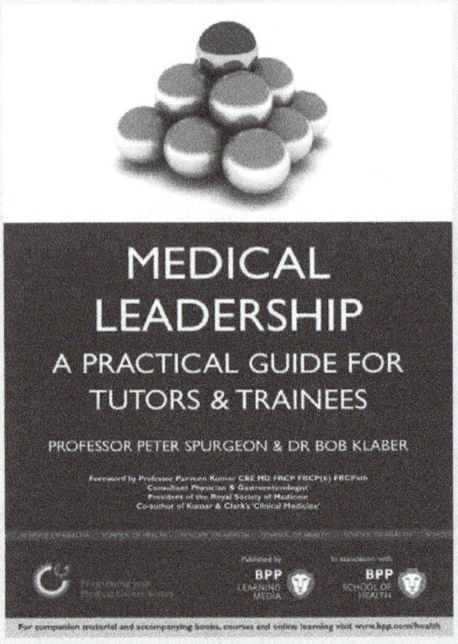

£19.99

November 2011

Paperback

978-1-445379-57-9

Are you a doctor or medical student who wishes to acquire and develop your leadership and management skills? Do you recognise the role and influence of strong leadership and management in modern medicine?

Clinical leadership is something in which all doctors should have an important role in terms of driving forward high quality care for their patients. In this up-to-date guide Peter Spurgeon and Robert Klaber take you through the latest leadership and management thinking, and how this links in with the Medical Leadership Competency Framework. As well as influencing undergraduate curricula and some of the concepts underpinning revalidation, this framework forms the basis of the leadership component of the curricula for all medical specialties, so a practical knowledge of it is essential for all doctors in training.

Using case studies and practical exercises to provide a strong work-based emphasis, this practical guide will enable you to build on your existing experiences to develop your leadership and management skills, and to develop strategies and approaches to improving care for your patients.

This book addresses:

- Why strong leadership and management are crucial to delivering high quality care
- The theory and evidence behind the Medical Leadership Competency Framework
- The practical aspects of leadership learning in a wide range of clinical environments (eg handover, EM, ward etc)
- How Consultants and trainers can best facilitate leadership learning for their trainees and students within the clinical work-place

Whether you are a medical student just starting out on your career, or an established doctor wishing to develop yourself as a clinical leader, this practical, easy-to-use guide will give you the techniques and knowledge you require to excel.

BPP UNIVERSITY SCHOOL OF HEALTH

www.bpp.com/medical-series